the BIG fat conspiracy

MELISSA SWEET

the BIG fat conspiracy

ABC
Books

Published by ABC Books for the
AUSTRALIAN BROADCASTING CORPORATION
GPO Box 9994 Sydney NSW 2001

First published June 2007

National Library of Australia
Cataloguing-in-Publication entry

Sweet, Melissa.
    The big fat conspiracy.
    ISBN 978 0 7333 2181 8 (pbk).
    1. Children – Health and hygiene. 2. Overweight children.
    I. Australian Broadcasting Corporation. II. Title.
613.7042

Cover and internal design by Ellie Exarchos, Scooter Design
Illustrations by Mitchell Ward, Rock Lily Design
Typeset in 11.5 on 17pt Apollo MT by Kirby Jones
Index by Puddingburn
Printed and bound in Australia by Griffin Press, South Australia

5 4 3 2 1

Permission has been granted to reproduce quotes from Satter, Ellyn 2000, Child of mine.
Feeding with love and good sense, Bull Publishing Co., Colorado; Satter, Ellyn 1987, How to
get your kid to eat ... but not too much. From birth to adolescence, Bull Publishing Co.,
Colorado.Permission also granted from NHMRC 2003, Dietary Guidelines for Children and
Adolescents in Australia incorporating the Infant Feeding Guidelines for Health Workers
(endorsed 10 April 2003), NHMRC, Canberra.

For Lorna Cameron,
a wonderful woman

Contents

Introduction

You might think that the title of this book is a blatant attempt to catch your attention. You'd be right about that, but only partly. There is something universally appealing about a wacky conspiracy theory, perhaps because we all know that sometimes life really can be stranger than fiction. There's no doubt that if any of your ancestors from the last 40,000 years or so had been told about the subject of this book, they would have thought it sounded like a fine old fairytale.

But this book is most definitely not a work of fiction. It's about a real conspiracy that is affecting the lives of all of us now and compromising the health and wellbeing of our children into the future. Some experts believe that the current generation of children will be the first whose life expectancy is shorter than their parents'. That's how serious it is.

So what is this conspiracy? It's called the modern world. Many aspects of our environment conspire to make us overindulge in some things and underindulge in others. It is no coincidence that this is to the benefit of many powerful interests—the food, marketing, advertising, media and car industries, to name just a few. But often it's not to the benefit of our health.

The big fat conspiracy

Being caught up in this conspiracy is like being swept along by a fast-flowing river. All the forces are pushing you in one direction and it takes some effort and strength to go against the flow. It's much easier to drift along, even though you know there are hazards ahead. The most obvious of these hazards is the growing girth of many adults and children in many countries. Overweight inspires so much public health and media attention because it's the huge rock sticking up out of the water. It's so obvious that you can't miss it.

But the world's ever-increasing weight problem is just the tip of the rock. The not-so-visible bit under the water can also do damage. Overweight can be seen as the most obvious expression of broader underlying health hazards—unhealthy eating and inactivity. The growing incidence of overweight is a symptom of an environment which can make it very difficult for parents and families to follow healthy lifestyles.

Many children, whether tubby or thin, are not enjoying good nutrition or the self-confidence that comes with being fit and active. Many are overfed but undernourished. Many are developing unhealthy food and activity habits which have not shown up in their waistlines—not yet, at least—but which may affect their health later; poor nutrition and inactivity contribute to many diseases, including diabetes, heart disease, strokes and some cancers, and therefore to many premature deaths.

Which brings us to another conspiracy: this time, it's a little one between you and me, the writer and the reader. This book was prompted by my concern about the growing numbers of children and young people who are overweight, and I hope it inspires you to take some steps to protect yourself and your family from the big fat conspiracy of modern life.

Introduction

But the last thing I want is to make parents or children overly focused on weight. As anyone who has ever obsessed over the numbers on their bathroom scales can testify, worrying about weight is often entirely counterproductive. It encourages unhealthy anxieties and unhealthy eating patterns, such as dieting. Encouraging children to worry about their weight might just end up giving them a weight problem.

So our little conspiracy, in this book about weight, is to pretend that it is not about that at all. Let's focus on gaining health rather than losing weight.

One of the reasons for this approach is self-interest. I want you to read this book, but study after study has shown that the words 'obesity' and 'overweight' have magic properties. The mere mention of them makes otherwise sensible people close down, switch off and block their ears. This happens even with the parents of obese children. Many parents don't see fat as a health issue for them or their families—it is something that affects someone else's children. In the same way, many people think their lifestyle is more healthy than it really is— poor nutrition and inactive lifestyles are problems other people have.

But the main reason that this book does not focus solely on weight is that good health involves so much more than having a healthy weight. Children can be overweight but fit, active, and enjoying a nutritious diet. On the other hand, just because a child is thin, it doesn't mean their health is optimal. 'Thin does not necessarily equal health, and thin does not necessarily equal a healthy lifestyle,' says Dr Rick Kausman, a Melbourne doctor who specialises in treating weight problems.

A healthy lifestyle has many benefits other than helping to control weight. It helps make sure that children have plenty of energy, sleep well, feel good, and enjoy learning. It also means they are less likely to suffer from problems like constipation and headaches. Strategies to prevent childhood obesity are likely to benefit all children, whether they are at risk of weight gain or not.

Overweight is a huge issue for adults, but this book focuses mainly on children and families because, as someone wise once said, an ounce of prevention is worth a pound of cure. This is particularly so in the area of weight control, where treatment is not spectacularly successful—one of the reasons obesity is so difficult to cure is that our bodies are far more efficient at gaining weight than they are at losing it. Most overweight children and adults who lose weight return to their previous size.[1]

It is true that not all fat children grow into fat adults, and it is true that some fat adults were thin children. But fat children are more likely to become fat adults and, with studies showing that obesity is becoming more common even among preschoolers, prevention efforts need to start very early in life, perhaps even in the womb (more on that later, in Chapter 9).

Another reason to focus on childhood is because some experts believe that obesity that begins early in life is more likely to cause health problems than weight gain at a later age. Others say that childhood is the best time for obesity prevention because it is when weight problems are best controlled—thanks to children's rapid growth, we can help them 'grow into their weight' rather than striving for weight loss.

There are also ethical reasons to focus attention on childhood. Children are dependent on us—not only on their parents, but also on other adults who shape their environments.

Introduction

All of us owe them a duty of care. As well, the habits that develop in childhood may last a lifetime. Children who genuinely enjoy a healthy diet and being fit are more likely to grow into adults who do the same.

Although this book is about children's health, it is the family's behaviour that counts. This book is not about forcing children to eat their greens or run around the block. That sort of approach might do more harm than good (find out why in Chapters 7 and 10).

Have another look at that rushing river. What's the best way to get your children across safely? It's not by tossing them a pair of floaties and telling them to swim for it. You need to help make the journey across as easy and pleasant for them as possible. You do that by providing a helpful environment—the family boat which is chugging slowly and determinedly across the river. Everyone is on board and heading in the same direction. The parents are showing their children the way.

This is not an easy job, and it's no wonder so many struggle. It seems very unfair to blame parents or children for being swept downstream, when so many powerful interests are working towards exactly that result.

Yet there are plenty of people prepared to nail parents for the childhood obesity problem. They condemn parents for children's poor diets and inactivity. Broadly speaking, there are two types of people who make these sorts of comments. The first speak out of ignorance or prejudice. They have not studied the evidence coming in from around the world about the impact of the modern environment on health, and they see fat as a sign of personal failing. The second group includes those who have a vested interest in describing the issue as one of individual choice and responsibility, thus deflecting attention from their own role. This group includes governments that are reluctant to make hard decisions about town planning and transport policies or television advertising to children. And industries that spend a fortune flogging junk foods to kids.

Many experts believe it will be difficult to achieve widespread, lasting improvements to children's health without making that journey across the river easier for families. This means major environmental changes—like stopping the advertising of junk foods to young children, like making it easier and safer for children to walk or cycle to school, like making vegetables and fruit more affordable and accessible, like making workplaces more family-friendly.

However, these changes will not come quickly or easily, despite the determination of many in the public health sector and the broader community. In the meantime, I hope this book inspires families to make some of the small changes in their daily lives which might add up to sizeable improvements to their health, now and in the future. It's not about asking you to do the impossible. It's about trying, within your family or community, to make healthy choices easier.

It's also about different strokes for different folks. What works for one family or community may not for another. What works for one family when the children are young may not work so well when the children are older. What works for your daughter may not work for her brother.

Despite all the alarming headlines and statistics about childhood obesity, this is not a book of doom and gloom or shame and blame. It celebrates the achievement, imagination and creativity of many families and communities, often in the face of adversity. As some of the stories in this book show, many people have developed innovative strategies for countering what some child health experts have dubbed the 'toxic' or 'obesogenic' environment many children live in.

Read on, and find out about the wonderful Apple Slinky machine and how it is revolutionising school fundraising, the clever ideas being put into practice in remote Aboriginal communities (Chapter 12), and what children themselves think might be helpful (Chapters 6 and 8). If you don't already know about the importance of the 'division of responsibility' in helping children eat well, don't miss Chapter 7.

Above all, this is a book that says that enjoyment is the key to a healthy lifestyle and good health. You're so much more likely to cross that river successfully if it's an enjoyable trip.

Your survival guide to the Big Fat Conspiracy

This book is divided into three sections. It takes a broad and detailed approach, so don't feel you have to read it all. Just skip the sections that aren't relevant to your interests or needs.

The first section is called 'Understanding vs blaming'. Once you start to look at all the forces that affect children's health, you realise what a difficult job many parents face today. It also becomes clear that weight gain is an almost inevitable consequence of modern society, and that conscious action is needed to prevent it.

This section examines the issues affecting children's health in some detail, because there are so many sceptics—many of them in powerful positions, such as politicians and media commentators—who persist in seeing problems with children's health and weight as the sole responsibility of parents. 'If only parents would stop giving their kids lollies and chips, the problem would be solved' is their typical comment—if only it were that simple! I hope this section will help all of us understand how our actions can affect children's wellbeing. If it is too detailed for you, head straight to the practical advice in the next section.

The second section is called 'What you and your family can do'. It looks at some of the ways families can make it easier for themselves to enjoy good health. It is packed with tips about how to build regular activity into your family's life and how to really enjoy healthy eating. It also contains useful advice on how to develop a healthy relationship with television and other screen-based entertainment, and specific information for families who are struggling with weight issues.

The third section is called 'The power of many'. It examines how communities can work together to make a powerful difference to people's lives. It has many examples from across Australia of schools, local councils, community gardens, farmers' markets, businesses, and other groups working to improve the environments which affect children's health. This section is a treasure trove of ideas which you can adapt to your own needs and circumstances.

Reading this book may take some thought and effort. It does not promise quick or easy fixes. If it did, it would not be worth reading, because quick fixes are rarely helpful or sustainable solutions to complex problems.

The big fat paradox

If this book hadn't been called *The Big Fat Conspiracy*, it might have been called *The Big Fat Paradox*. Here are just a few that spring to mind:

• We are living longer and have more wealth than ever at our disposal, yet we feel under more pressure to do more things faster. At the same time, we are moving less and our bodies are becoming slower. We email someone in the next room because we think we haven't got time to take 10 steps.

• Time-saving technology is more widely available than ever before, but people feel more rushed and time poor than ever.

• We spend more time renovating our kitchens than using them, whether for cooking or sharing a family meal. And it sometimes seems that we also spend more time watching TV shows about cooking, or reading about cooking, than we do actually cooking.

• We don't cook because we don't have enough time because we're watching TV, where the ads tell us we don't have enough time to cook and should instead buy the easy foods. You know, the ones full of fat, sugar and salt.

• As the range of low-fat foods, bestselling diet books and the weight-loss industry has expanded, so have our waistlines.

• Eating on the run is almost certain to pile on the kilos.

• People are more health conscious than ever—research shows that even young children frown upon the fat and salt in chips—but many do not meet the dietary recommendations for vegetables and fruit consumption.[2]

• Many people are overfed but undernourished.

• Many parents do not realise their children are overweight, or that this might have health risks. At the same time, many normal-sized children judge themselves to be overweight.

The big fat conspiracy

- Many of the symptoms of 'affluenza', the over-consumption syndrome which sees Australians throw away more than $5 billion worth of food and drink in a year, are also contributing to expanding waistlines.[3] On the other hand, in wealthy countries like Australia, obesity is more common among the poorer groups in the community, where financial pressure encourages unhealthy eating.
- Children are growing up faster than ever before—and not just because they are hitting puberty earlier and earlier—and yet they are moving more and more slowly.
- Children today are so sophisticated in so many ways. They recite brand names, know about the latest product launch and speak in the universal language of TV sitcoms. Six-year-olds talk about 'dumping' their boyfriend. The internet and other electronic media let them explore the world in ways that previous generations could never have imagined. On the other hand, they are less independent than ever. Many are not allowed to travel or explore their neighbourhoods by themselves or enjoy freedoms that were taken for granted by their parents.
- Parents grow ever more fearful and protective of their children, although in many respects the world is a much safer place than it was when they were growing up. Ironically, many parents who worry about letting their children loose in the local park have no qualms about taking them to the playground at McDonald's or encouraging them to sit quietly in front of the TV.

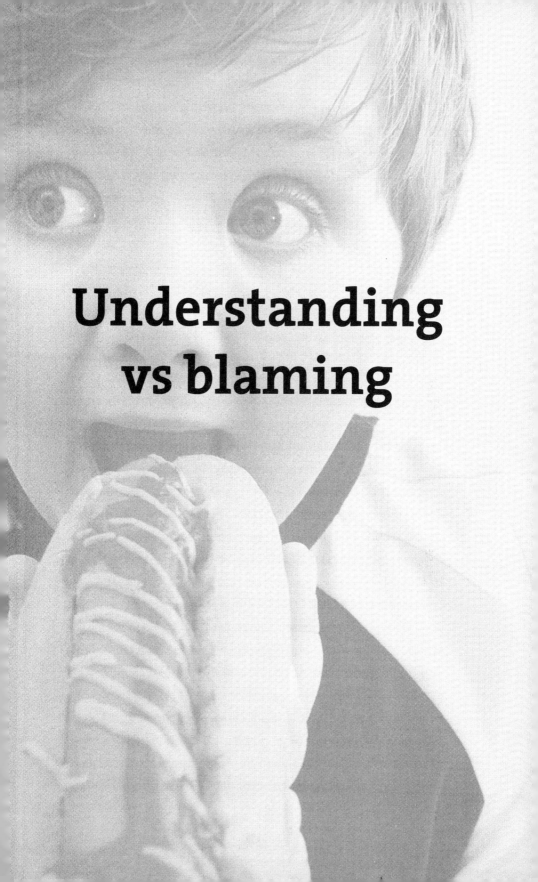

Understanding vs blaming

1. The big fat conspiracy

Many, if not most, people are at least a little sensitive about their shape or size. This is not surprising, considering the cultural and social expectations about how bodies should look, not to mention the deeply ingrained prejudices surrounding fat. Even health professionals who specialise in treating obesity share some of wider society's beliefs that people who are fat are lazy or greedy. Or both.

The rapid explosion in rates of obesity and overweight right around the world—in countries rich and poor—has forced a radical rethink of these stereotypes. The fact that so many people in so many different places are piling on so many kilos makes it clear that something much bigger than any single individual must be involved. Weight gain was once blamed on moral weakness, vulnerable personality types or bad behaviour, but it is increasingly being understood as a normal physiological response to a pathological environment.[1] Instead of being seen mostly as a medical problem, weight has become an environmental and an economic issue. Globalisation, industrialisation, urbanisation, environmental change and economic development are blamed for creating conditions which support and encourage inactivity and over-consumption of food.[2]

For Bob Volkmer, a child health researcher at the Children, Youth and Women's Health Service in Adelaide, the analogy with intensive animal production is obvious. 'How do you fatten up an animal?' he asks. 'You coop it up and you feed it a lot. That's exactly what our modern environment does.' Others talk about free-range versus battery-reared children. In a similar vein, many studies have shown that wild animals carry far less fat than their domesticated cousins.

Some observers draw comparisons between obesity and infectious disease epidemics.[3] Germs might have caused the infections, but it was urbanisation and industrialisation that created the perfect breeding grounds for outbreaks of disease. Similarly, obesity can be viewed simplistically—as a consequence of overeating and inactivity—or as the result of a complex interplay of environmental factors, many of which are associated with increasing affluence and the growth of cities.

Take a trip

Taking a quick spin around the globe helps illustrate this. The pattern of obesity in countries tends to reflect their stage of economic development. The overweight epidemic started to spread rapidly in the high-income countries of western Europe, the US and Australasia during the 1980s and 1990s, and even more recently in middle-income countries.[4] Obesity is becoming prevalent even in poor countries, many of which are caught in a situation known as 'nutrition transition', where significant proportions of their people suffer from either under-consumption or over-consumption. Within a population, obesity first becomes noticeable in middle-aged women, then middle-aged men, then teenagers and finally children.

In the early stages of the spread of obesity, the effects tend to be most obvious in the wealthy—those who are the first to enjoy the benefits of modernisation, such as cars, labour-saving devices, sedentary recreation, and the easy availability of rich foods. As economic prosperity spreads further, allowing ordinary workers to buy cars, TVs and takeaway meals, obesity becomes more prominent in the poorer groups. This is at least partly because their environments—which typically include much easier, cheaper access to fatty food than to vegetables and fruit—encourage weight gain.

The big picture[5]

The big fat conspiracy is not only a problem for Australia. It is an international problem, sometimes referred to as "globesity", as these figures show.

• Internationally, about 10 per cent of young people aged 5 to 17 are overweight, including 2–3 per cent who are obese. In 2000, an estimated 30–45 million worldwide were obese. Obesity is becoming the most common chronic condition in children in the Americas, Europe and the Near/Middle East. One study estimated that 3 per cent of preschool children in developing countries are obese.

• Data from Brazil and China shows that the rate of increase in obesity among children in some developing countries is similar to or even greater than in the US. Between 1974 and 1997, the prevalence of overweight and obesity in children in Brazil rose from

4 per cent to 14 per cent. In Chile, 12 per cent of 6-year-old boys and 14 per cent of 6-year-old girls were overweight in 1987; by 2000, the rates had jumped to 26 per cent and 27 per cent respectively.

- In the US, over the past 30 years, the obesity rate has tripled among children aged 2 to 5 (from 5 to 14 per cent) and youth aged 12 to 19 (from 5 to 17 per cent). It has quadrupled among children aged 6 to 11 (from 4 to 19 per cent) By 2010, it is expected that 20 per cent of children and young people in the US will be obese.
- The highest rates in Europe are found in the south. One survey found that 36 per cent of 9-year-old children in Italy and Sicily were overweight or obese, as were 26 per cent of boys and 19 per cent of girls in Greece, 27 per cent of children in Spain, and 39 per cent of teenagers in Crete.
- Several countries in North Africa, the eastern Mediterranean and the Middle East have high rates. More than one-quarter of preschoolers and 14 per cent of teenagers in Egypt are overweight or obese, as are 25 per cent of children in Cyprus.
- Even in very poor countries where obesity remains rare, it is on the increase. In Bangladesh, rates of obesity in preschoolers increased from 0.1 per cent in 1982–83 to 1.1 per cent in 1996–97. Mauritius and Tanzania are among the rare countries where obesity rates in children are reported to have fallen.

The rapid changes occurring in China show us a powerful case study of the impact of economic development on waistlines. Researchers investigated the impact of changing transport patterns between 1989 and 1997, when the car began to supplant traditional forms of transport—walking and cycling.[6] Those with access to cars also began to expand at the girth. Changes in transport were accompanied by changes in food habits, education, leisure time activity, computer and TV ownership, and urbanisation. About 7.7 per cent of children in China are overweight, but the rate reaches 12.4 per cent in city areas and 29 per cent among preschoolers in city areas.[7]

Even in remote villages in Papua New Guinea, the impact of modernisation has been linked to expanding waistlines.[8] Researchers developed an 'index of modernity' based on education levels, type of housing, occupation, use of TVs and cars and how much modern technology was used in a particular village. Several villages were then rated on the modernity index and the people's weight was measured. As the level of modernity increased in a village, so did the level of fatness. One of the researchers involved in that study, a diabetes expert from Melbourne, Professor Paul Zimmet, links the obesity epidemic to the 'coca-colonisation' of the world. For experts like Zimmet, that particular soft drink has become a metaphor for something other than the glamorous lifestyle portrayed in its advertising. It is no statistical coincidence that rates of obesity have risen as soft drink sales have soared.

Of course, ours is not the first generation to complain about the 'modern world'. It's been a constant complaint throughout history, just as every new generation has had to listen to its elders moan about all the things that are wrong with 'young people today'. Modernisation has indeed brought many benefits. Apart from enjoying great material wealth, children today—and perhaps even their parents—cannot even imagine the devastation of infectious diseases which were once commonplace. Childhood is in many ways safer than ever before. Nonetheless, there are other indicators that the news on modernity is not all good. Just pull out your old school photographs and compare them with your children's. You probably won't have to look too hard to spot what's changed.

On average, the kids in the colour photographs will be taller and chubbier than the ones in the black and white pictures. Not all of them, though. We are, as some wit once joked, all individuals, every single one of us. Everyone responds differently to the same circumstances or environment. Some people will be unlikely to gain weight no matter what's going on in their environment, while others will find it easy to pile on the kilos even when food is scarce. The majority fall somewhere between these two extremes, and will put on the odd kilogram if the environment encourages it. In experiments where people are deliberately overfed in closely controlled conditions, the amount of weight gain varies greatly between individuals. But identical twins tend to gain similar amounts, which suggests that much of the variation is genetically based.

Ancient genes a bad fit for a modern world

Our ancient genes are at the root of this modern epidemic. The human race adapted over millions of years to living in a world of scarcity, where you ate up when you had the chance if you wanted to survive. We developed a taste for sweet, fatty foods because they were rich sources of energy. There was little need for us to develop mechanisms to protect ourselves against overabundance.

Our bodies were programmed to respond to deprivation, not excess. No wonder it is so much easier to put on weight than to lose it. We were also programmed to conserve our energy for when it was really needed—in hunting food or defending ourselves. No wonder we now have such a great love affair with the couch and other energy-saving devices.

Our physiology hasn't changed much in thousands of years but our environment certainly has. The modern equivalent of hunting and gathering involves driving to a supermarket or, in the ultimate symbol of unhealthiness, a drive-through fast food outlet. Perhaps it doesn't even require that any more—now we can just pick up the phone to place an order, or do it over the internet. Our bodies' mechanisms for regulating appetite are not well equipped to deal with this world. When we are inactive, they are even less effective.

Aboriginal history holds the clues

Nowhere is the impact of westernisation more obvious and more devastating than among indigenous people such as Australian Aborigines.

Their traditional diets provided them with a wide range of nutritious foods. The wild animals they hunted were low in fat; the plants that they gathered provided fibre and carbohydrates that were slowly digested and absorbed. Wild honey was the only traditional source of carbohydrates loaded with calories.

Many of these foods were also rich in vital nutrients. A species of wild plum eaten in northern Australia has the highest vitamin C content of any known food, according to one study.[9] The nutty-buttery taste of the witchetty grub reflects a fat that has a composition very similar to olive oil, and a yam widely eaten in northern Australia boasts far more nutrients than its modern equivalent, the potato. Analysis of the composition of goannas, snakes, kangaroos, fish, wallabies, turtles, possums and other traditional sources of meat reveal low levels of saturated fats but a relatively high content of polyunsaturated fatty acids, and particularly omega-3 fats, which may protect us against cardiovascular disease and have other health benefits.[10]

Hunter-gatherer societies are thought to have worked hard—but not too hard—for their food. It has been estimated that such societies probably spent no more than three to five hours a day earning their sustenance, which is far shorter than the typical working day in agricultural and modern societies. However, finding and preparing food could involve bouts of intensive activity.

Their traditional diet and lifestyle protected Aborigines from many of the diseases associated with 'civilisation', such as diabetes and cardiovascular disease. They were fit and extremely lean, but studies found little evidence of malnutrition. If Europeans were as thin as Aborigines were, they would be likely to be malnourished. Aborigines' blood pressure was low and, like their weight, did not increase as they grew older.[11]

Professor Kerin O'Dea, a scientist who has documented the impact of westernisation on Aboriginal people in northern Australia and is now based at St Vincent's Hospital in Melbourne, says studies of Aborigines and other traditional societies suggest that increasing blood pressure is not an inevitable consequence of ageing. Instead, it results from the western lifestyle and age-related increases in weight. She says Aborigines had two key survival strategies to cope with an irregular food supply: they maximised energy intake and minimised energy output. Apart from gathering and preparing food, energy was not squandered. The notion of deliberately working up a sweat for no particular purpose would have seemed absurd.

When they had food, they ate it. If there was plenty, they feasted, sometimes eating two to three kilograms of meat each at a single sitting. They particularly valued meats and energy-dense foods such as honey. Their 'thrifty' metabolism also helped them make the most of their food during times of abundance: their bodies stored any excess as fat, so it could be drawn upon in times of scarcity. The 'thrifty genotype' hypothesis, which arose in the early 1960s, says that many indigenous peoples are extra effective at metabolising glucose, which is beneficial when food is in short supply.

But all these factors that were so advantageous to hunter-gatherers combined to ensure a health disaster when Aborigines moved to a western diet and lifestyle. This has been the case for many other indigenous people as well. Their thrifty metabolism, their traditions of feasting, and their preference for energy-dense food meant they soon put on weight in their new environment, and many developed non-insulin-dependent diabetes and cardiovascular disease. Feasting on lamb or other domesticated meats that have a high fat content means your calorie intake is two to four times higher than when eating the same quantity of kangaroo meat, which is very lean, according to O'Dea.

However, there are concerns that focusing on the 'thrifty genotype' hypothesis might distract attention from all the other factors which have made it extremely difficult for Aborigines to maintain healthy lifestyles in the modern world. The recent history of the Pitjantjatjara people in central Australia, as told by Stephan Rainow, the public environmental health officer for the Nganampa Health Council, which provides the area's health services, shows us a powerful example of this. He says local people first came into sustained contact with outsiders during the testing of atomic bombs in the region during the 1950s. They were moved onto missions or other settlements, and were given rations, mainly flour, sugar and tea. Later, community stores were established—at first they were run by government, then by the communities themselves.

Rainow remembers living in one remote community (in the late 1970s) which received a planeload of perishables once a week. They would be consumed within a few days, leaving limited supplies for the rest of the week. In many communities, people still relied on bush tucker for most of their food. They hunted and gathered, assisted by modern technology in the form of rifles and motor vehicles. And women who went out digging for rabbits inevitably came home with dozens, says Rainow.

Two events changed this hunting and gathering pattern. The Port Arthur massacre of 1996 led to tougher gun laws, which had a dramatic impact on locals' ability to hunt. The release of the calicivirus was also disastrous—the rabbits disappeared. Rainow says the end of rabbit hunting also affected women's health: they were no longer using as much physical energy as when they had to dig up rabbit burrows.

People began to rely more on the community stores. Many of these had limited ability to store fresh produce, so they tended to stock ready-to-eat foods that were high in fat, sugar and salt. Soft drinks have traditionally been one of their highest selling lines. Lack of housing and other infrastructure meant that even if fresh produce had been more widely available, many people wouldn't have had the facilities or skills to prepare it. Poor access to healthy food is reflected in poor health; Rainow says people in their 20s are being diagnosed with type 2 diabetes.

The Nganampa Health Council is now working at getting the community stores to stock foods that have a higher nutritional value and improving the management practices of the stores. They are also working closely with businesses to improve the range and affordability of their food supply. 'Our primary concern is to make sure people have access to affordable healthy food,' says Rainow.

The Pitjantjatjara story is not unique. Surveys have consistently shown that fresh food is extremely expensive and often of poor quality and variety in remote Aboriginal and Torres Strait Islander communities. In other words, some of Australia's poorest and most unhealthy people are expected to pay the highest prices for fresh food of variable quality. At the same time, junk food, takeaways and soft drinks are often readily available, widely promoted and relatively more affordable. Not surprisingly, studies have shown that in some Aboriginal communities fruit and vegetable consumption is much lower than it is elsewhere in Australia, and sugar consumption is far, far higher.[12]

Some studies suggest that the key to improving the health of Aboriginal people and other Australians lies in the past. Professor Kerin O'Dea was involved in a series of studies in the 1970s and 1980s that showed the benefits of a traditional diet and lifestyle for members of the Mowanjum community in Western Australia's Kimberley region. Small groups returned to a traditional lifestyle for periods ranging from 2 weeks to 3 months. The composition of their food was carefully analysed and the study participants were extensively tested before, during and after the studies. Their health improved markedly, even after just a fortnight in the bush. In one project involving 10 people with diabetes, the participants lost between 3 and 12 kilograms during the 7 weeks of the study and their diabetes control and cardiovascular risk factors improved markedly. O'Dea and her colleagues concluded that the hunter-gatherer lifestyle was effective in treating obesity, non insulin-dependent diabetes, high blood pressure and coronary heart disease.

The studies have been described as among the most important pieces of Australian health and medical research in recent decades. Apart from their scientific significance—showing that dietary and lifestyle changes could have a major effect in just weeks on a condition which takes years to develop—the work also had political and cultural impact. For instance, bush tucker was once prohibited in some areas, but now it is promoted in some indigenous health education campaigns as a way of managing chronic disease. O'Dea has spoken to all sorts of groups about how the traditional hunter-gatherer lifestyle can teach western communities how to treat and prevent many chronic diseases.

Running backwards

In 2000, 14 men were asked to wear a small device around their waists to measure their activity levels. It was sensitive enough to record even their fidgeting.

Seven of the men were actors at Old Sydney Town, a historic theme park north of Sydney, where they played the parts of Australian soldiers, convicts and settlers in the early 19th century. During the study, they agreed to avoid the use of modern technology as much as possible when not at work. Two took the project so seriously that they abandoned modern life altogether during the study, and stayed at the theme park all the time. The other seven men involved in the project went about their lives as usual, working as accountants, information technology buffs, doctors, and taxi drivers. One was an entertainer.

The researchers found that the old-timers were far more active than the modern workers; the difference was the equivalent of walking an average of 8 kilometres a day.[13] The difference for the two men most dedicated to the traditional lifestyle was equivalent to walking about 16 kilometres a day. This is about the distance people think our hunter-gatherer ancestors travelled each day, foraging for food.

The researchers concluded that the widespread use of labour-saving technologies means we are unlikely to be as active as our forebears unless we make a conscious effort. When you add these lower activity trends to our abundant, energy-dense food supply, say the researchers, it seems that obesity is 'almost an inevitable consequence of modernisation'.

Unintended consequences

Throughout history, people have aimed to build a better future for their children. They didn't want their offspring to go without, as perhaps they had done, or to work as hard as they had done to put food on the table. Their dreams have come true. Never before has food been so easily available, for so little sweat.

'We have spent thousands of years trying to create this environment,' says Garry Egger, Adjunct Professor in the School of Exercise and Nutrition at Deakin University in Victoria. 'We never thought of the downside. We applaud every advance in technology without thinking of the negative effects.' It's a reminder to be careful what you wish for. The best intentions can have unintended consequences. Here are a few examples:

• After the hardship years of World War II, many countries developed 'cheap food' policies, supporting farmers as they boosted production of crops and animals. One history has documented how this allowed even the poor to eat plenty of meat, butter, fats and sugar. Governments wanted to ensure children's growth and a strong workforce.[14] One of the consequences, however, was a huge epidemic of coronary heart disease, which emerged first in the more affluent and agriculturally innovative countries.

• Labour-saving devices have transformed our lives, and not only on the factory floor. Push-button technology saves us from getting off the couch to change the channel, from getting out of the car to open the garage, from beating eggs by hand, from walking to the clothesline to hang out the clothes. These days you don't even have to work up a sweat scrubbing the bathroom—a spray and wipe will do. These are small, everyday things, so you mightn't expect them to add up to much. But they do; research increasingly suggests that the loss of exactly this kind of everyday, incidental activity contributes to weight gain. Technology can also have other, indirect effects on health. Microwaves might be convenient but they also make it easier to eat on the run, rather than sitting down to the table as a family, a ritual that has been shown to promote healthy food habits.

• We want our children to have every opportunity. We send them to the best schools, which often means travelling further than the closest one—and the closest one is the one most likely to be within walking distance. We push schools to provide the best academic opportunities possible, even if this means there is little time left in the school day for running and playing. In 1999, a South Australian study documented how many schools reduced the time students spent in physical education classes to accommodate academic demands.[15] As one teacher told the researchers: 'How many parents complain in your parent-teacher interviews that their kids aren't doing well at fitness?' The study showed that dedicating time to PE did not harm academic attainment.

• We designed our suburbs with cul de sacs, thinking this would provide safer play areas for children. But what it also has done is discourage us from strolling around our neighbourhoods, because walking to the park or the shops became such a circuitous, unappealing exercise. We are much more likely to walk around our neighbourhood if the streets are in a grid pattern and there is a visible destination, such as a corner shop.

• The double or triple garage doors that dominate the face that many houses present to the street mean there are fewer windows facing onto the street and hence less of a feeling that children on the streets are being watched over. Dr Paul Tranter, a senior lecturer in geography at the Australian Defence Force Academy in Canberra, cites this as just one example of how modern urban design makes the streets less safe for children to use.[16]

Social changes

Many of the social changes which have accompanied economic development have also had a marked impact on children's lives. More families have both parents working—and single parents families where the single parent are also more likely to be working working—and often for long hours. One large study that tracked the lives of more than 10,000 Australian children and their families found that 40 per cent of children were younger than one when their mother returned to the paid workforce.[17] And two-thirds of 4 and 5-year-olds had a mother who had returned to paid work at some stage since their birth. In that same study, 47 per cent of working parents said they often or always felt rushed. Interestingly, so did 36 per cent of parents who were not in the paid workforce. Meanwhile, a national survey in 2004 found that about a third of full-time workers with children agreed with the statement, 'Your work means you currently neglect your relationships with family and friends but you plan to make up for it in later years'.

How ironic is that: technology was meant to give us more time, not less. As journalist Carl Honoré points out in his book challenging the cult of speed, that particular prediction was spectacularly off target.[18] Honoré cites Benjamin Franklin's vision of a world devoted to rest and relaxation. In the 1700s, Franklin predicted that men would soon work no more than 4 hours a week. Similarly, George Bernard Shaw predicted we would work less than 2 hours a day by 2000, and in 1956 Richard Nixon told Americans to prepare for a 4 day working week in the 'not too distant future'.

When Australian National University researchers recently asked 50 leading Australian experts why they thought obesity levels had skyrocketed, they nominated time as one of their top culprits. Or lack of it. When your days and weeks disappear in a frenzy of clock-racing, it's hard to find time to play with the kids or shop. Or is it? Australians spend hours each day in front of the telly, where many of the advertisements tell us we are too busy to cook, and should buy this or that convenient product, whether it's a processed meal, a takeaway, or the latest gizmo for saving our precious time and energy. Marketing surveys show that a third of the food budget in Australia is spent on foods prepared away from home, which tend to be much fattier than home-cooked meals.[19]

American journalist and academic Ellen Ruppel Shell argues that many people have been sucked in by industries with a vested interest in spreading the word about the scarcity of time.[20] People have been persuaded that spending a few minutes refuelling in a fast food outlet is 'fun', says Shell, whereas a family dinner at the kitchen table is an 'obligation'. Similarly, walking a few blocks a day is a dreary chore, while spending hours transfixed by a cathode ray tube is 'relaxing'. She says the image makers who produce and market TV have succeeded in convincing the masses that they are too exhausted to do anything after work other than collapse in front of 'can't miss' programming. Just savour the many delicious ironies in this image: the couch potato is ploughing through takeaway while salivating over the delectable celebrity chef Nigella Lawson, at work on the TV with her electric pepper grinder. Who needs to cook when you can watch someone else doing it? It's a bit like sex, according to the same logic. Apparently many of us are having less sex than our parents did, though there is more sex than ever on TV, billboards and in so many other parts of daily life.

It's not only adults who race the clock. Some children, if their parents can afford it, are also way too busy to kick a ball around a park. Academic coaching, music lessons, drama lessons and being driven from one engagement to another leaves little time for unstructured play, which is important for children's development in lots of ways. Young children talk about scheduling time to play with friends, sometimes weeks in advance. One study of Year 5 students (aged about 10) in western Sydney found one-quarter reported having no or minimal time for free play during the 3 days of the survey. Forty per cent of the children spent an average of 60 minutes or more after school doing homework.[21] Some education authorities recommend that 30–45 minutes would be more appropriate for 10-year-olds.

The fact that people are becoming parents at older ages today than they did 50 years ago is also having an effect, points out a 46-year-old friend with two young children and a demanding job. This friend is constantly running between her children and her work. She doesn't have much time or energy left for running around the backyard or park with her kids. Her partner's long working hours don't help. 'Older parents often don't have the physical stamina to run around with their kids,' she says. 'And because we're further into our careers than younger parents, we tend to have more responsibilities at work, and we are often expected to put in long hours.'

When parents don't have as much time or energy for their children as they or their kids would like, what do they do? Try to make everyone feel better. Often that involves buying a treat. Perhaps the latest computer game. Or, more likely, some junk food. It's not just dads who only see their kids on weekends who try to compensate for their absence with sweets. A Victorian Government report into nutrition in childcare centres describes parents sometimes using food as compensation for children attending childcare or as a means of dealing with their own guilt.[22] Parental guilt is, of course, well nourished by marketers, who make a living out of both cultivating it and preying upon it.

For many child health experts, the rising rate of obesity in children is just one effect of a whole set of social changes, including an increasing focus on the rights of the individual rather than collective responsibility. Other symptoms, according to Newcastle community paediatrician Professor Graham Vimpani, include increases in reporting of child abuse, and increasing concerns about behavioural problems in children. 'The group of people in society that has had responsibility for the care of children has shrunk from 80 people—if you think of clans in traditional societies and extended families—down to one or two caring for three or four kids,' he says. 'The support available for those caring for the kids has diminished considerably, so the stress of parenting is greater than it may have been once. The fragile nature of the modern family and the difficulty of achieving work–life balance for parents is a real challenge and struggle.'

The fear factor

Two marriages have put public health researcher Garry Egger in a good position to reflect on how the job of parenting has changed in recent decades. His first son is now in his 30s and has a young daughter. Egger also has two young children, aged 13 and 10.

'It's much harder now than when I was bringing my first son up,' he says. The most obvious change relates to heightened safety concerns, resulting in overprotective parents wrapping their children in 'cotton wool' or engaging in 'helicopter parenting', the term for when parents hover anxiously around their children. It's so different from when Egger was a lad, he says, when he vanished with his mates and roamed the neighbourhood all day, far from parental supervision. Just about every parent of a similar age tells a similar story. Professor Louise Baur, a paediatrician at Sydney's Westmead Hospital who specialises in treating and researching childhood obesity, reminisces over her memories of growing up in Sydney in the 1960s and 1970s. 'We had bushland at the end of the street where we used to disappear,' she says. 'There was the corner store where we got milk and bread. We rode our bikes to school. Today there is a motorway where the bush was. The shop has gone and the school bans kids from riding bikes to school.'

Fear rules many children's lives, in ways great and small. It seems a bit unfair, however, to blame parents for being so anxious when so many interests have a stake in promoting public fear or an exaggerated sense of risk. It helps to sell everything from soaps to medicines, from newspapers to government policies. Politicians, doctors, lawyers and many other powerful agents in society use fear when they want to influence our behaviour. It is very difficult for parents to resist such emotional blackmail and to dispassionately examine the reality of the risks facing their children. The media, in particular, has a huge impact in distorting the community's perceptions of risk. Relatively uncommon events, such as a child abduction, are more likely to attract headlines than more everyday events such as traffic accidents. Most people believe crime is becoming more common, for instance, when the opposite is true, according to research cited by the Australian Institute of Criminology.[23]

Risk and its management has become a huge industry. It sustains an army of consultants, experts, researchers and bureaucrats. Charles Landry, an international authority on urban renewal, observes that risk has become a prism through which any activity is judged. 'It subtly encourages us to constrain aspirations, act with over caution, avoid challenges and be sceptical about innovation,' he says. 'It narrows our world into a defensive shell. The life of a community self-consciously concerned with risk and safety is different from one focused on discovery and exploration.'[24]

Many studies show that concerns about risk limit children's opportunities for play and adventure. 'The way the world is today, you don't let them play out in the street. It would be nice to let them just run around as we used to do, but you can't any more,' one parent told researchers who were investigating the influences on where children play.[25] People who worry about their neighbourhood's safety are also less likely to be physically active. Not surprisingly, people living in poorer areas are more likely to report safety concerns about their neighbourhoods. If you don't feel safe walking to the shops or in your local park, health promotion campaigns to encourage walking are less likely to have an effect. This is perhaps another reason why being overweight tends to be more of an issue for families struggling to make ends meet.

Parents are not alone in their worry that something dreadful will happen if they don't keep their children on a tight rope. Fear also motivates how schools, local councils, community groups, childcare centres and other institutions shape children's lives. It's an issue that often frustrates Sydney father Alan Barclay, who would like his children to have the opportunities for physical play that he enjoyed as a child. He has been fighting a losing battle to have their primary school replace playground equipment, which was removed a few years ago because of safety concerns. The school has also removed its bicycle racks, which makes it very difficult for his children to cycle to school as there is nowhere to safely store their bikes. Organisations' concern about safety risks can also affect children in other ways. Fears about liability and government risk management policies mean some childcare centres put far more resources and effort into preventing food poisoning than they do into ensuring that children have nutritious meals, according to one report. The Victorian Government's investment in food safety is limiting early childhood centres' ability to focus on healthy eating, that report says.[26]

Ironically, safety concerns may add to children's risks. Some parents prefer to drive their children to school to reduce the risk of 'stranger danger', and thus they add to traffic hazards. 'If all parents allowed their children to walk or cycle to school, they would be safer in terms of both traffic danger and stranger danger,' says Dr Paul Tranter.[27] 'They would be safer from traffic, as there would be fewer cars (especially near schools). They would also be safer from strangers because they would be in larger groups and hence could benefit from safety in numbers.'

Some experts believe the trend towards smaller families and older parents also contributes to 'bubble wrapping' of children. It means parents have a greater investment in fewer children. And it's not only children's waistlines that suffer when they are kept carefully cooped up. Professor George Patton, a child psychiatrist in Melbourne, warns that limiting children's independent exploration, risk-taking and physical activity may have profound effects on their physical, cognitive and emotional development.[28] Suffering—and surviving—scraped knees and other setbacks helps prepare children for the ups and downs that life will inevitably throw their way.

Unhealthy development

It's fair to say that children's health and wellbeing has not traditionally been a front-of-mind issue for town planners and developers. You can tell that is a fair comment just by looking around our cities and suburbs. So many aspects of urban design make it difficult for children to enjoy healthy, active lives. These include the scarcity of fresh produce outlets and public transport infrastructure in many new housing estates, and the lack of opportunities for children to safely walk or cycle to destinations in their neighbourhood such as school, the shops or a friend's place. Some researchers have gone so far as to suggest that much planning and development is designed, presumably unintentionally, to promote crime and reduce safety.[29] Even when planners have tried to do the right thing by providing open public spaces such as parks and ovals, their efforts have not always been productive, according to Ed Blakely, Professor of Urban, Regional Planning and Policy at the University of Sydney. These spaces might be useful for people wanting to play sport, but they are unlikely to engage a broad range of people in diverse activities, he says. People need to be 'seduced' to use such areas, by the use of paths, signs, aesthetic features such as lakes and the opportunity to undertake a variety of activities. Dog walkers as well as footballers, playground enthusiasts and power-walking grandmothers need to be welcomed.

However, healthier town planning means much more than better access to well-designed green spaces. Many experts believe our entire approach to town planning needs an overhaul. Everything from the pattern of streets to the size of pavements, the design of suburbs and community centres, and the placement of public facilities needs to be rethought so that it creates opportunities for physical activity, especially walking and cycling. People are more likely to walk when they have a destination. Planning that puts residential, commercial and public areas close together means people can walk to the doctor, to school or to the train station. 'You need to have paths that take you some place, whether to a shop or a lake,' says Blakely. 'Our footpaths are organised more as decoration at the front of the house than as something people would use. They are not wide enough, and when houses are set back behind fences and hedges, it's unfriendly. Most of our suburbs do not have interesting places to walk.'

While a few places, notably Western Australia, are implementing a more healthy approach to urban planning, this is still the exception rather than the rule. 'We live in cities that were designed to use energy—but not our own,' says Blakely.

Car crush

It's no coincidence that car advertisements appeal to our emotions rather than our reason. Australians' all-consuming love affair with our sleek, sexy, speed machines—whoops, that's the subliminal power of advertising at work—just isn't rational. If reason ruled, we'd be calling the whole thing off. Instead, in some cities cars are multiplying at a faster rate than people.[30]

Putting aside issues such as pollution and petrol prices, let's simply consider the impact of cars on kids. Children are spending more and more of their time in cars. Many are no longer allowed to walk or cycle to school because their parents are frightened of the traffic. So they are driven instead, adding to the traffic their parents are frightened of, and to the general congestion on the roads. Because there are fewer kids walking, the streets are emptier and don't feel as safe. Kids don't get to

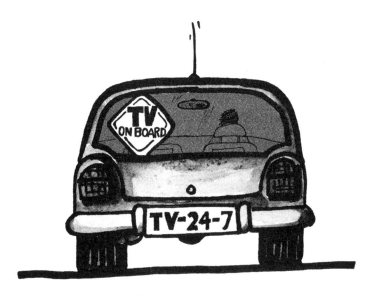

Telly-commuters

know their neighbours or neighbourhood, reducing the sense of safety that comes with familiarity. The closure of many local shops, because of the big shopping centres, also reduces the number of people pounding the pavements—and adds to the traffic jams. Many roads are busy even on weekends as parents chauffeur their children to sports. Our cars are driving us in ever more vicious circles.

In Britain, it has been suggested that the typical family now spends more time together in their car than at the family meal table. Which brings us to the ultimate in unhealthy relationships: the union of the car and takeaway. It is consummated, of course, at the junk-food drive-through. For those who might sniff in disapproval at such a partnership, Australian National University researcher Dr Jane Dixon points out that most of us, whether drive-through lovers or not, suffer from a 'car-centred diet'. She contrasts the Australian way of food shopping, which for most people involves a drive to a supermarket, with the traditional 'pedestrian-friendly diet' that involved a walk to local shops or markets. 'Very few of us can provide the household with food without the car, which is dispiriting,' she says, 'especially if you care about an active population and the environment.' One government planning department developed a 'litre of milk index' which showed on a map the locations where a litre of milk could be bought. This graphically revealed that shops selling milk in older suburbs were accessible by foot. But in the newer suburbs where many young families live, milk was sold in shops that were almost impossible to reach by foot.

Dr Mayer Hillman, an English authority on transport and the environment, offers a fresh perspective on 'stranger danger' too. The most dangerous strangers for children and young people are those otherwise harmless people behind a steering wheel. He argues that danger should be removed from children rather than vice versa, and suggests that cars have helped create an environment for children which shares many of the characteristics of a prison. Like prisoners, children have a roof over their heads, meals and entertainment provided— but they are not free to come and go.

The rise and rise of the motor car is helping to breed child-unfriendly cities and attitudes. One study found that children in Canberra and Sydney were far less likely to be allowed to come home from school alone, to travel to places other than school alone or to catch a bus alone, compared with children in German cities.[31] One of the study's authors, Paul Tranter, a geographer at the Australian Defence Force Academy in Canberra, says Australian cities are not as child-friendly as some other cities that are more materially deprived. Some researchers believe that one of the key characteristics of a child-friendly city is that its young have freedom to explore their environment, uninhibited by physical, social or cultural constraints. Australian cities do not rate highly on this scale, says Tranter, who blames both our culture and our urban design. In Germany, there is a greater sense of collective responsibility for children, and parents are more likely to trust that other adults will look out for their children. The higher population density also means children are more likely to be in walking distance of schools, friends' homes and community facilities. The other key factor, says Tranter, is the widespread use of public transport, by rich and poor, and the fact that it is generally perceived as safe and reliable. As well, Germans are more enthusiastic users of their public spaces. 'Our lifestyles are much more privatised here,' he says.

One way the car has contributed to the privatisation of formerly public space, Tranter argues, is by stealing residential streets from the children who once played on them. Growth in the levels and speed of traffic in residential areas means fewer kids gathering to play cricket or hopscotch on the roads outside their home. As the volume, speed and noise of traffic increases, children are forced off the street and onto the footpath; then into their front yards and then further, into the back or private parts of their home territory.

The 50 Australian experts asked for their views on why obesity rates were increasing were also quick to single out our obsession with cars.[32] The study's authors say strong government investment in the car industry and inadequate government promotion of mass transport systems have both contributed to and been driven by an increasing reliance on the car. Similarly, urban planners and developers have responded to and reinforced the dominance of the car. New housing developments are situated on major car routes rather than public transport routes, and new development approvals often require the provision of adequate car parking rather than the provision of walking or cycling facilities.

Cars are doing more than stealing children's freedom, argues Tranter. Children who are driven to school have less opportunity for the joy of exploring their natural environment, not to mention learning how to deal with the grumpy old woman on the corner who yells at them for picking her flowers. It's all part of developing a sense of place and an understanding of their neighbourhood. 'That's really important, not just as a feelgood thing, but for their health,' Tranter says. 'Feeling connected with people and having a good network of friends and community is probably far more important to your physical health than whether you drink, exercise, or eat well. We're very social animals.' In his book *In Praise of Slowness*, Carl Honoré cites studies showing a correlation between car ownership and sense of community. The less traffic that flows through an area, and the more slowly it flows, the more social contact there is among the residents. In suburbia, he says, many people know their neighbours' cars better than they know the neighbours themselves. Tranter believes that giving the streets back to children might also help their elders bond and develop stronger communities. 'Children are an effective way of breaking down the natural reserve between adults,' he says.

The saddest scenario for Tranter involves children who walk direct from their home into the car sitting in the garage. By the time the electric doors roll up, they are already transfixed by a small screen in the car and don't even look out the windows on their drive to school. Once at school, Tranter's research suggests, their environment is often structured and supervised to minimise their freedom and their contact with earth and nature. 'Adults restrict children's freedom in school grounds because this simplifies adults' lives,' he says. 'It keeps children out of the way, or easily supervised—it keeps children in their place.'

And if unforeseen circumstances meant these children had to walk home, there's a good chance they might not be able to find their way.

2. Commercial Time™

Random thoughts

• Pizza is home-delivered in just about every suburb and town across Australia. It's not nearly as easy to have fresh, affordable vegetables and fruit delivered to your door...

• A burger with chips and a Coke is sold at just about every blip on the map. But in many small country towns, fresh vegetables and fruit are expensive and limp, if they're available at all...

They're your little darlings. But that's not what some others see when they look at your kids. They see consumers, and they want to get their hooks into them and their spending power, now and into the future. The commercialisation of childhood has given new meaning to that old Jesuit saying, 'Give me the child until he is seven and I will show you the man.' The modern equivalent is more along these lines: 'Give me the child and I will have a customer for life'. It's a little like treating children as calves—brand them young and they will forever bear the imprint.

In a world which increasingly runs on marketing principles and which regards everything from schools to sports stars as brands, children have become the targets of some extremely clever, powerful adult persuasion. One problem with this is that the relationship between child and marketer is utterly unbalanced. Young children do not have the cognitive skills to pick ad-speak from adult speak which can be trusted. According to an investigation into advertising and children by the American Psychological Association, most children under 4 or 5 have little awareness of the concept of advertisements. They then start to recognise them as different—because they are funnier or shorter than normal television programs. Children younger than 7 or 8 usually lack adults' ability to understand that the source of the message has other perspectives and interests from them, or that the message intends to persuade and is biased and therefore needs a different interpretation from other messages. The Association cites research showing that fewer than 50 per cent of 8-year-olds understand advertising's persuasive purposes.[1]

What does this mean? It means that young children tend to accept commercial claims and appeals as truthful and accurate. Even when they grow older and wiser, they remain vulnerable to the power of the promo. After all, even the most sceptical and intelligent of adults can be sucked in. What chance do children have? They are bunnies caught in the mega-wattage of the marketers' spotlight. The American Psychological Association laments the use of child psychology in marketing. It cites books with titles such as: *Kids as Customers: A Handbook of Marketing to Children*; *Marketing To and Through Kids*; *What Kids Buy and Why: The Psychology of Marketing to Kids*; and *Creating*

Ever-Cool: A Marketer's Guide to a Kid's Heart. Researchers investigate how best to get kids to act as lobbyists. The target, of course, is parents and their purses. One marketing guru has identified a number of varieties of 'pester power'.[2] These include: the persistent nag, who begs, pleads and grovels; the demonstrative nag, who threatens tantrums or worse; the forceful nag, who is pushy and may use threats such as, 'Well I'll just ask Dad then'; the pleading nag, whose favourite expression is 'Please, please, please'; and the sugar-coated nag, who promises affection in return for indulgence.

It wouldn't be surprising if these descriptions sound like someone you know; the same marketing expert claims that 75 per cent of spontaneous food purchases can be traced to a nagging child. It's not only parents' wallets that suffer as a result. Parents often feel trapped: if they constantly refuse their children's requests, they feel mean; if they give in, they know they are paying an unhealthy price for peace. Some commentators argue that advertising-induced nagging is transforming relationships between parents and children.[3] Advertising often treats parents as obstacles for children to get around, they say, rather than as figures of authority whose opinions should be respected.

'Sometimes I feel that my main job as a parent is saying no to my children,' says a friend who is a father of five. He feels he is constantly battling the marketing and other social forces encouraging his children into unhealthy consumption.

Dream thieves

Market researchers intrude into every aspect of children's lives. They ask about their dreams and fantasies, and even study their artwork in search of inspiration for marketing campaigns. Cartoon characters have been shown to be particularly

42

effective at helping children recall and identify products. The American journalist Eric Schlosser describes how marketers conduct surveys of kids in shopping malls, organise focus groups for toddlers, hire children to run focus groups, and stage slumber parties where the questioning goes into the night. As well, he says, cultural anthropologists quietly and surreptitiously observe children's behaviour in their homes, at the shops and at fast food restaurants.[4] 'Making emotional connections and building relationships with kids' was the title of one talk given at a conference in the United States for those who market food to young children.[5]

Apart from the ethics of exploiting the cognitive vulnerability of young people, another problem with child-centred marketing is that so much of it is flogging products that many kids would be better off without. Children are developing 'emotional connections' and 'relationships' with foods rich in sugar and/or fat, as well as with the toys used to promote these foods. In the United States, about 80 per cent of all advertising directed at children is for toys, cereals, confectionery or fast food restaurants.[6] The food industry is the second largest advertiser in the United States, after the automotive industry.[7] In 2004, the fast food industry was estimated to have spent about $3 billion on advertising aimed at kids in the United States, while the food industry as a whole spent $10 billion in advertising and marketing aimed at young people.[8] Those figures come into perspective when you consider estimates that children in the United States spend about $36 billion of their own money each year, and influence another $200 billion in household spending. The market is obviously much smaller in Australia, but even so it involves billions of dollars. It is estimated that Australians spent $8.5

billion on fast foods in 1999. We also have the dubious distinction of being the world's fourth largest consumers of snack foods, behind the United States, Britain and Ireland.[9]

The price of food relative to incomes and other goods has dropped significantly in recent decades. The food industry is fiercely competitive, and has to fight hard for its customers. Its major weapon in this battle is advertising. Food lends itself to advertising because it is bought often, consumer views can change quickly, and it is one of the most highly branded items. According to University of Minnesota academics Mary Story and Simone French, a child's first request for a product to be purchased usually occurs at about 24 months, and three-quarters of the time this request occurs in a supermarket. The first such request is most likely to be for breakfast cereal; this is likely to be followed by requests for snacks, drinks and toys. Studies show that in such situations, parents say yes to children's requests for lollies and other food about 50 per cent of the time and for drinks about 60 per cent of the time.

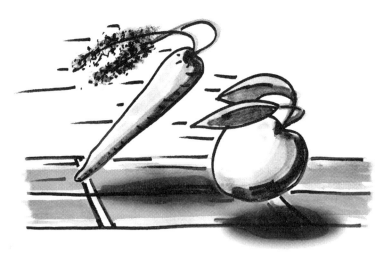

(Healthy) fast food

For those who might hope that the situation is different in Australia, the results of a 1996 study comparing international trends in advertising to children will be bad news. Consumers International monitored TV advertising to children in 13 countries over a 3-month period. Australia, the United States and the United Kingdom had the most food advertisements: between 10 and 12 an hour or about 200 in a 20-hour period. This was twice as many as in Denmark, Germany and France, and 6–10 times more than in Austria, Belgium and Sweden. Confectionery was the largest category, accounting for nearly a fifth of all food advertising.[10] When Victorian researchers asked parents about what influences the food choices of their 5 and 6-year-old children, the answer came back loud and clear: advertising of junk foods.[11]

The internet and other new media have opened up a whole new world for marketers. It is estimated that one website, nabiscoworld.com, attracts about 800,000 kids per month.[12] Sites like this have developed the concept of 'advergames'— games about the foods being promoted. At some websites, children earn points by playing marketing surveys to help industries finetune their strategies. Product placements in films and the use of Hollywood characters in food promotion are other marketing strategies. According to Eric Schlosser, the cross-promotion between Hollywood and the fast food industries means that the popular culture of American children has become indistinguishable from the fast food culture.

School rules

Schools these days have become so much more than places of learning and play. They are, from some perspectives at least, fabulous 'marketing platforms'. Not only is the audience captive, but any messages that become associated with the trusted environment of school are also more likely to be trusted.

Numerous investigations have revealed the infiltration of junk food marketing into schools, in the United States in particular. Soft drink and fast food companies have contracts giving them exclusive rights to market and sell their products in schools. Screensavers on school computers and scoreboards on sports grounds advertise fast foods. In some US schools, reading incentive programs give students a free pizza if they read a certain number of books. Then there's the McDonald's Spellit Club, which rewards good spellers with food from you can guess where. Food companies have also developed games and counting books for use in classrooms. According to one estimate, there are more than 40 children's counting and reading books featuring various food brands.[13] Some people call these teaching tools, others call them advertising. There seems no limit to the lengths to which some companies will go. In 2001, a multinational food company tested an advertising campaign which involved 10 primary school teachers in Minneapolis driving to school in cars plastered with advertisements for a sweetened cereal. The teachers earned $250 a month for their efforts as 'freelance brand managers'. The campaign was cancelled after 3 weeks because of public protest.[14]

If you're thinking, *Well that's America—it couldn't happen here*, think again. While many Australian schools are making great efforts to lift their nutritional game (and not a minute too soon), many remain at the front line of junk food marketing. This is not a one-way relationship; some schools are happy to work with these companies if it will boost their coffers. One Queensland home economics educator recently wrote about the negative influence of food companies on schools, and described a recent conversation with a high school principal who was proud of his canteen's profits.[15] The principal was delighted about making a deal to buy a certain cola drink at a much reduced price so the canteen would make even more money.

With so much media coverage about childhood obesity, you might hope that schools would be reluctant to promote Krispy Kreme doughnuts. But the company has had little difficulty finding schools and related organisations willing to enter into fundraising partnerships. Within 8 months of opening in Australia in 2003, Krispy Kreme had reportedly provided cheap doughnuts for fundraisers in hundreds of NSW schools.[16]

Meanwhile, when researchers surveyed 18 primary schools in Victoria in 2004, they found that of the 17 that had a food service, all sold meat pies but only five sold fruit regularly. The researchers concluded that most schools do not see providing food as part of their core business, and lack the inclination and resources to take on this added responsibility.[17]

The location of fast food outlets near schools is also cause for concern. A survey of teachers at a Perth school located directly opposite fast food shops suggested that the McDonald's outlet was being used as a 'babysitting' service before and after school. Parents rushing to work told their children to stay at McDonald's until school opened. A teacher of a Year 5 class told the researchers: 'I know some kids whose parents take them to McDonald's for breakfast on the way here, and often they will go on their way home from school as well.'[18]

Meanwhile, well-meaning teachers often use sweets as rewards in the classroom. Many parents do not realise how frequently this happens. One Sydney mother was surprised when her daughter Clare came home from primary school and asked if she could attend Scripture class. The family was not particularly religious and Clare had never shown such an interest before. It turned out that sweets were handed out in the Scripture class. Clare, who had been brought up to be conscious of the tricks of marketers and advertising, wasn't impressed with the use of lollies as 'bribes', she told her mother—she just wanted to join the class so she could be with her friends. Clare's mother was not impressed either.

However, many other parents have fallen for the advertisers' line that children need treats every day. Surveys of the contents of lunchboxes suggest that foods that used to be used as occasional treats, such as potato crisps and chocolates, have become everyday foods. One Australian study found that the majority of parents think daily food treats are acceptable.[19] Providing a new take on the notion of a 'balanced diet', a parent told the researchers: 'School lunch is only one meal of the day. If it's balanced throughout the day [by other meals], it's OK for kids to have treats in their lunch.'

Food industry marketing and promotions do more than normalise treats. They can make eating an apple or a piece of fruit seem a bit odd. Why would children need or want fruit when they can have a fruit bar or some other sugary concoction? Consider the message conveyed by a package of hot cross buns which were on sale one recent Easter. 'Specially made for kids,' said the label, 'NO FRUIT'.

As a senior cancer researcher, Dr Christine Paul is extremely aware of the importance of good nutrition for health. Even so, she sometimes finds it a struggle to ensure a healthy diet for her two young children because of the junk food culture. When she walks with her children around their local shops in Newcastle, NSW, friendly shopkeepers will often hand them a sweet. 'The kids are just used to being given things,' she says.

Christine feels guilty if she doesn't send her kids to school with a muesli bar or a chocolate in their lunchboxes, even though she's not happy about doing it. 'You feel as if you are starving them if you just give them a piece of fruit and a sandwich to take to school,' she says. 'That's not what children eat today. You feel like an ogre if you don't give them a bit more. I give them the treat even though I don't want to. It's the mother guilt. You just feel like you have to provide in the same way that other children are provided for. I hear about other people's lunchboxes all the time—"So and so has chips every day, so and so always has a chocolate bar".'

How unsporting

Australians' love of sport is legendary. Sport symbolises strength, fitness, skill, endurance, courage and many other admirable qualities. Thanks to the skill and power of marketing, sport has also come to be associated in no small way with alcohol. Advertisements, sponsorships, logos and many other techniques are used to reinforce the idea that sport equals grog. It's no wonder sporting successes tend to be celebrated with a six-pack or six.

Food companies have worked hard to expand the equation so that sport also equals their particular brand. Many children's sports and athletics clubs have proven eager partners. Sometimes these alliances have helped to promote healthy foods. But too often, they have not. The partnering of sport and junk food sends young children a powerful message, cementing in their minds a connection between fun and achievement on the one hand and foods that are high in fat and/or sugar on the other. This is not peculiar to Australia. British sport reportedly received more than £40 million from the fast food, confectionery and soft drinks industries in 2003. The only sectors which contributed more generously to British sport were the financial services industry and alcohol manufacturers.[20]

When Ben Ross took his two young sons to Little Athletics meetings not long after moving to Hobart, Tasmania, he was hoping it would give them the opportunity for exercise and to make some new friends. He was not impressed when he realised that McDonald's was a sponsor and, among other things, provided vouchers as prizes. At one meeting Ronald McDonald mingled with the kids while McDonald's representatives received a formal acknowledgement from the meeting's organisers for their sponsorship. Ben was horrified by the notion that taking his kids to athletics might lead to them wanting to go to McDonald's. He told the meeting's organisers his views and said that his family wouldn't be returning. The Little Athletics organisation in Tasmania seems quite unperturbed by such concerns. A spokeswoman insists that the relationship with the fast food company is 'absolutely not a problem'. 'Just because McDonald's are sponsoring us doesn't mean that we're promoting eating their cheeseburgers,' she says. She does add, however, that McDonald's now offers a range of healthy foods.

This comment encapsulates just why the association that McDonald's has forged with Little Athletics (and many other sporting and community groups) is so valuable for the fast food company. In the world of public relations and marketing, there is nothing more powerful than the so-called third party endorsement. For McDonald's, an endorsement from a trusted and valued community organisation like Little Athletics is priceless. It is far more valuable for the company than spending huge sums of money on more traditional forms of advertising.

What such an endorsement does for the credibility of Little Athletics—and the wellbeing of its young charges—is another matter.

It seems that even the spokeswoman must have considered this at some level; she admitted to being surprised that more people hadn't complained, particularly given the strong community support for Tasmanian potato growers, who had had a falling out with McDonald's. 'We thought we'd have more negative feedback,' she says.

But many parents are concerned by such blatant attempts to insinuate fast foods into children's lives. Brisbane scientist David Frazer is passionate about fostering a healthy lifestyle for his children, and was excited about taking them to a recent sign-up day for weekend athletics. He was horrified when each child was given a bag stuffed with soft drinks, potato crisps and vouchers to McDonald's. They were also expected to compete in a shirt that had a big M on it, signifying their sponsor.

However, David says it is his children's schools that are his major concern. Sausage rolls, pies and soft drinks are the main fare at school sports days, and one of his sons can buy soft drink for less than it costs to buy water from the canteen. His children regularly come home with bags of lollies from their teachers. 'I know my kids get junk foods 5 days a week just by going to school,' he says. David and his wife are seriously contemplating home-schooling for their youngest child, even though they don't think it's ideal socially, because they fear they cannot win the battle with the junk food culture found in many schools.

Karen Campbell, a dietitian in Melbourne who specialises in researching childhood obesity, often finds it difficult to juggle her roles as professional and parent. She is conscious that it is not appreciated when she raises concerns about the use of lollies as rewards in the classroom, or when she suggests to the tennis coach that he reward her children with a pack of tennis balls rather than soft drink. She was appalled when her son recently won a McDonald's voucher as a reward for a good game of footy. When she raised her concerns with the local football club, they were not taken seriously.

If health professionals, with all their expert knowledge and authority, have trouble swimming against the tide of junk food, the task must be even more daunting and difficult for others. It's another reminder of why parents need help—not accusing fingers—to combat the big fat conspiracy.

Food for thought

Unless you are old enough to remember what shopping was like in the 1950s, you may not appreciate the huge changes that have occurred to our food supply. Shoppers were once individually served in specialised shops such as the grocer, greengrocer, baker, butcher and milk bar. According to one history, the advent of supermarkets in the 1960s brought in self-service, reducing the requirement for staff and thus helping to make food cheaper.[21] Increased efficiencies in production and manufacturing also contributed to food becoming cheaper. Ever since, food companies have competed for market share by increasing their range of products. In the 1960s, it is estimated that Australians had access to 600 to 800 different foods, varying with the season. The average Australian supermarket now stocks 12,000 to 15,000 items, and many in the United States have up to 10 times that number.[22]

It is no coincidence that the range of products and the size of supermarkets have expanded at the same time as our waistlines. We are more likely to eat more when we are dizzied by choice. How many times have you left the supermarket with items you had no thought of buying when you arrived? Experiments show that even when people feel satiated by one particular food, they will continue to eat when a new food is presented.[23] As well, many of the new products are high in fat and/or sugar. The food industry knows our weaknesses. It is also where their profits lie; fats and sugars are extremely cheap inputs for manufacturers, and they make far more money from selling and promoting 'value-added' processed foods than they do from fresh produce. The advertising statistics reveal where the profits lie: nearly 70 per cent of food advertising is for convenience foods, confectionery and snacks, alcoholic beverages, soft drinks and desserts, and a mere 2 per cent is for the staples of a healthy diet—vegetables, fruit and grains.[24] Even in health magazines, the advertisements for foods high in fat and sugar far outnumber those for grains, vegetables and fruit.[25]

It's not only what we eat but how we eat that has changed so much in recent decades. Where once eating out of the home was reserved for a treat or special occasion, these days it has become the norm. According to figures cited by the National Heart Foundation, Australia now has more than 58,000 commercial food service outlets, including fast food outlets, restaurants, hotels, clubs and cafes. In 2004, Australians ate 4.8 billion meals and snacks out of the home, an average of four meals eaten out each week by each Australian. One in three people eat out almost every day, and this trend seems to be increasing. When it comes to fast food consumption, we're a world leader. Thirty per cent of Australians eat out at fast food restaurants every week, placing us in the world's top 10 fast food consumers. Hong Kong topped the list (at 61 per cent), followed by the US (35 per cent). Our favourite takeaways are sandwiches, hot chips, hamburgers, cakes and pastries.

It's not surprising, when you consider the size of the food industry, that it wields such power. It would be naive, says Dr

Tim Gill, Co-Director of the NSW Centre for Public Health Nutrition at the University of Sydney, to expect public health goals to dominate food policy, given the industry's political and economic clout.

'It's the second most powerful industry in the world,' he says. 'Policy on food is going to be driven by economics well before it's driven by public health.'

The eminent US nutritionist Professor Marion Nestle (whose name, it should be pointed out, is not pronounced like the food company's) first became aware of the food industry's influence on government policies and nutrition experts when she moved to Washington DC in 1986 for a new job. She was to manage the first (and only) Surgeon General's Report on Nutrition and Health, a comprehensive review of research linking dietary factors to chronic disease. It appeared as a 700 page book in 1988. The job was political dynamite. On Nestle's first day, the rules were made clear: no matter what the research suggested, the report could not recommend eating less of any category of food. Later Nestle wrote about the experience in her book, *Food Politics*. She said she had come to realise—through her work in academia, on government advisory committees and as a consultant to food companies, that many of Americans' nutritional problems, including obesity, could be traced to the food industry's interest in encouraging people to eat more. The industry's primary objective is to increase sales and income, not to encourage good nutrition, she says.

However, nutrition claims are often used to promote foods. Many observers have raised concerns about the close relationships between the food industry and nutrition organisations and researchers, and the potential for these links to influence and distort research and policy.[26] These connections also result in a proliferation of commercially motivated nutrition messages, some of which contradict others, creating unnecessary confusion about what constitutes a healthy diet. Yet the basic messages about healthy eating have not changed for years, despite a new nutrition controversy appearing every other week. Some commentators argue that the food industry deliberately creates controversy as a marketing strategy; first it creates the confusion, and then it sells the solution in the form of a product. Using nutrition claims to market foods also encourages people to focus on a particular aspect of their diet rather than on the overall picture. It's not surprising that the explosion in low-fat items coincided with widespread weight gain. People were so busy worrying about their fat intake that they didn't realise that many processed foods marketed as being low-fat are also high in sugar and calories. Filling your shopping trolley with low-fat foods can be very fattening.

Nestle also documents how food companies work hard to oppose and undermine advice to 'eat less'.[27] Messages to eat less meat, dairy and processed foods upset a host of interests, including primary producers and the many other industries which rely for their living on the promotion and consumption of these foods. Other experts point out that health messages promoting increased vegetable and fruit consumption also challenge the status quo. Economists from the US Department of Agriculture say that eating more fruit and vegetables and fewer animal foods would upset the existing 'volume, mix, production and marketing of agricultural commodities' and would require large 'adjustments' in international trade.[28]

Buyer beware

When doing my grocery shopping, I tend to buy the same old things while keeping an eye for a bargain. I'm interested in health, of course, but I'm usually most interested in trying to escape the supermarket as quickly as possible. Recently, I decided to take a different approach, to see what happens when I linger in the aisles, searching out products promoted on some sort of health basis.

I zoom past the fruit and vegies, there's nothing telling me to stop there, but am waylaid in the health food section which offers an impressive range of confectionery and mixed messages. Finally I settle upon a chocolate bar marketed both as 'decadence double chocolate' and 'a fast and easy way to lose weight'. It is also promoted as a good fibre and protein source, and for having a low glycaemic index (GI).

Next stop is the spreads section where I can't resist the Nutella. Not only does it contain 12 small packs, perfect for popping in a school lunch box, but it also bears a reassuring low GI symbol. Must be good.

There I also meet Mr Fluffy, the cartoon character used to sell Fluff, 'the delicious American marshmallow spread'. Fluff is packed with sugar but you have to look hard to work this out. It's the 'fat free' star on the front which is so eye-catching.

I am reminded of some of my favourite pieces of dietary advice: never eat anything which has a cartoon character on the front, don't eat anything your ancestors wouldn't recognise as food, and if something sounds too good to be true...

The cereals section is another minefield of dietary confusion. You wouldn't believe from looking along this aisle that, technically speaking at least, the only high-level health claim currently allowed on food relates to folate reducing the risk of having a baby with a neural tube defect.

Whether something amounts to a high-level health claim in the legalese of food regulation is, however, all in the detail and interpretation. Just because Uncle Tobys has a cereal called 'Healthwise, for Heart & Circulatory System' and bearing a tick from the National Heart Foundation does not mean that we should interpret this as 'eating this cereal might help reduce your risk of heart disease'. Of course not.

Naturally, I can't go past Kellogg's Coco Pops, that outstanding example of successful nutritional marketing. The adult equivalent must surely be 'Wild Oats Cluster Crunch': 'wholesome, wholegrain crunchy oat clusters oven-baked with pieces of hazelnut & chocolate'. The front of the packet boasts a low GI stamp and on the back is an extensive blurb about the health benefits of breakfasting on something that tastes like dessert.

By the time I finally check out, my trolley is reeling from the massive sugar and fat hit accumulated from so many 'health' foods.

For doubting Thomases who think my random supermarket survey was too unsystematic to warrant drawing sweeping conclusions, I'd have to agree that it was more about having a bit of fun than serious science.

Consider this though: in late 2005, three dietitians spent six weeks trawling through the shelves of a large supermarket in Sydney. Of the 7,000 different foods on the shelves, they analysed the nutrition and marketing claims of 4,200 packaged items.

Alan Barclay, a dietitian currently doing a PhD at the University of Sydney, and his colleagues found that 63 per cent of these foods carried some sort of nutrition or health-related marketing claim. 'The chances are that a significant proportion of those are not what you might call "everyday foods",' says Barclay.

One-third of those carrying a health or nutrition claim breached either the Food Standards Code or Code of Practice on Nutrient Claims. One of the most common offences was to imply a product was low-fat by saying it was, for example, 92 per cent fat-free, when a low-fat claim is allowed only on products that are at least 97 per cent fat-free.

Barclay says the study's results reflect Australia's lack of an adequate surveillance system for food marketing, and claims regulators have traditionally been more focused on ensuring safety of the food supply than truth-in-marketing.

'There is an onus on our governments and regulatory authorities to provide better surveillance of the food system particularly in this current environment of overweight and obesity', he says.

It's an issue which is about to become even more relevant thanks to moves to allow a greater range of health claims on foods. Food companies argue they should be allowed to tell their customers if their products have health benefits. But many public health experts fear that such labelling will encourage distorted eating patterns and will only exacerbate the marketing advantage of processed and packaged foods (which we mostly need to eat less of) over vegetables and fruit (which most of us should eat more of).

'Health claims are a big misnomer', says Associate Professor Mark Lawrence, a public health nutritionist at Deakin University in Melbourne. 'Health claims aren't about health; they are primarily about creating commercial opportunities for food manufacturers.'

Needless to say, I've resumed my normal supermarket routine, which means spending most time in the aisles with the least 'health claims' marketing the vegetable and fruit section. Happily, this usually also means a quicker, easier exit from the supermarket.

Super-size you

It is not only the range of food products has expanded. Food portion sizes have been steadily increasing since the 1970s and are an effective strategy for attracting customers and boosting profits. Paying only slightly more for a lot more food or drink is a bargain which few of us can resist. One study examining the consequences of super-sizing found that an average 12 per cent increase in purchase cost increased calorie intake by 23 per cent, while fat intake rose by 25 per cent and 38 per cent more sugars were consumed.[29] Super-sizing might sound like a bargain, until you remember that old maxim of retailing: the customer always pays, one way or the other.

In the United States, serving sizes of hot chips, hamburgers and soft drinks are now two to five times larger than they were in the 1970s. Ironically, even pre-prepared meals for the weight conscious now come in bigger serving sizes.[30] Restaurants are using larger dinner plates, bakers are selling larger muffins, pizzerias are using larger pans and fast food companies are using larger drink and french fries containers. Nestle and colleagues have also documented how recipes for cakes and desserts in new editions of classic cookbooks specify fewer servings, meaning that portions are expected to be larger. In the United States, one super-size serve of a popular soft drink contains the equivalent of more than one-third of many people's daily energy requirement.

The United States may be the world's heavyweight champion when it comes to super-sized portions, but we've also done our share of super-sizing in Australia. In some restaurants, a child-sized meal might once have been considered standard fare. A University of Sydney study found large increases in portion sizes between 1995 and 2003 in a wide range of foods. These included pre-packaged foods sold in supermarkets and takeaway foods such as hot chips and pizza. A photograph illustrating a near-tripling in the size of muffins provided a particularly graphic example.[31] As part of the study, 100 people were shown bulk quantities of different foods and asked to estimate a standard portion size. Even some of the dietitians among the study's subjects struggled with this task. The researchers concluded that the food industry's move towards larger portion sizes had influenced individuals' knowledge about what is an appropriate amount to eat. It's not surprising that some research suggests serving sizes of home-cooked meals have also grown.[32] Once piling your plate in public becomes both socially acceptable and a habit, it makes sense that many people would automatically do it at home too.

Super-sizing takes many guises. Sydney journalist Jenny Tabakoff has described the 'super treat' phenomenon, in which foods leap the 'species barrier'. Ice creams interbreed with biscuits while Easter eggs cross with chocolate bars. The development of Double Coat and Chewy Choc Fudge Tim Tam biscuits makes wolfing down an old-fashioned Tim Tam suddenly seem like 'self-restraint', writes Tabakoff.[33] Now that's a sign of twisted times: when scoffing a biscuit rich in fat and sugar, which was once marketed as the ultimate in self-indulgence, becomes an act of self-deprivation. Interestingly, however, a recent US study found less than a third of adults believed that portion sizes at restaurants had increased over the past 30 years. They also tended to describe the portion size they usually ate as 'medium', regardless of how big it actually was.[34]

Then there's the super-sizing phenomenon which is the dream of developers and the nightmare of public health experts and environmentalists. In the new suburbs that are sprawling along our city fringes and growth corridors, which are often the most affordable housing option for young families, huge houses crowd their small blocks. They leave little room for gardens, trees or places where children can run and play. But there is plenty of room for super-sized TVs and super-sized cars.

According to one investigation, the average floor area of new houses increased by 31 per cent between 1985 and 2000, and the size of apartments increased by 25 per cent. In the mid 1950s, new houses were about half the size of houses built today. In 1970, an average new house had 40 square metres of floor space per occupant; today's has 85 square metres.[35]

Can it be a coincidence that waistlines are increasing as the size of houses expands to accommodate smaller and smaller households? Professor Brendan Gleeson, of the School of Environmental Planning at Griffith University in Queensland, argues that the modern suburban 'mega-house' internalises activity, allocating large amounts of space to passive recreation such as home theatres, lounges and computer games, as well as to 'monster' garages. They are part of the new 'sedentary residential landscapes' where children are not allowed to ride bikes, climb trees or go to the park by themselves.[36]

Environmental injury

Over-consumption hurts the environment as well as our waistlines, and not only through the obvious waste produced by packaging and promotions. Nutritionist Dr Rosemary Stanton says it takes 640 kilojoules of energy to produce a can of low-kilojoule soft drink that contains 4 kilojoules of energy and has no nutritional value. Fake fats use even more energy and resources. Over US$200 billion has been spent so far developing Olestra, a kilojoule-free sucrose polyester to use in place of fats. She says it is ecologically absurd and enormously wasteful of energy and water to grow crops to feed animals, which is what happens with feedlot beef. It takes 16 kilograms of grain to produce 1 kilogram of beef, she says.

'Is it morally right to use limited resources to produce a mind-boggling array of foods for people who already eat more than their health can handle while others starve?' Stanton wrote in a recent nutrition newsletter.[37] 'We do not need fake foods. We do not need more packaged goods. We do not need foods to be available out of season, when they invariably have less flavour and lower levels of phytonutrients. We do not need fortified foods bearing health claims. We do not need imported food products and we certainly do not need hormone-implanted, lot-fed cattle or intensively reared chickens.

'Australia faces huge problems of salinity due largely to the way we have pushed agricultural growth, forcing the land to support many times our own population. Rivers have become silted, blue–green algae generated by fertiliser run-off choke many waterways, erosion follows overstocking, and pesticides pollute groundwater as we strive to produce more from every patch of earth.'

Poverty amid plenty

For a country as a whole, the growth in waistlines comes with increasing affluence and consumption. But for some sections of society, the battle of the bulge is associated with the battle to make ends meet.

Professor Adam Drewnowski, of the University of Washington in Seattle, has been at the forefront of research into the links between poverty and weight gain. Many factors are involved: people living in poor suburbs typically have easy access to fast food, but may have fewer shops selling fresh produce or fewer safe, affordable opportunities to walk and exercise.

Drewnowski's research shows that energy-dense foods which are high in fat and/or sugars are cheaper on a dollar per kilojoule basis than nutritious foods such as fruit and vegetables. He argues that public health campaigns have often been elitist because they have failed to acknowledge that their recommendations for people to eat lean meats, vegetables and fruit tend to cost more. Being on a tight budget encourages people to maximise calories per dollars spent. According to Drewnowski's calculations, the cost per unit of energy provided by potato crisps is about one-fifth of the energy cost of fresh carrots. As well, foods which are high in fat and sugar are less filling than nutritious foods, which tend to be more bulky and thus more filling. This means it is easier to over-consume when your diet is full of fatty, sweet foods.[38]

These are very real issues for the many families who watch their budgets closely. A large study found that almost a third of Australian infants and children were living in families with a combined income of less than $800 per week in 2004.[39] The latest National Nutrition Survey, conducted in 1995, found that about 5 per cent of people over the age of 15 report having not enough food to eat sometimes or often.[40]

Fruity Friday

Sydney is the capital of consumerism in Australia, and a city of incredible material wealth. Yet in significant chunks of the city, many families are closely acquainted with hunger.

A recent study involving residents in Sydney's poorest suburbs—Villawood, Warwick Farm and Rosemeadow—found that about 1 in 5 households sometimes or often do not have enough food to eat. About half of all single parent households in Villawood reported what is known in public health jargon as 'food insecurity'. When the researchers investigated the local food supply, they discovered large areas of the suburbs that had no easy access to local shops. They also discovered that prices in some of the large chain supermarkets were higher than the same outlets in wealthy suburbs.

Public health workers in the area have been trying to build links between community and business groups to help make it easier for struggling locals. A café has been set up at Villawood offering a free healthy lunch to all comers once a week, and a food action group is also working to improve the quality of the local food supply.

Warwick Farm Public School, whose 250 students come from more than 40 nations, is also doing its bit to try to improve the community's health. About 35 children breakfast for free at the school each morning and food parcels are sometimes sent home with them. After noticing a falloff in students' fitness in recent years, the school introduced a daily fitness program, including activities such as power walking, cross-country running, aerobics and dance. 'Everyone does something every day,' says the school's principal, Lyn Flegg.

Teachers report that the children tend to be better behaved in class as a result and more engaged in their lessons. The school also takes the children on active outings each term, to give them a chance to experience activities that otherwise might not be available to them, such as ice skating, ten pin bowling and indoor climbing.

Every now and then a local fruit shop sets up a taste-testing stall in the playground, so children can try new flavours and sensations. Sometimes it's 'Munch and Crunch Wednesday', other times it's 'Fruity Friday'. As well, for 10 minutes each day, students are encouraged to eat a fruit or vegetable in the classroom while their teacher reads to them.

Ms Flegg says the canteen's fruit sales have increased. 'There's nothing nicer than walking into a classroom and smelling a fruit break,' she says. 'We're ensuring they have a clear knowledge of what they need to do if they want to lead a healthy lifestyle—that's the most empowering thing we can do for our children.'

Cost is also a barrier for many people living in rural and remote areas—fruit, vegetables and other fresh produce can be prohibitively expensive, if they are available at all. The Queensland Government regularly does a survey of the cost and availability of a standard basket of healthy food items that would be enough to feed a family of six for 2 weeks. In 2004, people living in very remote areas paid 29.6 per cent or $113.89 more for the basket than city shoppers, and about 1 in 10 of the healthy food items were not available in remote areas. The price difference between urban and remote areas was much less for tobacco and takeaway foods.

There is also evidence that the price of nutritious foods has risen faster than the price of other foods.[41] In Brisbane between 1998 and 2004, the price of bread increased by 17 per cent, the price of milk by 22 per cent, and the price of fruit and vegetables by 33 per cent. In contrast, the price of soft drinks, waters and juices dropped by 3 per cent. Drewnowski has documented similar trends in the United States, where the price of fresh fruit and vegetables rose by almost 120 per cent between 1985 and 2000, while the price of soft drinks increased by only 20 per cent.[42]

Looking forward

The commercialisation of childhood encourages an early start to many unhealthy habits. Apart from building relationships with unhealthy foods, it teaches children to search for happiness and fulfilment at the shops. While this may bring some people transient happiness, more and more people are realising that a life filled with rampant consumerism is not so full at all.

In late 2004, a survey of more than 1600 Australians found that four-fifths believed our materialistic society makes it more difficult to instil positive values in young children. The survey was conducted as part of research for Clive Hamilton and Richard Denniss' book *Affluenza*, which challenges the view that increased consumption and economic growth will deliver increased wellbeing for society as a whole. Their book also cites research showing that most young people want more time with their parents rather than more money (acquired through the longer hours their parents are working). It is a finding which resonates with many psychologists, psychiatrists and other health professionals working with troubled young people. And yet so many forces in society, including governments and employers, seem to be making it more and more difficult for parents to find a healthy balance between their work and their family.

A significant minority of Australians are voting with their feet, opting to downsize their incomes, stresses and material aspirations in exchange for what they hope will be a better quality of life for themselves and their children. Of course this option—known as the downshifting, tree-change or sea-change movement—is not a realistic or desirable alternative for everyone. But its popularity does suggest that many people are seriously re-evaluating their lives and what is important to them. Time and time again they find that the answer lies in their relationships and their family.

It might sound as if I've come over all nostalgic in these first two chapters, harking back to earlier, happier times when hunter-gatherers ruled or when kids were free to roam the streets before bringing home a healthy appetite for the cheerful occasion of the family dinner. Don't be fooled. Every era has its problems. Taking a rose-coloured view of the past will not help us deal with the present or the future. But understanding where we've come from and having a careful look at our modern lives does yield some helpful clues for those who are concerned about children's health.

The first step along the road to making any kind of change is awareness. We have to acknowledge and work with the realities of our lives before we can make change. If you are interested in creating better health for you and your family, it is important to be aware of some of the forces shaping your life and your aspirations. Anyone who tries to tell you that it's as simple as eating better and moving more is telling you only part of the story.

3. Time for some measurements

Have you noticed the food industry's habit of highlighting the importance of physical inactivity as a cause of weight gain? When it funds awareness campaigns and research about obesity, these tend to stress the benefits of exercising more, rather than suggesting that eating or drinking too much might be involved. Of course you can't blame the industry for this; it is just doing what business does—trying to maximise profits and maintain a favourable environment for its operations.

But there can be little doubt that debate about which side of the energy equation—energy intake or output—contributes most to weight gain has been more than convenient for those who profit from maximising our food and drink consumption. It helps distract public attention from uncomfortable questions about the industry's role in a looming health, economic and social crisis. It also gives false comfort to Joe and Josephine Public, who wonder why they should bother changing their ways when even the experts disagree about what's important.

Time for some measurements

However, the debate does raise some interesting questions. It is not as easy to work out the relative importance of food and inactivity in weight gain as you might think. Here are a few reasons why:

• People either cannot refrain from little white lies or are genuinely deluded about themselves or are just hopeless at measuring things. When research is based on people's own reports of how much they eat, it inevitably suggests that they eat less than what is found when their food intake is independently verified. Somewhere in the universe there must be a huge black hole sucking in vast quantities of food and drink—something has to account for the mismatch between studies documenting how much food is available per capita versus studies based on people's own estimates of their consumption. Waste and spoilage cannot account for the discrepancy. Heavier children and adults are more likely to under-report how much they eat.

• Similarly, people are not very accurate when they tell researchers their weight and height. Short people tend to overestimate their height, and overweight people tend to underestimate their weight. The fatter people are, the more they underestimate their weight.

• When researchers try to overcome some of these problems by conducting surveys which carefully and independently measure people's weight, their findings may also be biased— by the reluctance of overweight people to participate in such studies.

• It is time-consuming and expensive to accurately measure how much energy individuals expend each day, but surveys based on self-reports of how much people exercise can be misleading. Even if people are playing more sport than they did 10 years ago, their overall energy expenditure may have declined because there is less activity in their daily lives. With experts encouraging us to move more, people may well be tempted to exaggerate their sweat levels. Most people want to be seen to be doing the right thing, or at least to believe that they are. As well, the answers that researchers get depend on the questions they ask. Thus one survey found that the proportion of Australian adults who are sedentary rose from 13.4 per cent to 15.3 per cent between 1997 and 2000. However, the Australian Bureau of Statistics found a trend going in the opposite direction, with 31 per cent of adults being sedentary in 2001, an improvement from 1989–90, when 37.5 per cent were stuck to the couch.

• Physical inactivity is both a cause and a consequence of obesity. It can be difficult at times for researchers to disentangle one from the other.

So keep those caveats in mind when considering the rest of this chapter.

What are children eating and drinking?

The short answer is: too much of the unhealthy things and not enough of the right stuff.

Major changes have occurred in what children eat and drink in recent decades. Their energy consumption has increased significantly. They are scoffing more processed, unhealthy foods such as potato crisps and other snacks, lollies, soft drinks and takeaways. These foods tend to be energy-dense and high in fats and/or sugars. Some studies suggest that the more people eat of foods that are energy-dense and nutrient-poor, the less likely they are to eat nutritious foods. It is ironic that so-called health bars are a major source of saturated fats for many children; and we know that many are eating more saturated fats than is advised.[1] As well, many children are not eating anywhere near enough of the foods they need for healthy growth and development, particularly vegetables and fruit. Many are more likely to have soft drink than milk. It's often the cheaper option.

Children are not only eating different foods compared with previous generations of children. Like the rest of us, their patterns of eating have also changed, and often not for the better. Many skip breakfast, a habit that is linked to increased risk of weight gain and unhealthy eating. They are more likely to snack—one Swedish study suggested snacks contribute more energy to most teenagers' diets than their three main meals[2]—and are also more likely to eat out. Takeaways and restaurant meals tend to contain more fat and salt than those prepared at home. According to one report, some single portions of fast food have an entire day's worth of calories and fat.[3] One analysis of the economic factors underlying obesity trends in the United States calculated that the increase in the number of restaurants per capita accounted for 61 per cent of the population's weight increase.[4]

Many researchers moan that we don't have more comprehensive and up-to-date national data about children's eating, but most of the studies that have been done point in a similar direction. Rather than bore you rigid with pages of statistics, here is a summary of some key findings, from Australia and elsewhere:

• The best Australian data date way back to 1995 and the last National Nutrition Survey. It found that children were consuming significantly more calories, snacks, soft drink and

71

sugar than they had a decade earlier. The increase in their energy intake was much greater than that seen in adults over the same period. Boys aged 10 to 15 were consuming the equivalent of 15 per cent more calories; girls had an 11 per cent increase in their calorie intake. These increases equate to eating the equivalent of an extra three to four slices of bread per day.[5] Snacks, lollies and other 'non-core foods' made up about one-quarter of children's total fat intake and one-fifth of their total energy intake.[6]

• It seems unlikely that the situation has improved much since 1995. In 2003, WA researchers asked children to keep a food diary for 24 hours, and found that 45 per cent reported eating confectionery such as lollies and 30 per cent ate snacks such as potato crisps.[7] Meanwhile, Sydney research suggests that ice creams, potato crisps, lollies, chocolate and hot chips are typical after-school fare. Almost two-thirds of the children surveyed said they made their own choice about what type of snack they had after school.[8] And another study in New South Wales found that 7–12 per cent of boys (depending on their age) drink more than 1 litre of soft drink per day, and about half of all students drink more than a glass each day.[9]. Many children say they usually have soft drink with meals at home and with lunch at school.

• You couldn't have missed all the news about the fabulous health benefits of fruit and vegetables even if you've been living under a rock—which just goes to show that knowing what you should do doesn't make it happen. Study after study shows that many children are missing out on these essential building blocks for lifelong health. A Western Australian study suggested that children's fruit and vegetable consumption fell between 1985 and 2003.[10] A large national study in 2004 found that roughly 1 in 6 children aged 4 to 5 ate little or no fresh fruit or vegetables.[11] In 2001, a large study of NSW children found that well under 20 per cent were reported by their patients as eating recommended levels of vegetables. The news on fruit was more encouraging: at least 70 per cent were enjoying the benefits of a healthy dose of fruit.[12] In another study of children aged 6 to 18, 1 in 6 had eaten no fruit or vegetables in the 3 days before being surveyed. As well, 1 in 3 had either skipped breakfast or made do with a drink. Some even had cordial or soft drink for breakfast.[13]

• Teenagers are particularly vulnerable to unhealthy food habits. A Western Australian study found that almost one-third of adolescents skipped breakfast at least 4 days a week.[14] A New South Wales study of 15-year-olds found that more than 80 per cent did not eat enough vegetables, while more than one-third of boys did not have enough fruit.[15] Almost half of the boys and about a third of the girls had more than one cup of soft drink a day. In 1999, a national survey of children aged 12 to 17 found that three-quarters had eaten fast food in the past week. Ten per cent of boys and almost the same proportion of girls had eaten fast food at least four times in the past week.[16]

• Fast food plays a large part in many young children's diets. In 2001, more than two-thirds of New South Wales children under 13 were reported by their parents as eating at least one serve of hot chips a week. About one-quarter ate two or more serves a week, while 1 in 10 had hot chips at least three times a week. The survey also found that just over a quarter of children aged 2 to 4 reported drinking at least one cup of soft drink, cordial or sports drink per day, as did just over 40 per cent of children aged 5 to 12.[17]

• A study investigating the diets of more than 3,000 children and teenagers in the United States found that 16 per cent did not meet any of the dietary recommendations, and only 1 per cent (1 per cent!) met all of them.[18]

How fit are children?

It may sound confusing, but a few different issues are important here: how inactive are children, how active are they, and how fit are they? It is likely that the answers to these three related questions have the same worrying implications for children's health.

Many children are now spending more time watching TV, playing with computers or sitting in cars than being physically active. A large NSW study found that two-thirds of girls and three-quarters of boys in secondary schools spent more than 2 hours a day in front of a small screen in 2004.[19] These sedentary habits start very young—even babies spend long hours in front of the mesmerising screen.

Research on trends in children's involvement in sport and other forms of recreational exercise produces mixed results. There is little doubt, however, that fewer children are active as part of their daily life; for example, there has been a dramatic fall off in walking and cycling to school. It has been estimated that up to a quarter of children are not sufficiently active for their health, that 30 per cent are unfit and that 60 per cent have moderate to poor motor skills.[20] And activity and fitness levels tend to fall off as children get older—teenagers are the masters of lounging.

• When researchers asked more than 10,000 families to keep a diary of how their children spent a day in 2004, they found that 45.5 per cent of infants watched TV, a video or a DVD on that day, for a mean of 1.4 hours. About 90 per cent of 4 and 5-year-olds did likewise, for an average of 2.3 hours per day. This was more time than these young children spent walking, running or doing other exercise. In fact only 66 per cent of 4 and 5-year-olds engaged in these activities at all on the day in question. Another 25.6 per cent used computers or computer games for a mean of 1.1 hours per day.[21]

• Almost a third of children aged 5 to 14 reported skateboarding or rollerblading in a 2 week period, compared with 97 per cent who watched TV or videos, and 69 per cent who had played electronic or computer games.[22]

• Cars are taking over the school transport run. Although 60 per cent of primary school students in Western Australia live within a 20 minute walk of school, 60 per cent of these students travel mainly by car.[23] In 1981, 24 per cent of Adelaide children went to school by car, 42 per cent walked and 14 per cent cycled. By 1997, 60 per cent went by car, 20.5 per cent walked, and 4.5 per cent cycled.[24]

• Studies produce mixed results about whether children are exercising more or less. A South Australian study of children aged 9 to 15 found that 51 per cent reported at least three vigorous bouts of physical activity in the previous week. By 2004, 76 per cent said they were doing this.[25] A large NSW study found that in 2004, three-quarters of boys and girls aged 11 to 16 met recommendations to have at least 1 hour of moderate to vigorous physical activity each day. This was a significant increase from the proportion who reported these activity levels in 1985, although fewer were walking or cycling to school in 2004.[26] However, other researchers note that there are significant gaps in what is known about the trends in children's active play and participation in school physical education and sport.[27] A WA study found that almost 30 per cent of primary students and over 50 per cent of secondary students reported doing no physical education. By age 12, only about 50 per cent of young people engage in aerobic activity at least four times a week; by age 16, only about a quarter maintain this level of activity.[28]

• The aerobic fitness of children around the world is declining, and this is most marked in older age groups, according to one international analysis.[29] Studies in South Australia and Tasmania have documented similar trends.

• However, there is some good news. Recent efforts to promote activity in schools in New South Wales seem to have had an impact. A large study testing the fitness levels of children in Years 4, 6, 8 and 10 found that more students were fit in 2004 than in 1997. Even so, many children did not pass the test: about 40 per cent of boys and 20–30 per cent of girls were considered unfit.[30]

And what about children's size?

Children are taller and heavier than ever before. They also reach puberty younger. Their increasing height does not explain all their extra weight: their waistlines are expanding and they are getting fatter. Fatness is becoming more common even in very young children. The trend became noticeable in the 1980s, and some researchers believe it is accelerating. If current trends continue, it has been predicted that between a third and a half of all young Australians will be overweight by 2020.[31]

• In 2003, boys were on average 3.2cm taller and 5.1kg heavier than boys of the same age in 1985. Their waists had increased by a mean of 5.6cm. On average, girls were 2.8cm taller and 5.1kg heavier, and their waistlines had increased by

7.4cm. These figures come from a study comparing WA children's measurements in 2003 with a national survey in 1985.[32] Another study concluded that between 1899 and 1999, children's height and weight increased at an average rate of about 1.02cm and 1kg per decade.[33]

• In a large study involving about three-quarters of all 4-year-olds in South Australia, researchers examined what proportion were overweight or obese in each year from 1995 to 2002. In 1995, 3 per cent of boys were obese and 7 per cent were overweight. By 2002, 4 per cent were obese and 13 per cent were overweight.[34]

• A study conducted in the Barwon–Southwestern region of Victoria in 2003–04 found that 19.8 per cent of children aged 4 to 13 were overweight, and a further 8.3 per cent were obese. Girls were more likely than boys to be overweight.[35]

• A 2004 study of almost 5,000 children in New South Wales, aged from 5 to 16, found 25 per cent of boys and 23.3 per cent of girls were either overweight or obese. Some of the highest rates were documented in children aged 9 to 12 (in Years 6–8): 1 in 3 boys in Year 6 were classified as overweight or obese.[36]

• A study examining data on children's weight which was collected in South Australia, Victoria and New South Wales between 1969 and 1997 found that the results for each state between 1985 and 1997 were surprisingly similar. The proportion who were overweight increased by about 60 per cent, the proportion who were obese trebled, and the proportion who were either overweight or obese doubled. South Australian data showed that between 1969 and 1985, the proportion of girls who were overweight or obese did not change, but among boys the prevalence of overweight and obesity increased by 60 per cent. In other words, weight gain has been most pronounced in the last decade or so. 'These results should increase our sense of urgency in identifying and implementing effective responses to this major threat to public health,' the researchers concluded.[37]

4. What's the worry? Weighing up the health issues

A round the world, some rather eminent knickers are in a knot. Many authoritative organisations and experts—from the World Health Organization down—are alarmed about what the growing problem of children's weight might mean for the future. Problems once thought of as afflictions of middle age and beyond, such as type 2 diabetes and cardiovascular disease, will be diagnosed at younger and younger ages, they warn. Health services will be stretched and unable to cope with the burden of illness as more and more people begin to develop the complications of diabetes at younger and younger ages, they say.

The thing to remember when you hear these sorts of predictions is that they generally are referring to the impact of increased rates of obesity across the entire population. Looked at on this scale, even a relatively small increase in the incidence of a common health problem such as type 2 diabetes or cardiovascular disease can have large repercussions for society generally. It is much less clear what these sort of predictions mean for any individual child who is overweight. Some overweight children may suffer serious health complications because of it, but most will be perfectly healthy children, depending on how much excess weight they are carrying and whether or not their family history puts them at increased risk of future obesity and serious conditions such as diabetes.

For most overweight children, the most likely health issue is the strong probability that they will grow into unfit, overweight adults who are at increased risk of a range of potentially serious diseases, especially type 2 diabetes. However, not all fat children become fat adults; nor were all fat adults overweight as children. Similarly, most people who develop type 2 diabetes are overweight—but not everyone who is overweight is destined to have diabetes; they are simply at greater risk of getting it.

Any individual child's risk of suffering current or future health problems will depend on many factors. These can include: how overweight they are; how old they were when they put on excess weight; and their family history—for example, are one or both of their parents significantly overweight, or do close family members suffer from type 2 diabetes or heart disease? A child who is mildly overweight but has parents or aunts and uncles with type 2 diabetes may be at greater long-term risk than an obese child whose parents are trim and healthy. An overweight child who is physically active and has a generally healthy diet is likely to do better than a thin child who is inactive or has a poor diet. For many children, however, being overweight is a sign of a poor diet and inactivity, which are significant health risks in themselves.

Obesity and overweight are often lumped together as if they are the same. Generally speaking, however, obesity is far more likely to result in serious health problems. The health implications of simply carrying a few extra kilograms are still being debated by experts. On the other hand, with so many forces conspiring to add to our weight and with our bodies so clever at retaining weight gain, it is likely that many people who start off just a bit overweight may end up with the more serious problem of obesity.

It should also be remembered that the distinctions between being a healthy weight, overweight and obese are somewhat arbitrary. These categories provide a general guide to what are considered healthy or not-so-healthy weight ranges, but falling into a particular category is no guarantee that someone is healthy or unhealthy. A more intensive investigation is needed to establish this. According to Melbourne weight loss specialist Dr Rick Kausman, it is possible—and not uncommon—for someone to be overweight according to a chart but to be at the most healthy and comfortable weight that is possible for them.

None of this means that excess weight is not an important issue for children. It can cause current or future health and social problems for the individual. At a broader societal level, it seems likely that the growing incidence of overweight will put a huge strain on health services in the long term, especially given that health services already often struggle to provide appropriate care to those in need. An American study has already shown a huge increase in rates of hospital treatment for obesity-related conditions in children and teenagers over the past 20 or so years.[1] The epidemic may also have less obvious ramifications for the economy and society. Defence forces, for example, say the growing incidence of obesity is contributing to difficulties finding fit, healthy recruits.[2] It may also reduce productivity more broadly, with one report showing higher levels of absenteeism among obese workers.[3]

However, numerous studies show that many parents do not recognise the potentially serious consequences of their children's overweight; many simply see it as a matter of appearance. Indeed, many people equate chubbiness in children with good health, or see it as a phase that children grow out of. For most children, living in today's obesogenic environment, that is not the case. Many children will carry excess weight from their preschool, primary or high school years right through into adulthood.

Living with uncertainty

Many people do not acknowledge how much uncertainty surrounds some of these dire warnings about the impact of childhood obesity. Most people have difficulty dealing with uncertainty—we often prefer to be given concrete 'facts'. And when experts, governments and others communicate with the public through the media or other avenues, their messages are often simplified so that they will be easy to understand and have the most impact. This often leaves little room for the uncertainties to be acknowledged or explained.

Here are a few reasons why there is some uncertainty about the impact of being overweight as a child:

• The future can rarely be predicted with certainty. Most medical predictions are based on estimates of the probability that something might happen rather than a cast-iron guarantee. We are all individuals, and we all react differently to the same environment and circumstances.

• Widespread obesity is an extremely recent problem in terms of the long history of humanity. Many estimates about the health effects of obesity come from studies done decades ago, when the environment was not so obesogenic and obesity was far less common than it is today. So the results may not be terribly relevant to today's children; indeed, some experts fear that those studies may greatly understate the impact of the current levels of obesity. The epidemic is so new that long-term studies tracking its impact will not be available for decades.

• Rather than waiting another half a century to work out the impact of overweight on the future health of today's children—whether, for example, they will develop earlier or more serious forms of heart disease in middle and old age—researchers often look for 'surrogate' measures of poor future health. These might include increased levels of risk factors such as high cholesterol or high blood pressure. However, it is difficult to be sure what increased levels of these risk factors in children might mean for their future health.

• Because obesity tends to continue from childhood into adulthood, it can be difficult for researchers to separate the effects of obesity in childhood from its effects in adulthood. Similarly, it can be difficult to establish whether a problem that is more common among overweight people is a cause or an effect of weight gain. Unhealthy eating patterns, such as binge eating, might be both a cause and effect of weight gain, for example. In other words, people who binge eat might be more likely to put on weight; and people who are worried about their weight may be tempted to try fad diets, which can lead to unhealthy eating patterns. A similar problem arises because of the circular relationship between fat and lack of fitness: obesity can be both a cause and an effect of lack of activity. Researchers have had great difficulty untangling the contributions of overweight and unfitness to poor health—this issue is the subject of ongoing medical debate. Similarly, heavier girls tend to mature early, and early puberty is associated with poorer self-esteem. It can be difficult to distinguish between the relative impact of overweight and early maturity on girls' self-esteem.

• Many studies on the impact of obesity have involved children undergoing treatment at specialist clinics. It is likely that these studies are not representative of the broader population of overweight children, and they may underestimate or overestimate the impact of weight gain on children. Many of the studies of the psychological impact of obesity, for example, have involved children undergoing treatment for their weight, who might be expected to have more severe physical or mental health issues than children who are not undergoing treatment.

• It is relatively simple to measure a child's weight. Knowing when it signals a health risk is much more difficult. Body mass index (BMI)—the measure of a person's weight relative to height—is generally accepted as giving the best available correlation between body weight and increased risk of poor health. In adults, a BMI of 25 to 30 suggests that someone is overweight, and a BMI of above 30 signals obesity. BMI charts have been developed for children using comparable cut-off scores and taking into account their stages of growth and development. Like most tests, though, this one does not always give reliable results. Because the BMI reflects a person's weight rather than their degree of fatness, two people with the same BMI may have quite different physiques. One person may be heavy and muscular and the other may be heavy and fat. The interpretation of BMI scores should also take ethnic background into account. Asian children, for example, may be overweight at lower BMI scores than children of Caucasian background. People who are obese are not all the same; the degree and distribution of excess body fat varies greatly, and so do the associated health risks. Having a lot of fat concentrated around the stomach is particularly undesirable.

How does the child measure up to the adult?

Overweight tends to be a persistent problem—as mentioned in previous chapters, our bodies are particularly good at retaining weight gain. Fat children are more likely to become fat adults. This is especially likely if one or both of their parents is overweight, because parents and children share similar genetic and environmental influences. The later in childhood and adolescence that weight gain occurs, the more likely it is to be carried into adulthood.

Many of the studies investigating weight trends have been done overseas, but Victorian researchers have provided some local estimates of how children's weight changes over time.[4] In 1997, they examined more than 1,400 children aged 5 to 10, and found that 15 per cent were overweight and 4 per cent were obese. When they checked again in 2000, 20 per cent of the children were overweight and 5 per cent were obese. Of the 1,160 children who had a healthy weight in 1997, 125 had become overweight and 4 had become obese by 2000. Only 55 of the children who had been overweight or obese in 1997 had lost weight over the following 3 years.

Predictions

Many of the estimates about the implications of childhood weight come from a large study which has been running for more than 30 years in Louisiana in the United States, tracking the health of more than 16,000 children and adults. It centres on Bogalusa, a semi-rural community which lies about an hour's drive north of New Orleans; it takes its name from a creek which the local Indians called 'Bogue Lusa', meaning smoky or dark waters.

The Bogalusa Heart Study found that between 53 per cent and 90 per cent of overweight children become overweight adults (depending on how old they were when they became overweight), and that only about 7 per cent of normal weight children became obese adults. Only 20 to 25 per cent of obese or overweight adults had been overweight as children.[5] However, obese adults who had been obese as children were significantly heavier than those who only put on weight as adults.

Some other predictions about the future of fat children come from a study involving 854 people born in Washington State in the United States between 1965 and 1971. The researchers checked their vital statistics early in life, and when they were aged 21 to 29, and also examined their parents' medical records.[6] Their findings included that:

• Those children who were obese at 1 and 2 years of age were unlikely to be obese as young adults if their parents were not obese. Only 8 per cent of these children were obese in adulthood.

• At the other end of the spectrum, about 80 per cent of children who were obese between ages 10 and 14 were obese as young adults if they had at least one obese parent.

• Children were far more likely to grow into obese adults, whether or not they were overweight in childhood, if they had at least one parent who was obese. Among non-obese toddlers, 28 per cent of those with at least one obese parent were obese as adults, versus 10 per cent of those whose parents were not obese. Among obese preschoolers, 24 per cent of those with non-obese parents became obese adults, whereas 62 per cent of those with at least one obese parent became obese themselves in adulthood.

• The researchers cautioned against intervening to treat young children for obesity unless they also had at least one obese parent. After age 10, though, decisions about whether to intervene could be made primarily on the basis of the child's own weight. On the other hand, it is never too early to encourage healthy eating and activity in children and babies.

Health issues for children

Broadly speaking, excess weight has two major consequences for physical health: it puts an extra load on the body, and it causes metabolic changes which increase the risk of problems such as type 2 diabetes.

1. Orthopaedic problems

You only have to carry a bag of potatoes around the supermarket to realise what a strain it must be for the body to lug around an extra load all the time. Overweight children and teenagers are more likely to suffer ankle sprains and fractures, flat feet and other orthopaedic problems. In severe cases of obesity, this can lead to bowing of leg bones or problems with hip joints. Sore feet, legs and backs, heat rash, shortness of breath and general physical discomfort are common complaints. These things can have a marked effect on children's quality of life.

2. Disturbed sleep

Extra weight can also make it difficult for children to breathe normally while they sleep, which can result in heavy snoring, reduction in air flow or even temporary cessation of breathing (sleep apnoea). As a result of disrupted, poor-quality sleep, children and teenagers may feel tired during the day or have difficulty concentrating and learning. Their growth and development may also be affected. An American study found that obese children and teenagers were four to five times more likely to suffer from disordered breathing during sleep than those who were not obese.[7] Sydney specialist Professor Louise Baur says obesity and sleep disturbance can become a vicious circle; overweight children who feel tired because of poor sleep are less likely to feel like being active, which in turn affects their sleep and weight.

3. Other medical problems

Overweight can exacerbate other conditions, particularly asthma; weight loss can improve asthma management. Almost a third of obese children have asthma, and they use more medications, have more wheezing episodes, and more unscheduled visits to hospital than lean children with asthma.[8] And obese children and teenagers may be more likely to have difficulties with health care generally, because medical procedures and medicines may be more risky or less effective.

4. Risk factors for cardiovascular disease and diabetes

The Bogalusa Heart Study has helped show that many of the physical changes that lead to cardiovascular disease begin in childhood. Anatomical changes, such as thickening of artery walls, have been documented in children as young as 5. The study found that about 60 per cent of overweight school children had one risk factor (such as high blood pressure, cholesterol or trigylcerides) and 20 per cent had two or more risk factors. They were also more likely to have elevated fasting insulin concentrations, which is a risk factor for diabetes, as explained below in 'Old names no longer fit'.[9] Among the 5 to 10-year-olds, overweight children represented 7 per cent of the children with no risk factors, 22 per cent of the children with one risk factor, and 80 per cent of the children with three risk factors. Overweight children were about 10 times more likely than other children to have two risk factors, and 44 times more likely to have three risk factors.

Old names no longer fit

Diabetes, a long-term condition, has been described as one of the leading threats to the health of Australians.[10] It is a group of conditions characterised by too much glucose in the blood and urine, and broadly speaking, there are two main types. Type 1 occurs when the body's own immune system destroys the cells in the pancreas that produce insulin. Insulin is a hormone which is vital because it enables the body's cells to take up and use glucose and other nutrients that circulate in the blood. This type of diabetes is sometimes known as juvenile-onset because it usually affects children and young adults. It is treated with injections of insulin, and was once also called insulin-dependent diabetes; this name is no longer used because many people with type 2 diabetes also need insulin treatment.

Type 2 diabetes develops more gradually—symptoms often take years to emerge—and is called a 'lifestyle disease' because of its association with overweight, high blood pressure and high cholesterol. People with type 2 diabetes produce insulin, but their bodies do not respond to its action properly. Insulin resistance may develop because the person is overweight and has too many fat cells, which do not respond well to insulin. Also, as people age, their cells becomes less effective at responding to insulin.

Early warning signs for diabetes include high levels of insulin, when measured in a fasting patient. This may indicate that extra insulin is being released because of high levels of glucose in the blood or because the body's cells are less sensitive to insulin. Elevated levels of blood glucose in a fasting patient may indicate that not enough insulin is being released from the pancreas to lower the blood glucose, or that cells have become resistant to insulin action. Obesity almost always causes insulin resistance, but only some obese people with insulin resistance develop diabetes. It is more likely that they will if they have a family history of diabetes. Obesity and insulin resistance tend to cluster with other risk factors for cardiovascular disease, including high blood pressure and cholesterol. This clustering of risk factors is known as the 'metabolic syndrome', and it is associated with a greatly increased risk of heart disease and strokes. One study found that 30 per cent of overweight teenagers had the metabolic syndrome, compared with only 4 per cent of lean teenagers.[11]

People with type 2 diabetes or its precursors are generally advised to lose weight and become more active. The impact of such lifestyle changes was dramatically illustrated in the research mentioned in Chapter 1, which involved Aboriginal people in northern Australia reverting to a traditional lifestyle. In just a few weeks, their diabetes improved significantly.

Type 2 diabetes was once also called adult-onset diabetes, but that is no longer an accurate description—obese teenagers and even young children are now being diagnosed with it. Reports first began to emerge of adult-onset diabetes affecting young indigenous people in North America and Australia in the late 1970s and early 1980s. There have since been increasing numbers of reports in other obese young people. Twenty years ago, type 2 diabetes accounted for less than 3 per cent of all diabetes cases diagnosed in children and adolescents in the US. These days, it accounts for 30 to 45 per cent of diabetes diagnosed in adolescents and young adults.[12] One study of 167 obese children and adolescents in the United States found more than a fifth had impaired glucose tolerance, which can lead to diabetes. Even more worrying, 4 per cent of the adolescents had undiagnosed type 2 diabetes. In Cincinnati, the prevalence of type 2 diabetes in teenagers increased tenfold between 1982 and 1994—from 0.7 to 7.2 cases per 100,000 population. Similar increases have been noted elsewhere in America.[13] In Europe, type 2 diabetes and impaired glucose tolerance are also being reported among obese adolescents. A study of obese teenagers in Hungary found that about 2 per cent had type 2 diabetes and 15 per cent had impaired glucose tolerance; cases have also been reported in UK teenagers.[14]

It is difficult to get precise figures on the numbers of young Australians with type 2 diabetes, but there are several indications that it is becoming more common. One study found that 43 children and teenagers were diagnosed with type 2 diabetes at the Princess Margaret Hospital in Perth between 1990 and 2002. They were aged between 8 and 17, and just over half were of indigenous origin. The researchers said their findings suggested that there had been a significant increase in the rate of diagnosis rate of type 2 diabetes in children and adolescents in Western Australia, particularly over the past 7 years, and that this was in line with the increasing incidence of obesity.[15] The Mater Hospital in Brisbane is reported to have diagnosed 12 children with type 2 diabetes over a 2 year period, with the youngest patient being only 9 years old.[16] It is likely that some

91

hundreds of Australian children and teenagers are living with type 2 diabetes, and it is widely expected that diagnoses of type 2 diabetes in young people will become more frequent. A recent NSW study, which involved blood tests of Year 10 students in Sydney, found worrying levels of risk factors. 'Almost 1 in 5 adolescents have high insulin concentrations, which is a significant step along the path to type 2 diabetes,' the researchers said. The rate was much higher among obese teenagers, reaching almost 70 per cent among obese boys.[17]

The actual numbers of young people with type 2 diabetes are still relatively small, but the fact that there are any is causing great alarm—it means the disease's serious complications, which usually begin to emerge 10 to 15 years after the disease develops, will become more common in adults who would otherwise expect to be in their most productive years. These complications are the end result of the body's muscle cells being unable to take up and use the fuel they need to function effectively. They include cardiovascular disease, kidney failure, blindness and neuropathy, which sometimes leads to gangrene and limb amputations. It has been estimated that 10 per cent of overweight teenagers with type 2 diabetes will develop kidney failure in adulthood—they will require lifelong dialysis.[18]

Professor Paul Zimmet sees a bleak future for many of these young people. 'If a child or young adolescent gets type 2 diabetes, they could be faced with up to 60 years of drug therapy and they might only be in their late 20s when they start to get complications,' he says. The effect on indigenous, Pacific Islander and other ethnic communities which are at increased genetic risk for type 2 diabetes could be devastating, he warns. Other experts warn that the twin epidemics of obesity and type 2 diabetes mean that coronary heart disease could become a disease of young adulthood.[19] Another concern is that the effect of standard drug therapies for type 2 diabetes on children has not been adequately evaluated.

As if all this isn't bad enough, some experts suspect that the rising incidence of type 1 diabetes, which has been documented in children in Australia and elsewhere, may also be linked to the increase in childhood obesity.[20]

* Type 1 and type 2 account for most cases of diabetes. Another type is gestational diabetes, which develops during pregnancy. It usually disappears after the baby is born but is a risk factor for developing type 2 diabetes later in life. Other types of diabetes can develop as a result of a drug reaction, genetic defect or disease.

5. Fatty liver disease

Non-alcoholic fatty liver disease is a serious health problem which can eventually progress to fibrosis, cirrhosis and end-stage liver disease. It has traditionally been seen only in middle-aged and older people, but its very early manifestations are being found in obese children. Most will show no symptoms, but some may complain of feeling unwell, or fatigue or discomfort in the upper right abdomen.[21]

6. Puberty blues

Weight gain has a different effect on the timing of puberty for boys than it does for girls. Overweight boys tend to mature later, whereas increases in girls' weight and height are thought to contribute to earlier puberty for them. One American study found that on average, girls are experiencing the start of breast development when they are between 8 and 9 now; this is a year younger than 20 years ago.[22]

Another study, which tracked almost 200 girls from the ages of 5 to 9, showed a strong correlation between weight gain and early puberty.[23] It found that 89 per cent of girls who were early developers were overweight or obese at age 9; only 29 per cent of girls who hit puberty later were obese at age 9. The researchers said their findings were cause for concern, because there is other evidence that girls who reach puberty young are more likely to smoke, drink and have behavioural problems in adolescence, possibly because they are more likely to associate with an older peer group. Earlier puberty is also associated with an earlier start to sexual activity, an increased risk of eating disorders, and an increased risk of developing breast cancer in later life.

The social scene

Many experts believe that social stigma and related problems such as bullying are the most common immediate problems for overweight children. It is not only other children who are unkind. Sydney specialist Professor Louise Baur has seen young patients who have been given a hard time about their weight by family members, teachers and health professionals. She has even heard of strangers on the street passing derogatory comments in front of overweight children.

Several studies have shown that children seem to share broader society's negative views about overweight. Even young children who are not overweight say they want to lose weight. They are less likely to want to play with overweight children. Negative attitudes towards obesity have been documented in children as young as 3.[24] Children as young as 6 have been shown to associate obesity with things like cheating, laziness and stupidity.[25] When researchers asked 10 and 11-year-old children to rank who they liked best out of a series of drawings of children with various handicaps, they ranked the obese child last. They would prefer to be friends with children with a wide range of physical disabilities, including facial disfigurement, than with fat children. This study was conducted first in 1961 and again in 2001, and it seems that the increasing prevalence of childhood obesity has not softened attitudes. Another study, of 9-year-old girls, found they and their parents generally tended to attribute positive characteristics to thin people and negative ones to overweight people, even though many of the girls and their parents were overweight themselves.[26]

Given findings like this, it may seem surprising then that the evidence about the effect of obesity on young children's self-esteem and psychological wellbeing is mixed. Some studies suggest it has little effect; others suggest that it is damaging. Evidence about it being harmful for the psychological wellbeing of teenagers is much more consistent. Some researchers think that this may be because younger children's view of themselves is based largely on the messages they receive from their parents, but as they get older, it comes more and more from the broader culture and community.[27]

Debate has also raged about what comes first: poor self-esteem or a weight problem. One study, which followed 1,520 children for 4 years from the ages of 9 and 10, found no significant difference in their self-esteem according to their weight at the start.[28] By the time the children reached early adolescence, though, obese girls and boys were more likely to report lower self-esteem than other children. Those obese children whose self-esteem fell during the study were also more likely to report feeling sad, lonely and nervous. They were also more likely to smoke and drink than obese children whose self-esteem increased or remained unchanged during the study. One of the interesting findings was that many children's self-esteem fell as they grew older, regardless of their size. Overall, 69 per cent of obese white girls had a decrease in self-esteem over the 4 years of the study, compared with 43 per cent of non-obese white girls. By the early teenage years, 14 per cent of obese boys had low self-esteem, compared with 9 per cent of non-obese boys. The researchers said they could not be sure that obesity itself caused low self-esteem. Other factors associated with obesity, such as inactivity, depression or being poor, may contribute to lower self-esteem levels in obese adolescents.

An Australian study found similar trends in younger children.[29] It involved a representative sample of 1,157 Victorian children aged 5 to 10 who were examined in 1997 and then again 3 years later. At the start of the study, overweight and obese children were slightly more likely to have lower self-esteem than other children; this difference was much more marked 3 years later. The researchers said their findings suggested that weight gain played an important role in reducing children's self-esteem.

Obesity can have a lasting effect on psychological, economic and social wellbeing. One large study found American women who were obese as adolescents had lower education levels, earned less money, were less likely to marry and were more likely than women who had not been overweight as teenagers to be poor.[30] The researchers blamed discrimination against the obese for this, and concluded that overweight during adolescence has greater social and economic consequences than many other chronic physical conditions. A study in Britain produced similar results, leading those researchers to conclude that obesity may be the 'worst socio-economic handicap' for young women.[31] Other research has documented discrimination against obese people in the workplace, in medical and health care services, and in housing.[32] Obese adults are more likely than non-obese adults to suffer depression, anxiety, poor social relationships and generally worse mental health.[33] A survey involving thousands of Australian women found that those who were overweight or obese were less likely to report being satisfied with their work, career, study and close personal relationships, although the differences between the groups of women were not huge.[34]

Health issues for adults

Many experts believe that the most significant consequence of childhood obesity is its impact on coming generations of adults, who are likely to suffer higher rates of heart disease, stroke, type 2 diabetes, certain cancers, gall bladder disease, osteoarthritis, endocrine disorders and other obesity-related problems. The result, many warn, could be a significant fall in life expectancy.[35] No less an authority than the Surgeon General of the United States says that preventing obesity in children has the potential to prevent cardiovascular disease in adults. Meanwhile, the National Health and Medical Research Council suggests that in Australia, about 66 per cent of type 2 diabetes, 22 per cent of coronary heart disease, and 29 per cent of hypertension is due to obesity.[36] Being overweight can also affect women's ability to conceive, and being overweight during pregnancy can mean risks for both mother and baby.[37]

There is some evidence that obese adults are more likely to suffer associated health problems if they put on weight as children or teenagers rather than in adult life.[38] Dr Tim Gill, Co-director of the NSW Centre for Public Health Nutrition, based at the University of Sydney, says that overweight children who continue to put on weight as adults are more likely to develop type 2 diabetes than overweight adults who were trim as children. Research in Finland suggests that the metabolic syndrome is especially common among obese adults who were also obese as children.[39]

It may also be the case that being overweight early in life brings increased risks even for adults who have since trimmed down.[40] One US study found that men who were overweight as teenagers were more likely than those who weren't, to die prematurely and to suffer coronary heart disease and other problems, regardless of their weight as adults.[41] But other researchers believe that most of the health problems associated with childhood obesity are in fact due to its persistence into adulthood. Yet others suggest that the risk may be highest among normal-weight children who become obese adults.[42]

While it seems clear that obese adults are more likely to die prematurely, debate continues about the impact of simply being overweight. Some studies show increased rates of diabetes, gallstones, hypertension and heart disease in overweight adults,[43] but others have found no evidence that being overweight, as distinct from obese, increases the risk of premature death.[44] (You can find out more about the difference between obesity and overweight in Chapter 11.)

Risks of inactivity

Is it fitness or fatness that matters most? This tricky question has provoked many a heated debate. Because people who are overweight tend to be unfit, it has been difficult to work out the impact of each characteristic. The relationship between fitness and fatness is complex, too. Physical activity does more than simply burn up calories; it also helps sleeping, digestion and appetite mechanisms—all of which are important for weight control.

Many experts believe that being inactive and unfit is just as big a health risk—if not a bigger one—than being overweight. People who are lean and unfit may be more likely to have health problems than fit fat people.[45] Others say that even if obese people become fit, it may not make up for all the health risks associated with their weight, and that it is important to shed some kilograms too.[46]

People who are inactive are more likely to develop insulin resistance and type 2 diabetes, regardless of their weight.[47] According to Professor John Hawley, an expert on the effects of exercise on metabolism, based at the RMIT University in Victoria, exercise is one of the best ways of making the body's muscles more sensitive to insulin. And the International Agency for Research on Cancer, based in France, estimates that physical inactivity is responsible for 14 per cent of all cases of colon cancer and 11 per cent of postmenopausal breast cancer cases.[48] There can be little doubt that inactivity is a major health problem.

Rather than focusing on your family's weight, it makes far more sense to put your effort into encouraging everyone to be more active. And don't assume that because your family is lean, it doesn't matter if they don't exercise. Here are a few things to consider:

• Children who are overweight are less likely than others to develop the skills and confidence to participate in sport and other physical activities. They are also less likely to be fit.

• Being physically active has many benefits for children and teenagers, apart from weight control. It helps build and maintain healthy bones, muscles and joints, promotes the development of movement and co-ordination skills and self-confidence, and prevents and controls mental health problems such as depression and anxiety. A WA study found that physically active young people had higher self-esteem and reported fewer emotional problems than those who were sedentary. Seventeen per cent of teenagers who exercised regularly reported mental health problems, compared with 30 per cent of the couch potatoes. The study also found a link between regular exercise and better academic performance. On the other hand, children and teenagers who are physically inactive are more likely to smoke, drink, take drugs and have behavioural problems. Children and teenagers who are in the habit of being physically active are thought to be more likely to be active as adults.[49]

• Adults also gain many benefits from being physically fit. It reduces their risk of dying prematurely, and developing heart disease, stroke, high blood pressure, and type 2 diabetes. It is estimated that 30 to 40 per cent of cancers are preventable by appropriate eating habits plus physical activity.[50] Active adults are also less likely to suffer falls, and are more likely to have healthy bones, muscles and joints.[51]

Perspective

Childhood in the 21st century is, in many ways, safer than ever. Today's children are less likely than previous generations to suffer infectious diseases and accidents or to know the pangs of hunger and deprivation. Children living in wealthy countries such as Australia enjoy a standard of living their ancestors could not have imagined. But their physical and emotional health and development are under threat. Canadian researchers have coined the term 'modernity's paradox' in response to evidence of increasing rates of mental health, social and drug and alcohol problems in children and young people, despite the fact that they live in an era of economic growth and wealth.[52] Two of the most pervasive problems for children are physical inactivity and poor diet, and these are often seen in expanding waistlines. It is a terrible reflection on our society and its priorities that children born today may have a lower life expectancy than their parents' generation.

There are many reasons why encouraging weight obsession is not a good idea (more about this in Chapters 5 and 7). But helping families and children enjoy physically active lifestyles and tasty, nutritious food will have profound health benefits for current and future generations. It may help people who need to lose weight do that, and it may help others maintain a healthy weight. And as a Queensland Government report has noted, it would also help with all of Australia's national health priorities: asthma, cancer, cardiovascular health, diabetes, injury prevention, mental health, arthritis and musculoskeletal conditions.[53]

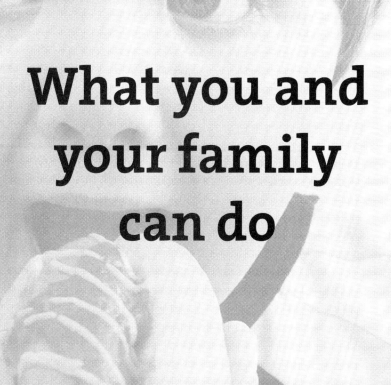

What you and your family can do

5. A family affair

People often react defensively when challenged about what they eat, or other aspects of their lifestyle. That's not surprising. It can feel like a personal attack when someone, or even some magazine or newspaper article, questions the way you bring up your family. As well, some people may be in denial, and others may not realise the impact their everyday decisions have on their family's health. So take a deep breath if you feel your hackles start to rise during this chapter—its aim is not to attack or criticise you, but to motivate and empower you.

But there's no point beating around the bush: this chapter is no picnic. It will challenge you to examine your own beliefs and behaviours. You can't lay the foundations for good health in your children without also working on your own wellbeing. Here are a few reasons why good health is a family affair:

• If a child is overweight or inactive or eating poorly, one of the worst things that can happen is for that child and their weight to become the focus of everyone's attention. This can make the child feel awful, and they may respond by maintaining their behaviour. It will be far more effective and better for the child if the whole family environment changes

104

in a way that makes it easier for everyone to eat well and be active.

• If a child is overweight or inactive or eating poorly, chances are some other family members have the same problems, which means that everyone will benefit from making some changes to family habits.

• Previous chapters have discussed how difficult the modern world makes it for children to achieve good health. This doesn't mean that parents are powerless. Parents have a huge impact on the micro-environment children grow up in, even if the task sometimes feels overwhelming.

• Children are like sponges. From their earliest days, they soak up what they see their parents, brothers and sisters and significant others doing. Parents are powerful role models. If you enjoy eating well and being active, your children are likely to do the same. Your children are more likely to do what you do, rather than what you say they should do.

• Of course making changes to your daily habits and routines is far easier said than done. Anyone who's ever tried to do it knows how hard it can be. This chapter will give you some tips for making change easier. It's about creating positive new habits, rather than obsessing about bad old ones.

The good news is that even relatively small steps can lead to big improvements in your family's health and wellbeing. The aim is not to create a perfect family with the perfect lifestyle and the perfect children. Striving for perfection can be soul-destroying, frustrating and not much fun. And it sets you up for failure. Far better to find a way to make a healthy lifestyle as enjoyable and as sustainable as possible for you and your family.

Five tips for a healthy family

Tip 1. Be aware

A father recently told me about how someone had described his teenage children as fat. He was shaking his head about it. His kids were not fat, he said. They were just a bit chunky, and it was nothing to worry about. It was an uncomfortable moment. I knew his children were more than just a bit overweight. Even though I hadn't seen them in their swimmers lately, I was pretty sure their BMIs would fall in the obese range. But I didn't speak up. No one likes to be told that their children are fat. Our society is so obsessed with thinness and so judgmental about fatness that it is not surprising many parents find it difficult to acknowledge when their children have a weight problem. It is especially difficult for parents who are self-conscious about their own size or lifestyle.

Many studies have shown that parents often do not recognise or acknowledge when their children are overweight or obese. They prefer to use words like 'heavy' or 'solid', and often do not see excess weight as a health issue. They are more likely to see it as a social problem. Parents are more likely to be concerned about their children's poor nutrition or inactivity than their weight.[1] When the NSW Health Department commissioned focus groups to research parents' attitudes, they found that parents typically see childhood obesity as an important issue—but not for them or their children. It is someone else's problem. A number of research groups, in Australia and elsewhere, have found that it is not always appreciated when they tell parents about their findings. Many parents do not welcome being told, by researchers or anyone else, that their children are overweight.

A family affair

Perhaps some are in denial, or feel guilty, as if their children's weight reflects poorly on them and their parenting. Well-meaning friends and family can reinforce this kind of denial: if you heard a friend wondering aloud whether their overweight child was carrying too much weight, how would you respond? It's often easier for everyone to look the other way.

As well, being overweight has become so common that it is now seen as normal. Children who once would have been considered a normal weight can now look thin in comparison with their classmates. And some parents worry that focusing on children's weight may encourage eating disorders or affect children's self-esteem.

Another reason many parents might not want to acknowledge their children's weight is their own waistlines. In 2000, just over two-thirds of Australian men and half of Australian women were overweight. But many adults who are overweight or even obese do not think they have a weight problem.[2] The rates are likely to be significantly higher among parents with overly heavy children. Why would parents be concerned about their children's weight if they do not recognise that their own weight may be a health hazard?

Awareness of a problem is the first step in making change of any sort. No one is going to be bothered to make a change unless they are aware that there is a problem that needs work and attention. Are you aware of the health and weight issues for you and your family?

Even if you and your family are already doing pretty well on this score, the obesogenic environment we all live in means you may face issues in the future. It's far easier and more effective to stop the problem arising than to try to do something once there is a weight problem—remember, our bodies are very determined to maintain the weight we gain. Scientists have calculated that someone who was once obese requires 10 to 15 per cent fewer calories to maintain their normal weight than someone of the same body composition who was never obese. This is because muscles become much more efficient after weight loss—they need fewer calories to perform the same amount of work. The body's metabolic processes continue to fight your attempts to maintain your reduced body weight for years after you lost the weight.[3] It's far better to avoid weight gain in the first place.

It is also important to be aware of your own attitudes and beliefs. Many parents believe it is all too hard, that weight is predestined, and that they have little influence over their children's lives. Many associate being a good parent with giving their children treats. They feel as if they are depriving their children if they don't give them sweets. Or they think their children are safer in front of the TV than playing in the park.

Taking some time to think about your family's beliefs and behaviours around food, activity, health and weight might give you some ideas about where change might be both possible and helpful.

Tip 2. Model behaviour

I know we haven't met, but I know at least three things about you (maybe this is a book of conspiracies after all...). One is that you probably underestimate how much you eat, just as I, and most other people, do. Researchers have called this the 'eye–mouth gap'.[4] Another is that you probably think your diet is healthier than it really is—something researchers call 'dietary optimism'.[5] One study of Melbourne families found that the more confident parents were about their children having a healthy diet, the more likely the children were to eat plenty of snack foods and few vegetables.[6]

The third thing we have in common is that we probably both overestimate how active we are—this one is called the foot–brain gap.

Keep these gaps between perceptions and reality in mind when you read the next section, which sets out three ways that parents and others who play important roles in children's lives can be healthy role models.

Modelling healthy eating

This is not only about what you eat; it's also about how you eat and how you feel about food and eating. Do you eat breakfast? Do you enjoy family meals at the table with the television off? Are healthy meals a pleasure rather than a punishment? Does the crunch of an apple make you salivate? Do you miss vegetables if you don't have them for a few days? Do you feel good about eating? Do you enjoy the occasional splurge on your favourite chocolate or ice cream without feeling a hint of guilt?

Don't feel bad if 'yes' is not your honest and instinctive answer to these questions. Many people are in the same boat. Many struggle with their attitudes to food and have difficulty meeting healthy eating recommendations. Only about 1 in 5 adults eats enough vegetables, according to a recent large NSW study. We do better in the fruit stakes but still less than 50 per cent of adults eat enough fruit.[7]

Mothers are a particularly powerful influence on children's food choices, and not only because they so often are responsible for shopping and cooking. They often are the family's authority on food and diet, so they wield extra clout as role models. A number of studies have shown that mothers who like soft drinks, snacks, sweets and fast foods are more likely to have children who like those foods. Research has found that a mother's liking for confectionery was the strongest predictor of whether children aged 9 to 11 ate sweets. Meanwhile, mothers who drink milk rather than soft drink are more likely to have daughters who do the same.[8] The researchers concluded that efforts to increase young girls' calcium intake should target mothers as well as daughters. And when parents eat fruit and vegetables, their children are more likely to do the same.[9]

Chapters 7 to 9 give detailed advice to help you and your family get a bigger health kick from your food.

Modelling an active lifestyle

Do you moan if you can't get a car park close to your destination? Does leaving home always mean hopping in the car? Does working up a sweat make you feel sick and miserable? Did you spend more time watching TV yesterday than walking or running? Do you automatically hop in the lift or jump on the elevator, rather than finding the stairs? Are you too busy most days to fit in a walk or a trip to the gym?

Don't feel bad if 'yes' was your honest and instinctive answer to these questions. Changes to our work and leisure have made it difficult for most adults to be active enough in daily life to benefit their health. Only 45 per cent of adults are physically active enough to meet health recommendations, according to a recent NSW study.[10] Meanwhile, a national study found that 15 per cent of adults do no physical activity at all.[11]

Some studies suggest that fathers who are physically active are particularly likely to influence children to be more active.

Chapter 10 gives detailed advice to help you and your family make physical activity an enjoyable part of your daily life.

Obsess not

It is no coincidence that an epidemic of weight gain has arisen at the same time as a flourishing weight loss industry promoting an epidemic of dieting. I include in the 'weight loss industry' those magazines, book publishers and others who make a profit out of promoting unnaturally thin figures and unhealthy, unnatural eating patterns—also known as the latest fad diets. Dieting inevitably leads to overeating, even in experiments on animals, and is associated with an increased risk of weight gain. A cynic might think that the weight loss industry keeps itself in business by promoting dieting— exactly the technique to ensure that customers always come back for more 'miracle cures' (which don't work).

Many parents, especially mothers, are caught in a vicious circle. They worry about their weight, which makes them try to restrict what they eat, which is difficult and leads to bingeing, which makes them feel guilty, which makes them eat more, which makes them worry about their weight, which means they are soon back where they started on this circle. And so it continues.[12] These eating patterns often lead to weight fluctuations or weight cycling, and these make it physiologically and psychologically more difficult to keep weight off. This vicious circle is often passed down from generation to generation. The world being the way it is, it tends to be women who are most worried about their weight, and so it tends to be mothers who often 'infect' their daughters with the dieting bug and body-image concerns. Some research suggests that this begins very early in girls' lives, even before they are old enough to go to school.[13]

Focusing on children's weight can have lifelong repercussions, especially for girls. Teenage girls who diet are more likely to feel worthless, and to be depressed and socially anxious. They are also more likely to be dissatisfied with their body, and to be heavier.[14] There are so many women and teenage girls who are unhappy with their body size and shape that some experts believe such discontent has become the norm, from very early in life. Preoccupation with weight can be crippling, leading to disordered eating as well as the less common but more serious eating disorders such as anorexia nervosa. Obsessing about your body's shape or size is not good for mental health or self-confidence. One study showed that the fear of being weighed was one of the most important factors in women postponing or cancelling medical appointments.[15] Another serious consequence of weight obsession is the use of cigarettes as a form of weight control.[16] But perhaps the worst thing about weight obsessing is that it is likely to encourage patterns of behaviour that promote weight gain.

Then there's the more general wellbeing issue: if you are spending so much of your life worrying about your figure or your weight, you have less space in your head and less time and energy for focusing on the things that really matter in life. Rather than encouraging children to worry about their weight, parents should set an example by not focusing on their own shape or size. If you tell your children that it's not their size or shape that matters, but at the same time you obsess about how you measure up to the 'stick insects' in fashion magazines, you know which message they will take in.

One expert who has specialised in treating eating disorders says there are two types of obese people: the emotionally healthy and the emotionally unhealthy.[17] Those in the second group see weight as their most important feature, and they put life on hold until they can get thin. An emotionally healthy obese person might prefer to be thinner, but doesn't let their weight dominate their life. The other key difference between the two groups was their parents' attitudes. Those in the second group had parents who were preoccupied with their children's weight.

Do yourself and your family a favour. Forget about fad diets and put away the bathroom scales. Counting kilograms or calories is a waste of time at many levels—for a start, it's time that could be spent more productively or enjoyably. Aim to be healthy and fit, rather than to be a so-called ideal body shape or size.

Instead of talking to your children about their weight, talk about the benefits of healthy eating and being fit and active. Think about what issues will matter most for them, at their stage of life. For example, many children may not be particularly inspired to know that eating fruit and vegies may help reduce their cancer risk; they might be more interested in knowing that healthy eating will help give them lots of energy, make them strong, and help them do better at school and sport.

What the research says

- Girls who put on weight between ages 5 and 7 were more likely to have mothers who put on weight, according to a study that examined more than 150 girls from Pennsylvania (in the United States) when they were 5, 7 and 9. It also found that girls who put on weight were more likely to have less active fathers who had a high energy intake. The researchers said their findings highlight the importance of the family, and thus of involving parents in treating childhood weight problems.[18]

- Girls who were heavier at 5 were more likely at age 9 to restrict what they ate as well as to eat to excess when they were not hungry, according to the same study. These girls were also more likely to be concerned about their weight and dissatisfied with their body, and to have put on weight. The researchers said their findings were consistent with other research showing that children's attempts to control their weight may promote weight gain.[19]

- The same study found that children as young as 5 are sensitive to their parents' perceptions of their weight: 5-year-old girls were more likely to think negatively about their body if their fathers were concerned about their weight. The researchers said this suggested that how parents and society deal with children who are overweight may affect the psychological health of children. 'Public health programs that simply raise parental awareness about childhood overweight without providing parents with concrete alternatives for addressing their concerns about their child's weight status may be harmful,' they said.[20]

- Five-year-old girls were more likely to think about dieting if their mothers had dieted recently, the same study found. More than 90 per cent of the mothers reported dieting recently. 'Women should be informed that weight control attempts may influence their young daughters' emerging ideas, concepts and beliefs about dieting,' the researchers concluded.[21]

- Another study, involving children aged 7 to 13, found that almost half were concerned about their weight, more than a third had already tried to lose weight and almost a tenth showed some signs of anorexia nervosa. Another study of almost 2000 high school students found that 11 per cent of girls could be classified as 'emotional eaters', meaning they binged and felt out of control about food.[22]

Against the odds: learning from the minority

It has become the norm these days for people to gain weight, adding a kilogram or two every year or so. But what about those who don't? Why are they different and what can we learn from them?

This was the thinking behind a study that followed 165 married couples, mostly in their thirties, over a 4 year period.[23] Only 13 per cent of men and 22 per cent of women were normal weight at the start of the study and stayed at or near that weight for the next 4 years. The women in this group ate fewer calories than other women, were less likely to diet or binge, and were more inclined to be active and participate in sports during leisure time. They were also more likely to have been lean as children, and their husbands were also more likely than other women's husbands to be active and lean.

The men who kept a healthy weight during the study ate less fat and more fruit and vegetables than other men, and were also less likely to diet or binge on food.

Although many people believe that some people can eat what they like, never exercise and stay trim, the researchers did not find evidence of that. Instead, they concluded that a healthy, stable weight reflected 'maintainable lifestyle behaviours' rather than conscious extreme efforts to resist weight gain. The findings also suggested that it's easier to maintain a healthier lifestyle if your partner is on the same wavelength.

Who's helping you?

When Karen Drayton rejoined the workforce after having two sons, she would never have guessed what a difference the new job would make to her family. For 18 months, Karen worked as personal assistant to Professor Kerin O'Dea, an international expert on the links between diet, lifestyle and health who was at that time the director of the Menzies School of Health Research in Darwin.

Through her work, Karen gained a better understanding of the effects of an unhealthy diet, and the benefits of exercise and eating plenty of fruit and vegetables. She also learnt, in graphic detail, about the many devastating consequences of type 2 diabetes. As a result of discussions with her boss, Karen made some changes to her family's routines. She and her husband Mark and their young sons Matthew and Alex became used to having water instead of soft drink or cordial with meals.

Karen became more conscious of reading food labels when shopping, and stopped putting packets of chips in her sons' lunchboxes. She also became more conscious of setting an example, and made a determined effort to squeeze exercise into her schedule.

Karen, who is in her early thirties, has a number of relatives with type 2 diabetes who are overweight. Looking back, she realised that she didn't have many healthy role models when she was growing up. But she was lucky, she says, to find a boss who was a role model. She credits Kerin with helping her make positive changes to her family's health. 'Kerin's so active and energetic,' says Karen. 'She doesn't deprive herself of food, but she doesn't eat rubbish.'

Not everyone has first-hand access to public health experts like Kerin O'Dea. But have a look around. Who can you learn from in your circle of friends, relatives and acquaintances? Who can help inspire and support you in making changes to your everyday routines?

Tip 3. Get real

By day, Tracey Wilson works to improve the health of her local community in Victoria's Central Highlands, around Ballarat. She manages a Primary Care Partnership, an alliance of health and welfare organisations. One of its top priorities is promoting physical activity and healthy eating.

Not surprisingly, these have also been priorities for Tracey and her husband Bernard in bringing up their two sons. The boys, now teenagers, both enjoy cooking, eating well and being fit and active. With both parents working full-time, this hasn't always been easy to do. A lot of planning and co-operation from everyone has been involved.

'The boys are a fantastic help,' says Tracey. 'They're interested in what we're going to have for tea, and will help out in the kitchen.'

But Tracey says the most important factor is that she and her husband have had a similar philosophy from their sons' earliest days: it is worth making some effort to support the family's health. 'If it's been a smooth ride for us it's because we have a shared understanding of where we're coming from', she says. 'Overall we are on the same page.'

Many parents are not so lucky; many do not get the personal or professional support that Tracey has had.

It is common for parents to have conflicting views about how to bring up their children or what changes might benefit the family. 'I'd be surprised if two people did agree on these things,' says Mary Pekin, who runs the Canberra and Wagga offices of Relationships Australia. 'Most couples, if you took any topic, like washing the dishes, how often you have sex, who takes the garbage out, whatever, are likely to have disagreements.'

The point is not that parents have to agree about the contents of their children's lunchboxes, Pekin says. But they should be able to listen to each other's point of view, express their own, and from there develop a solution that will work for everyone, especially the children.

Not every family has the skills to do this on their own. But we can learn and practise those skills until, like any habit, they become automatic. And developing these skills has lots of good spin-offs. Children are keen observers. If their parents yell at each other or stop talking to each other for days after having a fight, children won't take much notice if their parents' advice is that they should deal with conflict by talking about it.

And some families are struggling with more pressing issues: mental health problems, drug abuse, domestic violence or financial concerns, for instance. These generally have to be dealt with before it is possible to work on other health issues. But even families facing a bundle of serious problems can sometimes make small changes in their daily lives. This may help give them the confidence to try bigger changes.

Every family is unique, with different dynamics, history, beliefs and priorities. It has been said, not entirely in jest, that every family is dysfunctional in its own sweet way.

How people behave as parents is often influenced by how they were treated as children. What attitudes and behaviours have you absorbed, perhaps without even thinking about it, from your parents or other role models? Who tends to make the decisions in your family, and how?

Studies have shown that parents do not treat all their children the same way. The sex, age, birth order, physical appearance and abilities of the child can affect parents' attitudes and behaviours.[24] It is not uncommon for parents to encourage their sons to eat up and bulk up, but to encourage the opposite behaviour in their daughters, for example. The other side of the coin is that individual children will respond differently to the same parenting strategies.

What if the dinner table is full of unspoken and spoken hostilities and tensions? Some experts believe that children whose feeding difficulties cannot be resolved often come from homes where there are wars between the parents.[25]

What if your partner is, perhaps without even realising it, undermining you or threatened by what you are doing? Perhaps he or she doesn't want to stop having soft drink with dinner or eating snacks in front of the TV. Perhaps they come from a long line of couch potatoes and fast food addicts, and can't see any reason for changing their ways. Watch out for what some health professionals call 'silent saboteurs'—these are the people who break open the chocolate just as you're offering the kids a fruit platter.

Or perhaps you and your partner are separated; in this situation both parents may try to overcompensate by buying lots of treats or taking the kids to fast food restaurants. Children are always the losers when they become pawns in hostilities or power struggles between parents.

Dr Michael Carr-Gregg, a Melbourne psychologist who specialises in working with adolescents and their families, often comes across people who are resistant to change, or even actively working to sabotage it. Sometimes this goes back to deep-rooted issues such as unresolved grief or physical, sexual or emotional abuse. A child's weight or unhealthy eating patterns may be a symptom of other troubles. Many people turn to food in times of emotional distress. But as Carr-Gregg says, 'There's that wonderful old saying—you can't change what you don't acknowledge. We've got to acknowledge what lies under the problem first.'

The perfect family or relationship only exists in movie scripts. The rest of us have to live and work in the real world, where the barriers to changing family behaviour sometimes seem insurmountable. The first step towards developing solutions is awareness. Think about it: how might some of these issues be affecting you and your family and your health?

Ellyn Satter is an internationally recognised nutritionist and therapist (and author) who works with US families whose children are having difficulties related to food and eating. She says that the parents who are prepared to look closely at themselves and what they are doing are the healthy ones. The ones who don't question themselves but just blame the problem on the child are the ones who are likely to be in trouble. 'The blunt truth,' she says, 'is that you can't take your child any further than you have taken yourself.'[26]

Tip 4. Making change easier

Bad habits, it has been said, are like a comfortable bed. They are easy to get into, but hard to get out of.

Information does not translate into action. Just because we all know we should eat more fruit and vegetables doesn't mean we do it.

Here are a few reasons why people find it so difficult to change:

• Humans are naturally suspicious of change. In an evolutionary sense, habits may protect us. For example, having a routine probably helped our ancestors make sure they had enough food and drink to survive.

- People tend to filter out information that does not support what they already think and believe. Many people believe they are already doing the best things for themselves and their families. They may not see that there are beneficial changes they could make.
- Failure is demoralising. Many people don't try to change because they are afraid of failing. It's far less confronting to stick with the status quo.
- Changing habits can be uncomfortable, even painful. Starting to do some exercise, when you're not used to it or if you're carrying a bit of excess weight, can leave you sore and sorry.
- Sometimes people want to maintain the status quo, for reasons that are not obvious. 'When women are trying to lose weight, often really subtle things try to undermine that,' says Professor Ann Roche, Director of the National Centre for Education and Training on Addiction at Flinders University in Adelaide. 'It might not be seen to be in their partner's interests to have a slim, attractive wife, for instance.' She is suggesting that some men may feel threatened if their partner trims down and becomes more attractive to others.
- Sometimes, of course, it makes perfect sense to resist urgings to change your behaviour—many people and organisations have a stake in trying to make us do things that might not be to our advantage.

Stages of change

People who work in the drug and alcohol field have developed a model of the stages of change. This adaptation of that model may be useful for others.[27] The stages are:

1. *Precontemplation.* You are blissfully ignorant of or in denial about the need to change, and are not aware of the benefits it might bring. You think, *I hardly ever eat vegetables but it's not a big deal.* Ask yourself or your doctor or your friends what is known about the link between eating plenty of vegetables and a reduced risk of diseases.

2. *Contemplation.* You may realise the need to do something but feel ambivalent about it. You may see why it's a good idea, but you are also aware of what it will involve. People can stay in this stage for long periods of time. You think, *I know I should eat more vegetables but it's too much of a hassle and I can't be bothered.* If you are in this stage, think about what might help motivate you. Is there a family history of diabetes, cancer or heart disease? Would you like to have more energy? Think about what is stopping you making the change and how you might overcome those things.

3. *Preparing to make change.* You have found a greengrocer who will home deliver a box of vegetables every week. You've been meaning to place an order, but you're so busy that you just haven't got round to it. You think, *Once work settles down, I will get onto it.* If you are in this stage, do something concrete to make it happen. Write a note in your diary to remind yourself to ring the greengrocer next week.

4. *Action.* Your fridge is full of vegetables and you are learning lots of delicious ways to cook them. *It doesn't take that much time after all,* you think. It helps if family and friends are supportive of this change in your lifestyle.

5. *Maintenance/relapse.* You are cooking vegetables at least three times a week. When you unwrap the fish and chips instead on those nights when you really can't be bothered to cook, you try not to whip yourself and concentrate instead on the positive changes that have already occurred. After all, there are still plenty of vegetables in the fridge for tomorrow night.

6. *Mission achieved.* You don't even think about the vegetable issue any more. Cooking and eating vegetables has become part of your routine. You wouldn't dream of going back to the takeaway diet. *I feel so much better now,* you think.

That's the theory, anyway. Not everyone will move from stages 1 to 6, and not everyone will move through the stages in that order. When people are trying to give up smoking, for example, they typically go through this cycle several times before they quit. So don't give up if you get stuck in a particular stage or have trouble reaching the final goal.

Here are a few tips for making change easier:
• Think about what you want to change and why. If it is going to involve or affect others in the family, make sure they all have a chance to join in the discussion.
• Set your goals, and make sure they are achievable and realistic. Most people don't like being told what to do. They are far more likely to get involved in change if they have had a say in the goals and the strategies for achieving them. Everyone has to be part of the solution.
• Identify where you and the rest of the family are in the model of change. What would help you move to the next stage?
• What are some of the barriers to change? This might be people—perhaps grandparents who show their love by dispensing sweets—or environmental factors, such as the lack of a nearby park. Find ways to overcome or minimise the impact of these barriers.
• Triggers or incentives can encourage and support you in making change. What would work for you and your family?

• The most skilled experts in behavioural change—marketers—also have lessons for the rest of us. We can learn from how the junk food industry promotes its products. They give away toys with their food because they know this will encourage children to associate their restaurants with having a good time. Work out some similar strategies yourself. If your children get used to having fruit when you're all playing at the park, for instance, they may start to associate fruit with having a good time.

• Different things will motivate different people. What might motivate one family member might be a turn-off for another. Be aware of and respect these differences.

• Don't be put off by setbacks. They are normal. Don't throw your hands in the air just because you've taken two steps back.

• Conditioning is a powerful force. If you always buy a soft drink when you go to the movies, sooner or later you will start to crave that sugar hit as soon as you step into the cinema. Be aware of the emotions and cues that are associated with the behaviours you are trying to change. Try to decrease the negative cues and develop new, positive ones. Take a bottle of water to the movies or have one sitting on the table by the TV. Keep a pair of walking shoes by the door; just the sight of them might be enough to remind you to go for a walk.

• Identify problem areas and plan ways to deflect them. If your mother always arrives laden with chocolates and lollies for the kids, suggest that she might like to give them games instead, to encourage them to play outside—something as simple as a tennis ball, perhaps.

• Try to set up some structures to support the family during the period of change. Everyone may start off with the best of intentions, but we are all easily waylaid by the pressures of day-to-day life. It might help to put a checklist on the fridge to remind everyone of where they are at and what their responsibilities are. Or try scheduling a regular family meeting to review progress and help keep everyone involved and committed. This can also help spread the load, rather than making it all one person's responsibility.

• Do what the experts call 'cognitive restructuring'. Learn to identify, challenge and correct irrational thoughts. This means changing your 'self-talk', those silent conversations that go on in your head, so that they are positive rather than negative. Some examples of unhelpful and helpful ways of thinking include: 'I didn't go for a walk last night so I will never get fit (I didn't go for a walk last night but I can go for one tonight)'; 'I had a sausage roll for lunch so there's no point even trying any more (I had a sausage roll for lunch but tomorrow I will have a salad)'; 'I will never be able to get them to eat more vegetables (I will cook those vegetables a different way tomorrow and see if they will try them)'.

• Monitor the positives, not the negatives. Don't count how many days you couldn't drag yourself out of bed for a walk; count how many days you walked.

• Accept that change is rarely easy. Sometimes it requires discipline and sacrifice. But the more you can do to make it as easy as possible for everyone involved, the more likely you are to create lasting change.

• Pat yourself and your family on the back regularly. So many forces are working against your efforts to do the healthy thing. Taking a stand and starting to do things differently requires some courage and effort, and you deserve congratulations for it.

Tip 5. Small steps take you further than a giant leap

When you've finally decided to embark on change, it's tempting to make grand plans. It's also risky. Starting off with dramatic changes can backfire; they can be harder to achieve, and if you don't succeed, it may put you off trying again.

So start with small and realistic goals. They are more likely to be sustainable, to become part of your daily routine. It might be something as simple as making one change to your shopping list, or parking your car one block away from the shopping centre, or adjusting a favourite recipe. Brushing your teeth straight after dinner might deter late-night snacking. Gradual changes to your family's eating habits are likely to lead to better long-term results than big changes made all at once, say the experts.[28]

Small changes may be all you need to correct energy imbalances anyway. Some experts estimate that most of the population's weight gain could be prevented by changing the energy balance by the equivalent of walking for 15 minutes every day or eating a few bites less at each meal.[29]

Coaching for health

The psychological techniques that are used with sports and business people are also being used to help people improve their health and lifestyle. Here are a few pointers from some experts.

* **Dr Suzy Green**, a coaching and clinical psychologist in Sydney, has worked with many individuals and families wanting to improve their diet and lifestyle.

A family affair

Psychological coaching is different from therapeutic counselling: it is performance-enhancing rather than healing. Coaching is based on setting goals and monitoring achievements. This might mean setting a goal of trying a new vegetable every week or hitting the pool at least a few times a week. It also requires constant evaluation—looking to see what is not working and making changes to goals and strategies accordingly.

Dr Green encourages clients to set positive rather than negative goals—wanting to be healthy, rather than trying to lose weight, for instance. She also encourages them to focus on the benefits of achieving the goals, rather than the costs. Coaching is not suitable for everyone, Dr Green says. If someone is battling depression or anxiety, therapeutic counselling is more appropriate; these people should consult their general practitioner, she says.

* **Dr Tony Grant**, Director of the Coaching Psychology Unit at the University of Sydney, says that understanding the difference between self-control and self-regulation is the key to making change.

People who rely on self-control to make change say things to themselves like 'I should' or 'I must'. They are much more likely to achieve long-term change if they are capable of self-regulation—doing things they feel are the right things for them to do. He uses the following as an example.

The self-control approach: The chocolate is in the fridge. You think, *I should not eat it.* You walk away, willing yourself not to eat it and feeling deprived.

The self-regulation approach: As you walk away from the fridge you check how you feel about doing this. You feel really good about not having the chocolate.

Dr Grant says psychological coaching aims to help people shift from self-control to self-regulation by helping them get more in touch with their feelings and then using them in a constructive way. He calls this 'enhancing your emotional intelligence'.

Dr Grant has written a number of books about solution-focused coaching. Most are for business people, but many of the principles might be useful for families wanting to make change. Instead of dwelling on problems, he advises people to work on finding solutions. 'You may need to try several different solutions until you find the right one for you', he says.

Dr Grant also advises finding and using resources that can help you build solutions, and learning from previous situations where you found solutions to problems. 'By dwelling on the causes of problems we often perpetuate and exaggerate them,' he says. 'By looking for solutions we immediately shift the emphasis from the past to the future. If you start looking for solutions you start to find them.'

He also advises business chiefs to not expect employees to do something they wouldn't do themselves. Good managers know they will only win respect if they are prepared to do what they ask their staff to do. One could argue that it's the same with parents and children.

* **Dr Janette Gale** is a health coach and psychologist who has worked with children, families and entire communities in the Shoalhaven area south of Sydney.

She has some tips for what NOT to do when working on change: don't tell people what to do without asking for their opinions, and don't scare people into action without offering them hope, for example.

Instead, Dr Gale recommends setting goals that are specific, measurable, attractive, realistic and time-framed. In other words, to borrow some psychological jargon, setting goals that are SMART.

She suggests asking the following questions of yourself or other family members:

- What do you think you need to do in order to improve your health?
- If you were to do one thing to improve your health, what would it be?
- What could you do to make a small change in that direction?
- How would you feel about yourself if you were to do this?
- How different would your life be in one year from now?

She says fathers are often crucial in whether or not a family will be able to make change. 'If the father changes his behaviour, as well as the mother, the family will generally change,' she says. 'It is less likely if only the mother changes. Resistance from the father can undermine the whole process.'

A lot of Dr Gale's work involves helping women find ways to get their partners on board. Nagging is not helpful—it may make things worse. If women make the changes themselves, their partner will often follow. 'Some men need a lot of convincing,' says Dr Gale. 'They really want to know why change is needed. If they are not nagged, their resistance may dilute over time. They might even start to realise they are being stubborn and pig-headed. You need to figure out what will work in individual families.'

Dr Gale also recommends persistence. 'If at first you don't succeed, try again—but try a different strategy,' she says.

Making healthy choices the easy choices

Water will always take the easiest course down a hill. Humans are a bit the same; we tend to take the easiest option, even if it is going to mean that we eventually take a tumble over the waterfall. Maybe that goes back to the days when it was an evolutionary advantage to conserve energy.

That's why the mantra in health circles is that if people want to make lasting changes in their lives, the environment needs to support them by making healthy choices the easy choices. One of the most obvious successes of this approach has been in the field of smoking. It involved changing the environment to make it easier for smokers to quit—and more difficult for them to keep smoking—and included things such as introducing smoke-free workplaces and increasing the taxes on cigarettes.

My own experience with the power of such an approach began with the arrival in my letterbox of an advertisement for a new local business. For a modest sum, a large box of fresh fruit and vegetables would be delivered direct from the markets to my door each week.

It sounds such a simple thing, but it's had a huge impact. We are eating far more fruit and vegetables than before, just to work through our box before the next delivery. As a result, we are spending less (time and money) at the supermarket, and there is less room on our plates for processed foods. Where once we snacked on cheese and biscuits between meals, we are now much more likely to munch on fruit.

The best thing is that we are enjoying our meals more than ever. The produce is deliciously fresh and lasts much longer than the stuff we used to buy at the shops. One of the attractions is that we never know what will be in the box each week. It is always a surprise, and has encouraged us to try new recipes and ways of cooking.

It may just be a coincidence, but we now have more energy, and the fit of our clothes suggests that a few excess kilograms might have gone by the wayside, without any conscious effort on our part.

Parenting tips: Who's the boss?

Parents need knowledge, skills and confidence to bring up children. But many find themselves in one of the most important and challenging roles of their life with little preparation—and of course no training. They may end up relying on instinct or memories from their own childhood. Or the opposite: they may find themselves completely overwhelmed by a flood of well-meaning but sometimes conflicting and unhelpful advice.

Many experts believe that helping mothers and fathers improve their parenting skills is one of the keys to improving children's health and wellbeing.

Many organisations have a ton of information and practical advice to help you negotiate the parenting minefield (see the section in the Appendices, Further Resources, for their details). In the meantime, here are a few tips:

• Learn a little about the stages of child development. For example, don't try to negotiate with a 3-year-old; they are not little adults. They need you to set limits and boundaries. On the other hand, that authoritative approach may well backfire with teenagers.

• Be prepared to put in the hard yards, even though it's often easier to give in to a child who is whining for lollies, and to switch on the TV instead of supervising your kids at the park.

• Be consistent and clear, both in what you expect of your children and how you behave yourself.

• Learn to say no. Mean it when you say it. Don't be budged, or the word will lose its power.

• Develop ground rules for the whole family: no pestering in the supermarket, for example, or no TV while it's still light outside.

• Speak to children the way you would like to be spoken to. Behave the way you would like them to behave.

• Nurture your children's self-esteem and confidence. Many children have low self-esteem—it is not limited to those with weight problems. A recent study of Victorian children found 15 per cent of children of normal weight had low self-esteem. The rate was much higher in those who were overweight or obese (25 per cent and 47 per cent respectively). But roughly two-thirds of children with low self-esteem were not overweight or obese.[30]

• Encourage everyone in the family to adopt a positive, problem-solving approach rather than a blaming and shaming approach.

• Everyone makes mistakes. Don't even think about trying to be the super parent. Notice the small steps forward that you are all making and pat yourself on the back for them. If you are stressed, anxious or tired, parenting will be more difficult. Take some time out for yourself regularly.

Dr Michael Carr-Gregg says the single most important thing parents can do is to stay emotionally in touch with their child. 'Keep on knocking on their emotional door,' he says. 'Fight over things that matter, not an untidy room. No kid ever died of an untidy room. Know where your kids are. Take an interest in their lives. Don't allow them to push you away.'

...and some general tips, from the Triple P Positive Parenting Program at the University of Queensland:[31]

• When your child wants to show you something, stop what you are doing and pay attention to your child. It is important to spend frequent, small amounts of time with your child doing things that you both enjoy.

• Give your child lots of physical affection—children often like hugs, cuddles and holding hands.

• Give your child lots of descriptive praise when they do something that you would like to see more of, such as, 'Thank you for doing what I asked straight away.'

• Teach your child new skills by first showing the skill yourself, then giving your child opportunities to learn the new skill. For example, speak politely to each other in the home. Then prompt your child to speak politely, saying 'please' and 'thank you', for instance, and praise your child for their efforts.

Discipline versus punishment

Everyone can benefit from a little discipline. It is essential for children's wellbeing as they grow up and it helps make the job of parenting less stressful and more successful. Children need to know what is expected of them—and the consequences of breaking the rules.

The Australian Childhood Foundation draws a clear distinction between discipline and punishment.[32] Discipline comes from the Latin word 'to teach', whereas punishment is reactive and focused on penalising unacceptable behaviour. Children rarely learn correct or acceptable behaviour through punishment.

Why is discipline important?
Children need discipline to feel safe and secure while they are learning about themselves and their world. It helps them take responsibility for their own behaviour by teaching them acceptable ways to respond to situations. As they grow, children become more self-disciplined. They understand how to behave and can control their behaviour

themselves. Self-discipline develops through adults teaching and nurturing children's confidence. Successful discipline relies on a good relationship between you and your child and builds on your child's wish to please you. Successful discipline involves understanding the rules and what happens when rules are broken.

What about physical punishment?

Effective discipline can be achieved without using physical punishment. Physical punishment causes pain and does not communicate care or respect to a child. It can undermine a child's sense of love and security, and can lead to them becoming anxious, fearful or rebellious. Physical punishment teaches children that violence can be an acceptable way to solve problems. Hitting a child does not teach acceptable ways to behave. Instead it may result in a repeat of the misbehaviour. Often children are so upset or angry after being hit that they forget why they are being punished.

And the same goes for parents. Taking steps to improve your own and your family's health and lifestyle will require some self-discipline; punishing yourself won't help anyone.

6. The big turn-off

The travel writer Bill Bryson is responsible for one of my favourite quips about television. The best thing that can be said about Norwegian television, he once wrote, is 'that it gives you the sensation of a coma without the worry and inconvenience'. But it seems a tad unfair to single out Norway, given that the television-induced couch potato is such a universal phenomenon.

Eighty-odd years ago, when a Scottish inventor called John Logie Baird gave the public its first taste of television, few could have guessed how great its impact would be. Television surely has become one of the most powerful cultural and commercial forces in the modern world. It influences everything from global and national politics to the conduct of individuals' and families' lives. It has been estimated that by the time we turn 75, many people will have spent more than 12.5 years of 24 hour days doing nothing but watching TV, and that many children now have more eye contact with television characters than with their own parents.[1] By age 18, the average child has spent more time watching television (14,000 hours) than attending school (12,000 hours).[2]

Television has become such a constant in our lives that its presence is mostly taken for granted and its impact is often unquestioned. Yet there is more and more evidence that the box which has come to dominate most lounge rooms—and many kitchens and bedrooms, as well—is not a benign force, especially when it comes to young children. Many parents are happy for their children to switch on the television, because they think it is safer than many other activities. But TV, dubbed 'the other parent' by some researchers, is not the trustworthy babysitter that many parents assume.

Sure, it is convenient and almost guaranteed as an effective method for calming children's natural exuberance, occupying their attention or confining them indoors. But it also brings some significant health risks. One medical review concluded that television viewing affects children and adolescents' behaviour, academic performance, body image, nutrition and substance abuse, amongst other things.[3] In April 2006, a special issue of the American medical journal *Archives of Pediatrics and Adolescent Medicine* was devoted to exploring the impact of television and other media on the health of children and adolescents. 'Given the enormous influence that electronic media in all of their forms exerts on the lives of children, it is astonishing how little parents, researchers and policymakers have been spurred to action', commented an editorial in the journal.[4]

Weight gain is one of the most obvious risks of a television diet. Watching television affects both energy intake (by increasing the likelihood of snacking), and energy expenditure (by discouraging activity). Many scientific reviews have concluded that there is frustratingly little evidence about what interventions would be most effective at preventing rising levels of childhood obesity.[5] The epidemic is new, so there are no long-term studies that could provide such answers. But the one thing that most experts agree upon is this: television is a key culprit and regulating the time children spend in front of screens is one of the most important measures families can take to promote their children's health. Some studies have shown that rewarding children for not watching TV or engaging in other such sedentary activities is more effective at promoting weight loss than rewarding their involvement in exercise or sport. Many children who are encouraged to reduce their inactivity end up liking exercise more than those who are put into regimented exercise programs.[6]

Of course television is only one of an ever-increasing array of media technologies which are dramatically altering the way children spend their spare time—compared with previous generations. And it is likely that computer and other screen-based games, the internet, and interactive mobile phones represent only the beginning of the technological transformation of childhood.

This chapter examines how a screen-based diet affects children, and also gives some tips for regulating their exposure to television and related activities.

Reality TV

What is recommended:

• Medical experts recommend that children under 2 should watch no television at all because of its potential to harm their development. Older children should watch no more than 1–2 hours per day of quality screen time.[7]

The big fat conspiracy

What happens:

• Australian children begin watching TV from an early age: 4-month-olds watch an average of 44 minutes a day, building to an average of 2.5 hours by the time they are 4 years old.[8]

• When parents were asked to record their children's activities in a diary, the results showed that 45 per cent of infants watched TV, a video or a DVD for a mean of 1.4 hours on the day of the diary recording.[9] About 90 per cent of 4 to 5-year-old children watched TV, a video or a DVD for an average of 2.3 hours. This was more time than was spent walking, running or doing other exercise. About a quarter of these children also used a computer or computer games for a mean of 1.1 hours per day.

• According to a Victorian study, boys of primary school age watch an average of 15.7 hours of television a week, and girls an average of 14.8 hours.[10]

• TV ratings surveys show that Australians watch an average of 3.5 hours of television per day, with 5 to 12-year-olds watching about 2½ hours, and 13 to 17 year olds watching about 2 hours 40 minutes. Adults in the typical parental age range (25 to 34) watch more than 3 hours per day on average.[11]

• A 1999 survey found that 14 per cent of boys and girls watch at least 5 hours of television a day, and another 34 per cent watch 3–4 hours.[12]

• In Western Australia, a study found that only 4 per cent of boys of primary and high school age met the recommendations for time spent in front of a screen—no more than 2 hours per day. Almost a third of primary school girls said they preferred to watch TV or play electronic games than do physical activity.[13]

• A large NSW study conducted in 2004 found that 80 per cent of high school boys in cities and 64 per cent of those from rural areas spent more than two hours each day in front of a TV or computer

138

screen. So did 66 per cent of high school girls from cities and 57 per cent of those from rural areas.[14]

What is recommended:

• Families should have firm guidelines on time in front of the TV and on other screen-based technologies. Parents should also monitor children's viewing and use of media technologies.

What happens:

• About 40 per cent of parents in households with TV had no rules about what children watched or how long they watched, according to a study conducted in the Barwon area in southwestern Victoria.[15]

• A great deal of children's TV viewing and use of media technologies goes unmonitored by parents. Parents often do not know the details of their children's activities on the internet (including in chat rooms).[16]

What is recommended:

• Children should not have a TV, or access to other screen-based forms of entertainment, in their bedroom—it increases the likelihood of excess viewing and weight gain, and reduces parental control.

What happens:

• Nineteen per cent of children lived in a family where there was a TV in one or more of the children's bedrooms, according to the Barwon area study.[17] Another study found that more than a third of older children had a TV in their bedrooms.[18]

What is recommended:

• Switch the television off during mealtimes and don't eat in front of it. People are more likely to eat too much and to have unhealthy eating patterns if they eat in front of the TV.

> **What happens:**
> • Forty-one per cent of families eat their evening meal in front of the TV every night, according to the Barwon area study.[19] In a study of Victorian families, a third reported watching TV while eating the evening meal more than 4 times a week. A further 22 per cent reported doing so 1 to 3 times a week.[20]
> • Almost 40 per cent of teenagers reported eating dinner in front of the TV at least 4 nights a week.[21]

Potential harms of TV

Don't get me wrong: television and other screen-based technologies have the potential for good. They entertain, inform and help connect us to people and parts of the world we may otherwise never have known. Screen literacy has become a vital skill and is an important aspect of children's social and intellectual development. It will become ever more important as media technologies become more diverse and sophisticated. One study found that children who watched educational television programs in preschool performed better in school when they were teenagers.[22] Studies suggest that selective television viewing can help academic performance, and that video games involving information, academic content and problem-solving can boost children's learning.[23] One video game has even been credited with improving children's diets; players, who were rewarded in the game for tasks related to fruit and vegetables, were more likely to eat more fruit and vegies in the real world than children who did not use the game.[24] Researchers who find apparently conflicting study results—that exposure to media makes children both more aggressive and more socially skilled—say these findings reflect differences in what children watch and the time spent in media use.[25]

And it's not all about the kids. Television can also be a sanity-saving tool for parents in desperate need of some quiet time away from children's demands. Even Associate Professor Tim Olds, an expert on child fitness at the University of South Australia, acknowledges just how convenient television can be for parents. 'If it weren't for *Thomas the Tank Engine*, I don't think my wife and I would have had sex in the first five years of having children,' he jokes.

But there are also some downsides:

1. Impact on activity and weight

Many studies have shown that children who watch lots of TV are also more likely to eat poorly and to be overweight. The fattening effects of a TV diet are evident even in preschoolers.[26] One Australian study also found that children who watch lots of television are less likely to participate in organised physical activity.[27] Similarly, overweight children are less likely to succeed in shedding weight if they spend a lot of time in front of the TV.[28] Reducing children's television time is one of *the* most effective weight-busting strategies. At least two studies have shown that reducing children's time in front of television leads to weight loss.[29] Some experts argue that reducing children's time in front of screens may be more effective for weight control than encouraging children to play sport and get involved in other physical activity.[30]

Many explanations have been suggested for why television is so fattening. Here are some:
• There is less time available for physical activity. This is the suggestion of one study showing that teenage boys who

watch TV for less than 2 hours a day are far more likely to be fit than those who watch it for more than 4 hours a day.[31]

• Children who spend hours glued to the box fall into sedentary habits. They become used to lounging around rather than being active. This may help explain the findings of one study in which scientists were asked to identify people from an analysis of their daily activity patterns. When shown the activity patterns of Scottish children aged 3 to 5, they wrongly picked them as desk-bound office workers.[32] This suggests that children are becoming so sedentary that they are growing old before their time.

• There is some evidence that watching TV burns less energy than other sedentary pursuits. One study of children aged 8 to 12 found that their metabolic rates were lower when watching TV than when they were resting or sleeping. However, other studies have not shown such an effect.[33] Nonetheless, perhaps Bill Bryson's coma joke was not so far off the mark after all.

• Television viewing may be a marker of a lifestyle that promotes weight gain in a number of ways. In other words, children who watch a lot of television may also be more likely to have parents who are not particularly health conscious or who do not have the knowledge and skills to promote a healthier lifestyle.

• Eating in front of the television is likely to lead to overeating for a number of reasons. It may distract people's attention from the internal cues that tell them they've had enough to eat.[34] Children who watch a lot of television are also more likely to have poor quality or insufficient sleep, which can also contribute to disordered eating patterns. There is also the Pavlov's dog issue: people who are in the habit of snacking in front of the television are likely to crave something to eat as soon as the screen lights up.

However, one of the main reasons that television is so fattening is because it continuously bombards us with advertisements for foods, and usually foods that are high in fat and/or sugar. Many studies have shown that children who watch more TV are also more likely to consume fast food, energy-dense snacks and soft drinks, and are less likely to eat fruit and vegetables.[35] It is surely no coincidence that this pattern also reflects the content of television food advertising.

Many studies have shown that advertising is effective in influencing children's beliefs, preferences, purchasing behaviour and consumption patterns. It also contributes to their misconceptions about food; research has shown that many young children are convinced that fast foods and other heavily promoted junk foods are nutritious.[36]

It is not only the on-screen advertisements that encourage unhealthy eating. Films do the same, according to one study.[37] Researchers analysed the portrayal of nutrition and exercise in the 10 top-grossing films in America in each year from 1991 to 2000. Foods high in fats and sugars featured heavily, but fruit, vegetables and dairy products were seldom shown. The branded goods most often shown were soft drink, beer, confectionery, chips and pretzels, and alcohol. The researchers noted the common practice of companies paying to place their products in movies. Another US study found that alcohol, tobacco and illicit drugs feature widely in prime time TV drama, movies and music videos.

The cruel irony is that while TV is encouraging unhealthy lifestyles and weight gain, it is also promoting unrealistic beliefs and perceptions about body image. The people who inhabit TV-land tend to be thinner and more beautiful than those in the real world. Television characters who are overweight or obese are often portrayed as unattractive, unpopular or unsuccessful.

So the TV diet puts young people in an impossible position. It tells them they must be thin to be loved and successful, but at the same time it makes it more difficult for them to achieve a healthy weight. At least one study has linked television to the creation of eating disorders. Before television was introduced to Fiji, eating disorders in young women were unknown. Three years after TV arrived, dieting and vomiting to control weight had become relatively common.[38]

What the research shows

In 2005, researchers from the NSW Cancer Council spent long hours analysing the content of food advertisements screened during 672 hours of television viewing time. The footage was shown by Channels 9, 7 and 10 in Brisbane, Sydney, the NSW town of Tamworth and Ballarat in Victoria.

A quarter (25 per cent) of all advertisements were for unhealthy foods, while just 6 per cent were for healthy foods. The advertisements for unhealthy foods peaked during times and programs when children were more likely to be watching. Fast foods and takeaways accounted for the biggest proportion of advertisements for unhealthy foods, followed by confectionery, chocolates, snack foods and sweetened breakfast cereals.

According to Ms Kathy Chapman, a senior policy officer and nutritionist at the Cancer Council, the study's preliminary results suggest that if children watch an average of 2 hours of commercial television a day, they see about 11 advertisements for unhealthy foods. 'The big implication is that food advertising really is contributing to the obesogenic environment', says Ms Chapman. 'When children are sitting down to watch TV, they are not seeing ads that reflect the Australian Guide to Healthy Eating. Instead, unhealthy eating is being normalised.'

When the Australian Division of General Practice did an audit of advertising during children's programs in the January 2003 holidays, they found that:

• children received no 'healthy eating' messages;

• there was an average of one food advertisement per break (sometimes three); and

• over 99 per cent of food advertisements were for junk food.

If children watched an average of 2½ hours of television per day during their summer holidays, the researchers estimated they would have seen more than 400 junk food advertisements, lasting almost 3½ hours.[39]

Children also are influenced by TV advertising directed at adults. One study by a media buying agency reportedly showed that advertisers do not need to advertise in children's time slots to have them take notice. Carlton Draught and Hahn Premium Light beers ranked among the most popular TV ads with children aged 8 to 14.[40] Meanwhile, other research by the NSW Cancer Council shows that point-of-sale promotions in supermarkets, using cartoon characters, competitions and other such marketing gimmicks, are used mainly to sell unhealthy foods. That study found that 94 per cent of those promotions involved unhealthy foods, while just 6 per cent were for healthy foods.

2. Impact on growth, development and learning

Infants and young children need interaction with other people to help them develop relationship skills, language, and social skills. Television can interfere with this development, according to the advocacy group Young Media Australia:

> The infant who has learned that he can engage his parent in play and make objects do what he wants them to do acquires a fundamental belief in his ability to affect the world around him...Television is not capable of collaborative communication—where verbal and non-verbal signals are directly responded to by the other and which help infants develop healthy, secure attachments and the ability to self-regulate emotional and behavioural responses. This means TV is a very poor babysitter for infants and can hinder rather than help their most important developmental task, of attaching to their primary care giver.
>
> Infants learn that if I am hungry and cry, Mum will usually pick me up and feed me. Visual media does not respond to an infant's expression of their needs. Attempts to elicit emotional responses from a TV or computer will fail and can be very confusing for infants and very young children. Infants need to be able to indicate when they are tired and want to rest from further interactions. TV is intrusive and can overload neural circuitry. The infant can't switch off the images and rest when they have had enough.[41]

Parents' and carers' TV viewing may also be an issue. If you are regularly absorbed in a program while feeding or playing with your baby, you may miss emotional cues that need your response. If the program is disturbing or upsetting, the infant may pick up on your distress. Listening to music may be a more relaxing option, according to Young Media Australia. The Royal Australasian College of Physicians cites research showing that having the TV on in the background has a detrimental effect on children's play: infants and toddlers spent less time playing with toys and had a shorter attention span when the television was on.[42]

The possibility has been raised that television viewing may interfere with children's neurological development. Some researchers believe that banning all screen time during the formative years of brain development may reduce children's subsequent risk of developing attention deficit hyperactivity disorder (ADHD). However, this issue is controversial, and the Royal Australasian College of Physicians says there is no evidence to support a link between TV viewing and ADHD. One study which followed children for 26 years from birth found that those who had watched a lot of television in childhood and adolescence had poorer educational achievement.[43] The researchers concluded that excessive television viewing early in life 'may have long-lasting adverse consequences for educational achievement and socio-economic status and wellbeing'. However, such a study may also reflect that children who watch a lot of television are disadvantaged in other areas of their lives as well.

3. Impact on behaviour

If television simply reflected the real world, it would be a lot more boring—and less watched—than it is. Television news and general programming competes for our attention by providing viewing which is sensational, compelling, and far removed from the reality that most of us experience. Even so-called reality programming is engineered to be nothing like the daily humdrum that most of us know.

Young children, however, do not understand that what is shown on TV is a skewed picture. They cannot be expected to know that the behaviours and attitudes they see on the screen are not necessarily appropriate for the real world. One can only speculate how reality television shows such as *Big Brother* would have been perceived by those who drafted Australia's first television code in 1956, which stated that children's programs should impart a real appreciation of the spiritual values and of courage, honour and integrity. The code also specified that programming should respect the sanctity of marriage, and that heroes, heroines and other sympathetic characters must be portrayed as intelligent and morally courageous.[44]

One of the most disturbing lessons that TV-land teaches children today is that violence is an acceptable way of dealing with conflict. The content of programming has changed dramatically since television was launched in Australia in 1956. It has been estimated that by the time they turn 18, the average child in the United States has witnessed 16,000 simulated murders and 200,000 acts of violence on TV.[45] And that does not include all the shooting, fighting and killing they see on computer games. Many children's health experts are concerned about the impact of such exposure to violence. The Royal Australasian College of Physicians says there is now 'compelling' evidence that it does harm, with potential long-lasting effects.[46]

In the United States, a coalition of leading health organisations issued a joint statement concluding that media violence makes children more likely to:

- become emotionally desensitised to violence;
- avoid taking action on behalf of a victim when violence occurs;
- believe that violence is inevitable;
- believe that violence is an acceptable way of solving conflict;
- believe that the world is a violent place (which leads to greater anxiety, self-protective behaviours and mistrust of others); and
- use violence themselves.[47]

Parents and teachers are only too familiar with examples of children mimicking bad behaviour they have seen on TV or computer games. Even Hollywood executives believe there is a link between television violence and the real thing.[48] Some researchers argue that if television had never been invented, violent crime would be half as common as it is.[49] Media technology also exposes children to other undesirable behaviours. A US study found that about a fifth of children who use the internet regularly had been approached, usually in chat rooms, for sexual contact. The children in the study were aged 10 to 17. Most did not tell their parents about such approaches.[50]

Media content can make children frightened and anxious about the world, but this can also be a chicken-and-egg issue. Some children may turn to TV or other media technologies as a way of escaping difficult family environments, depression or other stresses. The Royal Australasian College of Physicians cites research showing that the more TV a family watches, the less likely family members are to communicate with each other, which of course means the family has fewer opportunities to solve any problems.[51]

...and some more reasons to switch off

• The easiest way to get children active is to switch off the TV. Often just doing that is enough to encourage them to start playing. Even if they turn to other sedentary pursuits, such as reading, they will probably burn off more energy than if they had stayed stuck to the screen;[52]

• The fewer food advertisements your children see, the less pestering you will get; and

• In a randomised controlled trial conducted in the United States, children at one primary school reduced the amount of time they spent in front of TV, video and video games. They were encouraged to have a 10 day turn-off with no screen time at all, and then to limit TV time to 7 hours per week. At the end of 6 months, children at this school had cut their average screen time from nearly 30 hours a week to 20 hours. They also gained half as much weight as children at another school where there had been no such intervention.[53]

How to switch off

The first and most important step is to think about the role of television and other screen-based entertainment in your family. Parents who understand that media exposure can have harmful effects on children are more likely to take steps to regulate their family's viewing. So the fact that you are even reading this chapter is a hugely important first step in the right direction. Here are some other possible steps:

1. Set rules

Work out some household rules about the use of television and other screen-related activities. The earlier you introduce these, the easier it will be for everyone. The following ideas have been helpful for some families, but remember, what works for other households might be different from what works for yours:

• Set some screen-free times. Mealtimes and homework times are crucial periods when the television and other screens should be off unless, of course, the computer is needed for homework purposes. Children often sleep better if they have a screen-free, quiet period just before bedtime. Some families have a no-screen rule during the school week, or before school, or on weekends when the sun is shining. Or declare at least one day a week 'technology free'—no TV, no videos, no DVDs, no computer games and no internet, unless it's really needed for homework. Set realistic limits: some parents will find it easiest to go 'cold turkey' with these rules, but others think it's more effective to introduce them one at a time. Setting a family TV Challenge or making a family pledge to reduce viewing time may help provide some motivation and goals.

The main point is to create an environment where the television is not automatically switched on, or left on continuously. Establish the habit in your children of asking for permission to switch on the TV or computer. Screen time should be a privilege, not a right.

Discuss the benefits of having this sort of household policy. Talk about how it might help different people in the household in different ways. There might be more time for family activities, for conversation, for games. Children might find they feel fresher in the mornings or have more energy for school or for playing. Parents might feel less stressed or cranky if everyone has more time to help with household chores. Try to involve everyone in discussing and developing your household's approach to screen time. Encourage older children to be aware of the issues for younger children, and to take some responsibility for them. Work out strategies together for resolving arguments about screen time.

• Be especially tough on commercial television. Young Media Australia advises not letting preschoolers watch any commercial television at all. Before age 7 or 8, children cannot understand the intention of advertising, which means they are particularly vulnerable to it. They don't know that what looks good to eat might not be good for them. When they get older, teach them to hit the 'mute' button during ad breaks. Advertising often relies on making people feel inferior if they do not have a certain product, and this can make young children feel insecure and anxious, says Barbara Biggins, of Young Media Australia. She recommends that parents start talking to their children about what advertisers are trying to do when the children are 6 or 7. Instead of watching commercial TV, borrow or rent videos and DVDs.

• Plan your week's viewing. Look at the television program and plan what to watch. Make it a conscious decision to turn on the television for selected shows and then to turn it off afterwards. Some researchers have called this 'intelligent viewing' rather than 'vegetative viewing'.[54] Or tape the programs you want to see so you can watch them together as a family. Decide, together, before anything gets switched on how long the child can have on the computer or in front of the television. Try to restrict viewing to short blocks of time. The longer children are transfixed, the more difficult it is to drag them away.

• Don't allow snacking or eating in front of the TV. If children want a snack, get them into the habit of turning off the television and having it in another room.

2. Walk the walk

Many parents complain about how much time their children spend in front of screens, even though they spend long hours in front of the box themselves. Be conscious of your own screen habits. Don't expect the children to do anything you are not prepared to do yourself.

3. Talk the talk

Know what your children are watching on TV or doing on the computer. Talk about the programs or games and the goals of advertisers, and help your children develop skills in critical thinking. Explain the different types of programs—news stories, dramas, documentaries, for example—and what this means in terms of how viewers should think about them. The Royal Australasian College of Physicians recommends that you discuss with your children the techniques being used by advertisers. You could also try turning off the sound during ads.

Don't just listen to what your children say about a program; look at their body language and be aware of the impact of different programs on their mood. Barbara Biggins says that parents can only be effective media educators if the television and other media are kept in a public space where parents can stay in touch with their children's viewing and activities. 'Parents need to choose their children's media experience as carefully as they choose their education and food,' says Biggins.

4. Encourage awareness

Encourage children to monitor how much time they spend watching TV or playing on the computer. Dr Kylie Ball, an academic at Deakin University in Victoria who has used this approach in research, thinks it can be useful for children from about the age of 10. Some families find it helpful to keep a diary of screen time in a prominent position, such as on the fridge. Often children and parents are surprised by how much time they spend in front of the screen—this on its own can help lead to a change in habits.

5. Rewarding behaviour

Don't use TV as a reward. Find healthier alternatives, such as spending some time together, visiting the park, playing a new game or reading a book.

6. Be consistent

Don't give into the grizzles (whenever humanly possible!). Enforce the rules that the family has agreed on and don't make exceptions. When you say no, stick to it. Many children will be happy to play or do something else once they've had their whinge about the TV or computer being switched off. Weather the storm and enjoy the calm that follows.

7. Do your sums

How many TVs or computers or video games does your household really need? The more you have, the more they will be used. Think about reducing or limiting the number of screens in your home.

8. Play on

Television can become a habit. If your household is used to having the TV on all the time, develop a substitute habit—put on the radio or CDs instead. Encourage the kids to dance along.

Try to create a family habit of quiet activities that do not involve TV, such as reading, drawing or writing. Improve everyone's skills in listening to stories, whether it's through reading to each other or listening to a tape or CD.

Support your children if they show an interest in hobbies. Don't worry if they complain about being bored. According to television critic Aric Sigman, boredom is one of the greatest gifts parents can give children—it does good things for their imagination, resourcefulness and intellectual and creative development. Children need time to read, write, explore, build, create, and fantasise, he says.

Don't feel that you have to always organise their games or play. Encourage children to be independent in their play from an early age. Take an interest in what they are doing and set aside time to play with them, but let them lead the way. 'I see young parents today wearing themselves out trying to entertain their children and keep them from being bored,' says Ellyn Satter. 'Don't do that. Let your child be bored. If he gets bored enough, he will think up something creative and wonderful to do.'[55]

9. Active alternatives

When appealing alternatives are on offer, children are often happy to switch off the TV. They may even do it without being asked.

'This generation of children will choose physical activity if it's packaged in a way that is more attractive than the sedentary alternative,' says Dr Jim Dollman, a researcher at the University of South Australia who was involved in a study which showed exactly that. When children aged 6 to 13 in an after school care service in Adelaide were offered a chance to participate in a range of non-competitive, inclusive games, many left the TV room to go and play. 'These kids do not innately resist physical activity,' Dr Dollman says. 'It's not a question of laziness. We need to get that out of the rhetoric. It's about them having a wider menu of choice for their leisure activity. Physical activity has to market itself in a way that competes for their leisure time. It's all a question of access and enjoyment.'

10. Out of sight

You know what they say about out of sight, out of mind? Keep the TV in a cupboard so that it is not constantly on view. Only allow it out during agreed viewing hours. Or hide it under an attractive cloth. Same with the computer and associated games.

Or put it out of sight—permanently. Families who have gone cold turkey often say they now have so much more time for talking, reading and doing things together.

11. Whatever works

Public health researcher Julie Leask is fed up with being warned about the perils of TV. Sometimes it's the only thing that gets her through those crazy times of the day when she is trying to juggle chores with the demands of two young children. She flicks it on to occupy them when she needs a few minutes to herself in the morning to have a shower or when she is trying to make dinner. 'It mesmerises them,' she says. 'It works incredibly well to take the pressure off me so I can get a few things done. I feel terribly guilty about it but I am not sure what else I can do when I don't have friends, family or husband around at the time when I need the space.'

Julie's solution is to restrict her children's screen time to those critical times of the day when it's a sanity saviour. Other households work it differently—it depends on their needs.

The point is to figure out what works for you. And throw away the guilt.

The TV-free diet

Soon after we begin chatting, Dr Annette Katelaris excuses herself briefly to deal with the background noise. 'Turn the volume down,' she instructs her kids, before returning to the telephone.

If you didn't know better, you might assume Annette wants the TV volume to be lowered. In fact, she is just asking her children to speak more quietly. Her household must be one of the few in Sydney, if not Australia, that doesn't have a TV.

Annette and her husband Dr John Downie are both doctors, but health concerns are not their main reason for choosing to be TV-free. They are so busy with work and family demands that they want to make the most of the family time they have. 'To me, time spent goggle-eyed in front of the TV is time not doing anything else,' says Annette.

She has noticed many benefits to their TV policy. Their three children—two teenage girls and an 8-year-old boy—are keen readers and have more time for active leisure pursuits, including music lessons. They are not as influenced by commercial trends and pressures as some of their peers, and their teachers report that they tend to think 'out of the box'—literally. They tend to be lateral and critical thinkers who have not been brainwashed by the worldview and values promoted on many TV shows.

Annette says the lack of a TV also helps family members engage with each other rather than just veging out in front of the screen. On holidays, if there's a TV, the family dynamics change noticeably. 'When they've been sitting in front of the telly, they can get really irritable and cranky', she says.

It isn't always easy to take a different road from the majority. Annette knows her children sometimes feel under pressure from friends, and left out of schoolyard conversations. They have sometimes longed for a TV.

As well, Annette often receives well-meaning offers of a TV from relatives and friends who cannot imagine why anyone would choose to be without one. She has no problem declining such offers, and says other families shouldn't be scared to try the TV-free life. 'They should relish the time they can spend doing other things,' she says. 'For our family it's been a very positive choice.'

Reality check: some questions to ask yourself[56]

- Do your children have a TV/computer with internet access in their bedrooms? If so, how do you monitor how they use this?
- Do you know what they are watching/using? Who decides what your child watches? Do you watch programs with them?
- Do you make rules and stick to them?
- How many hours does your child spend with the TV, video games or the internet? On weekdays? On the weekend?
- How much time are they spending being physically active?
- Have you talked about internet safety with them?

An insider's view

Gillian Hehir has a better idea than most parents of the techniques used in advertising and marketing to young people. Many years ago, and much to her regret now, she helped a tobacco company market cigarettes to teenage girls.

Now a marketing lecturer at the University of Ballarat in Victoria, Gillian has tried to bring up her son, 12-year-old Stuart, to be aware of advertisers' ploys.

She tells him about why they use celebrities to sell their products (because it works) and how breakfast cereals are often associated with sports stars and fitness despite sometimes being of dubious nutritional value. Gillian also encourages Stuart to study food labels while they are shopping, and to be aware of how a well-balanced diet well help him enjoy his sport even more.

Even so, she has seen him fall under the sway of marketers. 'I certainly talk to him about TV advertising, but even with that I find that he is influenced by what he sees on TV,' she says. 'When something new comes out, he wants to try it. I have the most problems with breakfast cereals.'

Gillian says her task has become even more difficult thanks to cross-promotion on the internet. Stuart often wants to buy products so he can link into online competitions and games.

She is a realist, so she can't imagine that companies will stop targeting children unless they are forced to do so. In a world where it is virtually impossible to shield children from advertising, Gillian believes the best option is to educate children to be critical consumers. 'There needs to be a degree of parental responsibility,' she says, 'not just in what children watch on TV, but also in how parents talk to them about it.'

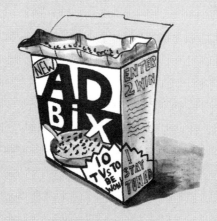

Breakfast serial

Listen to the experts

Teresa Orange and Louise O'Flynn are experts at using the media to influence behaviour. Teresa, a psychologist, has worked on campaigns targeting children for one of the world's largest advertising companies, and Louisa once promoted the United Kingdom's biggest consumer brand, the National Lottery. But these British women began to look at the media with new eyes when they became mothers and started worrying about how much time their children were spending in front of screens. The more they investigated the issue, the more concerned they became.

The result is a book, *The media diet for kids: a parent's survival guide to TV & computer games*, which gives parents some strategies for reducing their children's dependence on screen-based entertainment. The authors interviewed a stack of experts, parents and children as part of their research. Some of the most interesting tips came from children themselves.

Many children felt that too much screen time was a bad thing and looked to their parents to provide some guidance. 'If you don't get told to come off, it's hard to know when to come off,' said one 11-year-old boy.

Most children thought their parents were far too weak. 'They say no and don't mean it' was a frequent comment. When they became parents, these children said, they would be stricter than their parents had been. They said they would be upset, guilty, annoyed and cross if their own children ended up being media bingers.

Many children had become skilled at negating the parental switch-off. 'I just keep on going, "Please can I go on the computer" every five minutes, until she gives up,' said a 9-year-old boy.

Flex your muscles

Parents often underestimate their power. Anyone who has ever worked in a politician's office, the bureaucracy or the corporate sector can vouch for the impact of a well-timed and carefully worded letter, phone call or email.

For parents with the time and energy to get involved in advocacy around media issues, there are many opportunities. Here are a few which might be of interest:

1. Coalition on Food Advertising to Children

A number of leading health, medical and consumer groups formed the Coalition in 2002 to press policy makers and governments to ban food advertising to children. The Coalition's chair, Kaye Mehta, a lecturer in the Department of Nutrition and Dietetics at Flinders University in Adelaide, says Sweden bans all advertising, including advertising for food, to children under 12, and Quebec bans food advertising to children. The Coalition lobbies governments and trains parents to become advocates. 'You don't bring about change just through health experts lobbying,' says Mehta.

For more information, go to http://www.chdf.org.au.

Popping some myths

Dietitian Paul Jones discovered that the now-infamous Coco Pops ad, featuring ABC TV's *Playschool* presenter Monica Trapaga, was effective even before he'd had a chance to see it. This soon became apparent when he arrived at a primary school in the southeast Queensland town of Warwick, to give a talk on nutrition to a Year 6 class.

Paul had great difficulty convincing the children that Coco Pops are not the healthiest choice for breakfast. They told him about all the minerals and vitamins in the cereal, as described by Trapaga.

The children weren't as familiar with the cereal's other vital statistics, the ones that show it is high in sugar and low in fibre.

For Paul, the experience was a great reminder of the power of advertising, particularly on children. One more Australian study found that 54 per cent of Year 3 students believed that Ronald McDonald knew what was 'good for kids to eat'.[57]

Paul now belongs to The Parents Jury, an advocacy group founded in 2004 by Diabetes Australia (Victoria), The Cancer Council Australia and the Australasian Society for the Study of Obesity. The Coco Pops ad subsequently won the Smoke and Mirrors category in The Parents Jury's inaugural Children's TV Food Advertising Awards. The Parents Jury also wrote to Trapaga's agent and to Kellogg complaining about the ad.

The Parents Jury has also been lobbying the Australian Competition and Consumer Commission to investigate some of the health claims made in advertising of breakfast cereals and snack bars. Craig Sinclair, a Parents Jury founder, and director of the cancer education unit at Cancer Council Victoria, says the group is also lobbying supermarkets to provide confectionery-free aisles at checkouts.

Sinclair says parents can be a powerful force in bringing about change, whether in schools, school canteens or supermarkets. 'Parents have the most important role to play in changing the environment,' he says. 'We have seen that in the sun protection programs in schools, which have been largely driven by parents demanding action at a local level.'

For more information, go to http://www.parentsjury.org.au.

2. Young Media Australia

Young Media Australia is a community-based organisation which provides information and advocacy about the impact of media on children.

See http://www.youngmedia.org.au.

3. TV-Turnoff Network

Millions of people all over the world have participated in TV-Turnoff Week since it began in the United States in 1995. It encourages children and adults to watch much less television in order to promote healthier lives and communities.

For more information, go to http://www.tvturnoff.org.

4. White Dot

White Dot is a British-based organisation that supports TV-Turnoff Week and also runs a number of campaigns to discourage TV use. One of its campaigns involved promoting Zocolos, the Mexican word for town square, by encouraging residents in neighbourhoods to sit outside their houses for a night instead of watching TV.

For more information, go to http://www.whitedot.org.

7. The pleasure principle, food and other psychological issues

Let's start with a sweeping generalisation: the world contains just two types of people. The first is those who choose their food according to the nutrients it contains and how healthy it is (or is not). This is a fairly small group, including mainly nutritionists and dietitians, as well as that minority of the population known as health food fanatics.

The second group is the rest of the world. We choose what we eat because it tastes good, or because of habit, or convenience, or cost, or whatever. We might think about how healthy it is, but if we are honest with ourselves, this is not usually the most important criterion. Often, we choose what we eat because of how it makes us feel or because of how we are feeling, even if we don't make this connection consciously. We might feel happy when eating a particular cake because of the delicious flavour or because it reminds us of a cake that Mum used to make when we were kids. Or we might feel guilty when eating the cake because we have fallen into the trap of thinking some foods are bad, and that we are bad when we eat them. We might then feel so bad that we help ourselves to another few slices to try to make ourselves feel better.

If you stop and think about it, few aspects of our lives arouse more complex and deep emotions than food and its rituals. A thousand tortured soap operas could be written about our relationship with food and eating. People cook for each other to show their love and affection. They may also be trying to exert control over themselves or others. The ritual of eating together can forge deep connections. Or divisions. The whole gamut of emotions can be expressed and aroused when people prepare food or sit at the table—dislike, irritation, ambivalence, boredom, exhaustion, jealousy, rivalry and insecurity, to name a few of the more negative ones.

But for most people most of the time, food is associated with a far more positive experience: pleasure. A hedonistic streak runs deep in most of us, and we are seeking something far more gratifying than just fuel when we pick up a fork. In wealthy countries like Australia, where food is so abundant, eating has become something we do for pleasure rather than survival.

Unless you acknowledge and exploit the pleasure principle, you are unlikely to reach first base when trying to influence your family's food choices. It's all very well to tell your children—or even your partner—about the health benefits of fruit and vegetables. It is important that they understand these things. But they are unlikely to change their food preferences and eating habits purely on the basis of a food's health benefits. A far more effective strategy is to try to make sure that eating healthy food is associated with pleasure and good times. One study found that children and adolescents who have a healthy diet generally do so because they like the food they are eating.[1] The researchers suggested that promoting foods' taste and flavour, rather than their health benefits, will be most effective at encouraging people to eat them. The best way to convince children that healthy foods taste good is to really enjoy eating them yourself.

The last thing you want is for your children to associate healthy food with self-deprivation, punishment or feeling miserable.

Applying the pleasure principle

The Harry Potter phenomenon shows that the best way to engage children in reading is to enchant them. The same goes when it comes to developing children's interest in food, says well-known chef Stephanie Alexander. In recent years, Alexander has devoted much of her time and energy to bewitching young children with the creativity, thrill and discovery that comes with growing and cooking fresh produce.

In 2001, Alexander helped set up a kitchen garden at Collingwood College, a relatively disadvantaged school in inner-city Melbourne. As part of their lessons, students from Years 3 to 6 learn to tend and harvest the garden, as well as prepare meals. Raspberry canes, an almond tree, fruit trees, vegetables, flowers and herbs were planted, and a chicken run was built. Within a few years, the produce was so bountiful that the children were learning to make preserves and to bottle tomato sauce and pesto.

Alexander rarely talks to students about whether foods contain fibre or vitamins or other nutrients. 'They're taboo words,' she says, 'because I believe they are the way to turn children off.' Instead, she is more likely to ask the children to describe a flavour or a texture. She encourages their curiosity and helps them develop their new skills, such as rolling pastry or shelling peas.

Alexander became involved in the project because of her concern that so many young people lack basic cooking skills and exposure to fresh food. She also knew how much she had been influenced by her own childhood, when she and her siblings were actively involved in food production and preparation: working in the garden and milking the cows.

'All of us still retain a more than average interest in what we eat,' says Alexander. 'What happened when we were young has stayed with us all forever. The earlier children learn about food through example and positive experiences, the better their food choices will be through life.'

The Collingwood children are learning much more than how to grow and prepare food. They are also getting plenty of exercise—turning the compost, pushing the wheelbarrow, spreading the mulch and digging— and learning about the environment. They are also developing new social skills, including how to behave at the table. It is clear, says Alexander, that many are used to eating in front of the television.

The garden has shone a media spotlight on the school, which has been good for the children's self-esteem. 'Their sense of importance has grown astronomically,' says Alexander. 'They realise they're involved in something very special.'

In 2004, the Stephanie Alexander Kitchen Garden Foundation was established—its aim is to encourage and help other schools to establish similar projects.

The Foundation's manifesto states:

'We believe that the best way to encourage children to choose food that is healthy is to engage them in fun, hands-on experiences in growing, harvesting, preparing and sharing such food from the earliest possible age.

We believe that no-one embraces change in their behaviour if they think it will be unpleasant, uncomfortable or too difficult. Cautionary messages that food is 'good-for-you' or 'bad-for-you' do not resonate with young people.

We believe that children are more likely to experiment with foods they have grown or prepared themselves.

We believe that lifelong eating habits are developed early. We believe that children need positive models in their lives to reinforce that eating with others is a joyful activity, and one that they can enjoy as long as they live.

We believe that many young children do not receive such positive experiences at home, and therefore schools should consider including rich and interdisciplinary programmes that will fill this gap, as well as giving practical skills that will enable young people to take more responsibility for their own physical wellbeing.

We believe that the causes of obesity are complex and there is not one single solution, but we also believe that children who are encouraged to take a broad and active interest in food and the table from a very young age are rarely obese.'

Not everyone has access to a kitchen garden. But Stephanie Alexander's philosophy—about making the preparation and consumption of fresh produce an enjoyable experience for everyone involved—is invaluable advice for the rest of us.

Trusting your child

Babies and young children are smarter than adults in at least one important way. They usually know when they've had enough to eat. Their brain–stomach link is strong. After a big feed, they instinctively reduce their next food intake. This has been shown in a number of experiments, and helps explain why toddlers' consumption at mealtimes can be so erratic. They will adjust how much they eat according to how much they've already had that day.[2]

In one experiment, children were given a drink before having free access to snacks. They consistently ate more when the drink was low on energy than when they were given a drink loaded with calories.[3] In another study, young children were allowed to eat as much as they wanted over 6 days, choosing from a menu containing foods they liked. The number of calories they ate at each meal varied widely, but their total daily energy intake was relatively constant.[4] The researchers concluded that children, despite having little knowledge of nutrition, are able to keep their energy intake relatively stable when they have control over what they eat. Another study found that when babies' milk is diluted, they rapidly adjust how much they drink to maintain their energy intake.[5] Indeed, some researchers believe one of the reasons that breastfeeding seems to protect against later obesity is that breastfed babies learn to self-regulate their intake from an early age. When a baby is bottle-fed, they have less control over their milk intake.[6] This may also help explain why babies fed on formula grow more quickly than breastfed babies. (See Chapter 9 for more about breastfeeding.)

But in many older children, and perhaps most adults, the stomach–brain link has been corrupted. One study suggests that the connection starts eroding at an early age, as children start to take more notice of environmental cues than of what their body is telling them. Researchers found that 2 and 3-year-olds ate roughly the same amount whether or not they were given a regular size or a large portion. But children aged 4 to 6 ate 60 per cent more when their portion size was doubled.[7] We learn, as we get older, to start eating whether or not we are hungry, and to keep on eating even if we are no longer hungry. Perhaps that explains why so many parents don't trust their children to eat only as much as they need: the adults are so out of touch with their own internal cues and their stomach–brain link that they cannot imagine their children are any different.

Plus they have the weight of history on their shoulders. They come from a long line of parents who have struggled to raise children when food was scarce and who have encouraged children to clean their plates. They grew up being told, 'Be a good boy and eat up', so they pass this advice on to the next generation. Many parents and other family members equate expressing love with heaping a child's plate.

It is not surprising that many children lose the ability to know when they've had enough. Cultures and societies may vary in their traditions and rituals, but many share a deep-seated belief that children should be encouraged to eat up. According to University of Queensland parenting expert Professor Matt Sanders, many people define how well they are doing as a parent by whether their children are eating well. For many parents in many different cultures, this equates with children eating a lot.

It can be extremely hard for parents to resist these cultural and societal pressures, whether the pressures are stated or unstated. But being aware of them and their impact can make it easier for parents to help their children keep their stomach–brain connection. One way to do this is through the so-called division of responsibility, a now widely adopted concept that was developed by American paediatric dietitian and therapist Ellyn Satter (see breakout).

It holds that parents are responsible for the 'what, when and where' of feeding, and children are responsible for the 'how much and whether' of eating. In other words, parents are responsible for what food they serve their children and when and where they serve it, but children are responsible for how much of that food they eat—and whether they eat any of it at all.

This is not a cop-out for parents. It doesn't mean they should abrogate all responsibility for their children's eating or let them have as much junk food as they want. Parents have a crucial role in this process: ensuring that their children have a selection of tasty, healthy food served at the table at regular times. But they must also recognise that children will learn to eat a variety of foods and develop their self-regulation skills only when they are allowed to make their own choices about what they eat from their plate and how much they eat. It is about parents learning to trust their children, and children learning to trust their own skills.

Not surprisingly, parents who strongly encourage their children to eat up have heavier children.[8] Many studies have also shown that children who are poor at regulating their energy intake are also more likely to gain weight.[9] They are also more likely to have parents who are overly controlling about food. This control can take many forms. It might mean restricting 'forbidden' foods or encouraging consumption of 'healthy' foods. Or it might mean forcing, cajoling or even tricking children to keep eating even when they have clearly lost interest.[10] Whether children resist or comply with parental pressures, they are likely to end up eating more or less than they really want and losing touch with their body's internal cues.

Parents might be overly controlling about what their children eat because they are used to controlling and worrying about their own weight and diet, or because they do not believe children have the ability to self-regulate, or because they are worried about their children's weight. But this can become another one of those self-perpetuating vicious circles: these sort of concerns lead to controlling feeding practices, which leads to children developing unhealthy eating patterns and losing their stomach–brain connection, which leads to weight gain, which leads to parental concerns.[11]

Parents who respect this division of responsibility at mealtimes will be doing far more than helping their child develop healthy eating patterns. For a start, mealtimes will be more pleasant and involve less tension and conflict, and this may have other benefits for the parent–child relationship. Ellyn Satter's long experience in working with families has taught her that feeding is a metaphor for the parent–child relationship more broadly. Parents who adopt this approach will probably treat their children the same sort of way in other areas of their lives. As well, children learn about themselves and the world from the way they are fed, says Satter. When eating becomes associated with coercion, arguments and conflict, it sends a powerful message about what to expect from the world and how to interact with others.

The power of words

Never underestimate children. They hear the meaning behind what you are saying, even when you don't know what it is. Studies have shown that praising or rewarding children for polishing off their plate interferes with their ability to regulate their intake. In fact, many of the approaches parents and other carers use to try to get children to eat weaken children's stomach–brain connection:

• Experiments have shown that children learn to dislike foods when they are offered rewards for eating those foods. Telling children to 'eat your vegetables and you can watch TV' encourages them to dislike vegetables.

• Telling children to 'eat your vegetables and you can have a treat' is a double whammy; it teaches children that vegetables are no fun, and it reinforces the attraction of so-called treats.

• One experiment found that children who were rewarded for trying a new juice with a trip to the playground were less likely to sample that juice the next time they were offered it than children who had simply been allowed to experiment with it on their own.[12]

• Praising children for being 'good eaters' will encourage them to ignore the internal cues that tell them they have had enough to eat.

• Telling children who have left food on their plate to 'think of all the starving children in the world' will not only help them associate food with guilt, but will also encourage them to keep eating whether or not they are hungry.

• Telling children to eat certain foods because they are 'good for you' is likely to be ineffective and perhaps even counterproductive.[13] Like adults, children are more likely to eat healthy foods if they enjoy them. Who wants to feel as if they are taking medicine when they sit down to a meal?

• Saying, 'Johnny doesn't like spinach' in front of Johnny is a surefire way to ensure that Johnny doesn't develop a taste for spinach. If you say nothing about his refusal to eat spinach in the past, he may decide to try it next time it is offered.

Breaking free of the control factor

When Ellyn Satter started writing a book about feeding children, based on her personal and professional experiences as a parent and paediatric dietitian in the United States, she realised that she was angry. She was angry at all the people who had given her bad advice over the years, angry at herself for having followed that advice with her own children, and angry at all the bad advice that was still in circulation.

As she researched the first edition of her book, *Child of Mine. Feeding with love and good sense* (1983), Satter came to see that one theme has recurred throughout the history of child feeding: the perceived need for authorities and parents to exert control over children's feeding and, in so doing, to ignore children's own needs, behaviours and capabilities.

During the 1930s, for instance, parents were given rigid guidelines about feeding infants with formula every 4 hours. Failing to follow this regimen would, they were warned, have dire physical and emotional consequences. More recently, the control tactics have continued under a different guise. Satter cites parents being admonished to get small babies to eat more and grow faster, while big babies were starved to slow their growth. Much 'well-meaning abuse' was continuing in the name of feeding, Satter concluded.

Satter, who has retrained as a mental health therapist and published an updated edition of her book in 2000, is responsible for developing the 'principle of division of responsibility' which gives children back appropriate control over their food. She says it fits with the principles of the authoritative style of parenting, which is associated with parents setting limits and enforcing rules while also listening to children's requests and supporting them in surveying and

174

mastering their world. This parenting style is associated with children being self-reliant, self-controlled, inquisitive and content.

Authoritarian parents, on the other hand, are more likely to insist that their children stay at the table until their plate is cleared. This style of parenting, expecting immediate and unquestioning compliance with parental directives, is associated with obedient but unhappy children, who are more likely to be anxious, withdrawn or distrustful.

At the other extreme are permissive parents, who indulge the child's demands and do not set expectations or limits on the child's behaviour at the table or anywhere else. This parenting style is associated with aggressive children who lack self-control and are often disobedient or disrespectful.

Satter is concerned that the latest control tactics being touted by policy makers and health professionals involve instructions for parents to restrict their children's fat intake and weight. Such negative messages lead to struggles between parents and children, and feeding difficulties.

Healthy eating, says Satter, is not about restricting, controlling and avoiding. Rather, it is about enjoying food and learning to trust your children's ability to regulate how much they eat.

Harnessing hunger

Hunger has been an unpleasant and dangerous enemy throughout human history. When our ancestors went hungry, they felt weak and ill, and were vulnerable to illness and attack. Not surprisingly, humans came to fear hunger, and to do whatever it took to keep it at bay.

The recent dramatic changes in our environment mean that for many of the world's people, hunger is no longer the enemy. Instead, it is our unfamiliarity with hunger that causes problems. Not surprisingly, studies show that when children learn to eat when they are not hungry, they are more likely to put on excess weight.[14] Other studies have shown that obese children are less in touch with their internal satiety cues—they are more likely than other children to eat at a constant, quick pace, not slowing down as they reach the end of their meal.[15]

We have to become reacquainted with our former foe to ensure that children know what it feels like to be hungry, as well as what it feels like to satisfy that hunger. This doesn't mean starving or depriving children and making them miserable. That is likely to be counterproductive. Instead, try just asking them simple questions, to help them focus on whether they feel hungry or full.

In one study, US researchers found that with this approach, preschoolers' ability to regulate their energy intake was improved in just 6 weeks. Three and 4-year-old children were introduced to concepts of hunger and fullness (satiety) via a video, adult role playing and interactive play with dolls. The children were also encouraged to take note of how hungry or full they felt during and after their regular snack periods. Most children's ability to self-regulate improved: they became less likely to eat when they were not hungry or to refuse food when they were hungry. Finicky eaters who had previously over-responded to fullness cues benefited, as did heavier children who were used to overeating.[16]

Comforting kids

Had a bad day at the office? An argument with your partner? A fight with a friend? In such situations, many people do one of two things: they reach for a soothing tipple or a comforting nibble.

Most people learn very early in life that when they are upset, something nice to eat or drink will make them feel better. It's a message that parents, carers and advertisers are quick to reinforce. Just drink up/eat up and your blues will be banished.

Marge Overs was lucky that she learnt another positive association at an early age. Growing up in a country town, where she had to walk 3 kilometres just to get to the oval where she played sport every weekend, Marge came to associate feeling good with being active. She learnt that if she was having a tough day, a long walk would help boost her mood and give her space to think through her problems.

It is a lesson that is also helping her two children negotiate growing up in Sydney. When her 12-year-old daughter Clare is upset, Marge gives her time to settle down and then suggests they have a walk and talk; 9-year-old Patrick also enjoys his special walking time with Mum and insists on walking to school so they can talk.

Marge says she didn't deliberately set out to encourage her kids to walk when they were upset—it just evolved from them watching what she did. 'If I don't exercise, I'm more prone to getting down, so I use it as a physical and a mental boost', says Marge. 'It's my quiet time, my thinking time. When I'm cranky, I go out for a walk and try to sort it out in my head.'

Marge wouldn't want you to get the wrong idea—Clare and Patrick also enjoy their share of treats. Only saints can get by without occasionally using food as a comfort or reward for their children, she says.

The point is to be aware of the comfort habit and the impact it will have. Sometimes, this might be just the opposite of what you would like: if you give lollies to a child throwing a tantrum in the supermarket and demanding sweets, you are teaching the child that bad behaviour yields delicious rewards.

It is probably impossible, especially in this day and age, to avoid using food for comfort, at least sometimes. Even dietitians admit to doing this sometimes with their own children. But if children are given healthy foods for comfort from an early age, they may be more likely to reach for these foods as they get older.

You can also help your children associate other behaviours with being comforted—like going for a walk, doing a drawing, picking up a book, or having quiet time doing something together. Starting such habits early may bring lifelong benefits.

In years to come, when your children have had a rotten day at the office, they may be more likely to make themselves feel better by picking up a tennis racket than a six-pack.

Treats and other traps

Mention treats to children these days, and they will most likely think of chips, lollies or other unhealthy snacks rather than a trip to the zoo or a game in the park. The use of food as a treat has become so widespread that it has virtually changed the meaning of the word 'treat'.

Indeed, treats have become so common they are hardly treats any more. Instead of being an occasional indulgence for special occasions, they have become everyday foods. Many children expect to open their lunchbox and find biscuits, muesli bars or a packet of potato crisps. Many children have more than one such treat at school each day.[17] They also know that similar snacks will be available after school.[18]

As nutritionist Dr Rosemary Stanton says, abnormal eating patterns have become the norm. 'I regard it as normal to have all kinds of junk food at a party', says Stanton, 'but it is abnormal to have party food every day after school.'

The normalisation of treats is bad news for children, because such foods, by their very nature, tend to be high in fat, sugar and/or salt. The rise of treats has had two harmful consequences for children: it is one of the main reasons their energy intake has increased and is an important contributor to expanding waistlines, and it means that children are less likely to eat the nutritious foods they need for healthy growth and development.

Children, it could be said, are at risk of being 'treated' to poor health.

The second uncomfortable theme that emerges from the research is that there is no simple solution to the treat issue, especially when so many aspects of children's environment— their friends' lunchboxes, the advertisements they see on TV, the supermarket aisles and so on—are saturated with treats. These days many children would be unlikely to go through a normal day without being exposed to treats in some setting or other.

At the same time, research shows that many parents believe that restricting or forbidding certain foods will make their child less likely to want that food. They are wrong. The opposite is true. Many studies have shown that children are more likely to want foods that are restricted or forbidden. They are also more likely to eat them even when they are not hungry.[19] Forbidding children to eat junk food may only encourage them to do so.

You could be beginning to feel like throwing in the towel about now. It's starting to sound as if you're damned if you put sweets in the lunchbox and damned if you don't. What to do?

179

The big fat conspiracy

How can you try to reduce children's consumption of unhealthy treats without making the problem worse?

Here are some things to think about:

• Why do you give your children treats? Do you feel you are depriving them if you don't? Is it because all their friends are getting treats and you don't want them to miss out? If so, it might help to try to rethink what treats really mean for you and your children. Too much junk food is not really a treat at all—it may be depriving them of good health. If you want to give yourself or your children a treat, can you do it with something other than food? If you start to change the way you think about treats, it might just rub off on those around you.

• Treats are a valid part of a normal, healthy diet—but only if they truly are treats. Ellyn Satter recommends being matter of fact when talking to kids about treats and why they are fine as occasional or 'sometimes' foods.[20] Taking care to remove the emotion and special attention from treats will help your kids keep them in their proper place—something to enjoy occasionally.

• Dr Clare Collins, a lecturer in nutrition and dietetics at the University of Newcastle, suggests families make an agreement about how many treats they can have each week; she also recommends making gradual changes. She cites one survey showing that primary school children in the Hunter Valley area of New South Wales were having an average of five treats a day. Moving to five treats a week would be a significant improvement. She says some families have put aside the money they save through reducing food treats, and used it on other treats—such as a trip to the pool—and this has worked well for them.

One parent's solution

Professor Stephen Leeder, Director of the Australian Health Policy Institute at the University of Sydney, has some memories from childhood he would rather forget. He was overweight in the days when it was unusual for kids to carry extra kilos.

Teased mercilessly about his weight, Leeder learnt to dread swimming carnivals. Almost 60 years later, the memories remain acute. 'The embarrassment of the whole pudgy package was something awful,' he says. 'I wouldn't wish that on anyone.'

Leeder has battled all his life with weight. He was at his trimmest in the 1960s when he was in Papua New Guinea, working hard physically and eating mainly vegetables. 'Genes, environment, stress— you name it, they all conspire,' he says. 'How nice it would be if my addiction was not "fed" by people always wanting to feed me and food being so readily, bountifully, beautifully, cheaply available.'

Leeder's public health background gives him a broad perspective on society's weight problem. He sees it as the result of a complex interplay of urban design, societal, and food production factors. 'There are no quick fixes or magic bullets,' he says. 'It's a complex problem with multiple players.'

But in his own home, Leeder has found one low-key strategy particularly helpful for encouraging his teenage son James towards healthy snacks. When James or his friends complain about being hungry, Leeder doesn't ask what they want. He just cuts up fruit, makes an attractive platter, and puts it in front of the teenagers without making any comment.

'The fruit goes,' he says.

8. Five practical strategies for eating well

If you're sick and tired of being told what not to eat, you are in good company. The nutrition industry has a long and not particularly endearing history of tut-tutting. Years of negative messages—'You shouldn't eat this', 'You shouldn't eat that'—have left their mark. Many people have tuned out, or become irritated and confused by advice which is conflicting, complex or difficult to incorporate into their lives.

This section aims to give you some practical strategies for improving your family's eating habits. Wherever possible, these are put in positive terms—some things that you can try rather than lists of what not to do. Not every idea will appeal, or suit you. Just have a read and see what might work for you and your family. Remember that the goal is not perfection; it is to find small changes that can be sustainable long term.

1. Wonderful water

There are many reasons to encourage children to drink more water. They often forget to drink up, so remind them. Making water a regular part of the daily routine helps stop dehydration, and dehydration can lead to irritation and headaches. By the time children feel thirsty, they are often already dehydrated.

But perhaps the best reason is that making glasses and cups and bottles of water a normal and expected part of children's everyday life will make them less likely to reach for soft drink or cordial. Many studies have connected increased consumption of sweetened drinks with expanding waistlines. Soft drinks have been called the 'quintessential junk food' because they are high on calories and low on nutrients.[1] It has been estimated that a 600ml bottle of soft drink contains about 17 teaspoons of sugar and 200 calories, which takes about 45 minutes of moderate physical activity to burn up.[2] Australian children are drinking more and more sugar; about a third of all the sugar they consume is in sweetened drinks.[3] There is also some evidence that sugar in drinks or liquids is more likely to lead to weight gain than sugar ingested in solid form.[4] Many children also drink too much fruit juice, which can contain just as much sugar as soft drinks. It is generally advised not to give children fruit juice, or to give them a maximum of one glass per day.

Apart from the calorie issues, sweetened drinks are also bad for children's dental health. And when they fill up on soft drinks or other sweet drinks, they have less room for nutritious foods, which can lead to problems such as calcium deficiency, anaemia and failure to thrive.

It also means children are less likely to have milk. Not drinking enough milk can increase the risk of calcium deficiency and long-term problems such as osteoporosis. Around three glasses of milk a day provides enough calcium for children's bone development. Some research also suggests that soft drink can increase the risk of such problems in later life because of its effect on bones.

Milk is a healthy and tasty alternative for meals or snacks. However, children should not have cow's milk until they turn 1, because a baby's kidneys cannot cope with it. For 1 and 2-year-olds, full-cream milk is suitable. Hi-low milks are recommended for children aged 2 to 5. Low-fat milks are recommended for children over 5 who are eating well and enjoying lots of different foods.

Getting your family into the habit of having a jug of water on the meal table, or helping themselves to a bottle of cold water from the fridge is a relatively simple but important step towards better health. It will probably also help your budget.

Recommended consumption per day is:

• 5 glasses* (1 litre) for 5 to 8-year-olds;
• 7 glasses (1.5 litres) for 9 to 12-year-olds; and
• 8–10 glasses (2 litres) for 13+ years.

  * a glass is 200ml[5]

Children will need more if they are exercising or sweating due to heat.

Some tips include:

• Stop buying soft drink and cordials. It is much easier to promote water if there is no sweet alternative lurking in the fridge or cupboards.
• Cut up fruit and encourage your children to have that rather than fruit juice. Many children drink way too much juice and suffer diarrhoea and tooth decay as a result.

• Make water and milk attractive options. Make sure they are easily accessible in the fridge. Serve water with slices of fruit or ice blocks, or in decorated jugs or bottles. Freeze water bottles for taking to school. Always have fresh water in the car or in your bag on outings.

• Give children their own water bottles, and make sure they are not too big for a small person to handle.

• Lead the way. Quench your own thirst with water. Get the taste for it. Make a habit of it.

2. Vegetables first

The phrase 'fruit and vegetables' rolls off the tongue more easily, but it is 'vegetables and fruit' that we need to talk about, because vegetables need to be given much higher priority than they usually get. Many children do not eat nearly enough fruit or vegetables but they (and their parents) are particularly likely to be deficient in the vegetables stakes. The sweetness of fruit tends to make it more appealing to many palates.

It would be almost impossible to have missed all the positive news about vegetables and fruit in recent years. Study after study shows that people who eat plenty of vegetables and fruit are also less likely to develop a stack of serious diseases and are more likely to enjoy better health. Of course this could at least partly reflect that people who eat plenty of vegetables and fruit are also more likely to enjoy healthier lifestyles in other ways— they are probably more likely to be physically active, for example. But the more that scientists investigate the thousands of compounds that are found in vegetables and fruit, the more health-giving properties they discover. For children's developing bodies and brains, these nutrients are extra important.[5]

But there's another side to vegetables and fruit which isn't so widely appreciated. It involves the energy-density versus nutrient-density concept. Foods that are rich in fat and/or sugar are called energy-dense because they pack a hefty calorie count per gram. They tend to be less bulky than some other foods, meaning it is easy to consume a lot of calories before you feel full. It is particularly easy to overeat when fat and/or sugar are involved, because they taste so good. Humans evolved in times when there was an advantage to preferring energy-dense foods, and the food industry encourages these tendencies because fatty, sweet foods also involve higher profit margins.[6]

Nutrient-dense foods, on the other hand, pack a lot of nutrients into every gram but have fewer calories. They also tend to be bulkier, because of their higher water content. Several studies suggest that water in foods has a greater effect on our feeling of fullness than water consumed in drinks. You can feel full on fewer calories by eating foods with a high moisture content, such as vegetables and fruit.[7]

If your family eats plenty of nutrient-dense foods—such as vegetables, fruit and whole grains—they will not only reap the benefits of health-promoting nutrients. They may also feel more satisfied because of the bulk, and will have less room for foods rich in fat and sugar. This means they may be able to reduce their energy and fat intake without having to work at it—thus reducing the feelings of deprivation and self-denial which so often accompany efforts to cut back and are so counterproductive. This may be one of the reasons why people whose diets are based on nutrient-dense foods are less likely to be overweight.[8] They have discovered that they can eat a greater volume of food while eating fewer calories. Doesn't that sound so much more satisfying than your typical self-denying diet?

Victory with vegetables

'Many people do not like to eat vegetables—and the feeling is mutual.' That memorable line comes from a scientific article explaining that the reason vegetables are so good for us is also the reason that many people prefer sweets to spinach.[9] Plants protect themselves against being eaten by secreting natural pesticides and other toxins, which are usually bitter, acidic or astringent.

In the small doses found in plants, many of these compounds are beneficial for human health. But their flavour does not naturally appeal to human palates because we have evolved to be suspicious of bitterness as a way of protecting ourselves against poisons. Humans are much more sensitive to bitter flavours than to sweet ones—we can detect bitterness at much lower concentrations than we can detect sweetness.

Adults often develop a liking for bitter or acidic flavours—this is especially easy when the bitter flavour is associated with a pleasing effect, as with the jump-start of caffeine in coffee. But babies and young children have an instinctive aversion to such flavours, and need time and opportunity to learn that it is safe to eat them.

Professor David Laing is a neuroscientist at the Sydney Children's Hospital who has spent many years investigating the mysteries of human preferences in taste and smell. His experiments with newborns show that they make distinctive facial expressions in response to different flavours. They make a smile-like expression when a few drops of sucrose solution are put on their tongue, purse their lips in response to sourness, and gag in response to bitter flavours.

Laing's research has also shown that 8-year-old boys need twice as much sugar as adults before they detect sweetness, which indicates that their sensory system is still developing. Sensitivity to flavours varies greatly between individuals, but such findings might help explain why some children seem to have such a sweet tooth—

it could just be that their sensory system is still immature.

Laing's work has also shown that taste preferences develop early in life, and are fairly well established by age 4 or 5. The main implication of this, Laing says, is that a variety of foods should be offered to children from an early age. 'Our advice would be to get as many different fruit and vegetables into your children as early in life as possible', he says.

Most children will reject most new foods when they are offered them. They may need to see a food several times before they will taste it, and they may need to taste it several times before they eat it. They are just following their instinct for self-preservation—they have to learn that a new food is safe to eat. 'Don't give up on the first or second go', says Laing. 'Most children will accept it by the fifth try. Some may take ten times.'

Apart from persistence, patience is the other virtue required. When a child repeatedly rejects food that you have bought or prepared or perhaps even grown, only a saint would not feel a twinge of annoyance and frustration. It can be tempting, especially if the family budget is stretched, to give up and offer your child something you know they will eat, such as a muesli or fruit bar.

If you can resist this urge and avoid making a fuss about a refusal to try the new food, there is a better chance that they might try it next time. Children are quick learners: if they see that rejecting a certain food provokes an emotional reaction or leads to them being given something else that they like, they may continue to reject it.

Ellyn Satter says that generations of parents have been taught that children don't like vegetables, and have themselves created that reality by forcing, enticing and rewarding their children to eat vegetables. Children should be allowed to learn to like vegetables at their own speed and in their own way, she says.

Of course all this is far easier said than done. If it is too hard to stick to your guns today, try again tomorrow. Don't give up. And don't feel you've failed because of a setback or three.

How much should children eat? [10]

The National Health and Medical Research Council recommends that:
- children aged 4 to 7 should eat at least 1 serve of fruit and 2 serves of vegetables or legumes each day;
- children aged 8 to 11 should eat at least 1 serve of fruit and 3 serves of vegetables or legumes each day; and
- youth aged 12 to 18 should eat at least 3 serves of fruit and 4 of vegetables or legumes each day.

One serve of vegetables is: 1 cup of dark green leafy vegetable such as spinach or lettuce; or 1 cup of orange or yellow vegetables such as carrot; or 1 cup of legumes; or 1 potato. One serve of fruit is: 1 medium-sized piece of fruit such as an apple or orange; or 1 cup of diced fruit or canned fruit.

Helpful hints

• Eat more vegetables and fruit yourself (only about 1 in 10 Australian adults meets even the minimum recommendation for both vegetable and fruit consumption).[11] And eat a greater variety. Enjoy them and make them part of your daily routine. Establish habits: try having fruit with your breakfast every day, or a piece of fruit after dinner. Create a family tradition—that everyone tries a new food at the start of every month, for example. Make these a fruit or vegetable sometimes.

• Don't let your own preferences narrow your child's palate—don't assume they will share your likes and dislikes. If you don't like carrots, don't let this stop you serving them to your child. And don't make disparaging comments.

• Offer vegetables and fruit in a casual manner, assuming the child will enjoy them. Don't serve them loaded up with emotion and expectation—this will be counterproductive. Don't pressure, force or bribe your child to eat them.

• Telling children to eat their greens because 'they are good for you' is likely to be unhelpful. Instead, show that you like eating greens yourself.

• Involve your child. Get them to help in selecting what to buy at the shops or what to harvest from the garden, and then involve them in food preparation. If they are too young to use a knife, they can wash the produce.

• Keep offering a variety of vegetables and fruit in small portions. Don't be put off by rejection. Familiarity may lead to acceptance.

• Offer vegetables and fruit as snacks as well as at mealtimes. Deakin University researcher Dr Kylie Ball is used to hearing parents say, 'My child doesn't like fruit or vegetables.' Often she has seen that same child help themselves to fruit and vegetables when they are not given any other options for snacks.

• Offer them in different forms: raw, cooked, canned, dried or frozen. Stewed fruit is delicious for breakfast, dessert and snacks. Many children prefer their vegetables raw. Or dress them up with a splash of olive oil or a squeeze of lemon or a grating of cheese.

• In difficult times, many parents find it helpful to disguise vegetables and fruit—for example, by putting grated zucchini in mince patties or bolognese sauce, or making a vegetable dip or fruit smoothie.

• Present and store vegetables and fruit in a way that makes them attractive and easily accessible. Let your child know there is a special place in the fridge where they can find small bags or containers of diced carrots, apples and other produce. Thread small pieces of fruit and/or vegetables onto a kebab stick.

• Young children are more likely to enjoy vegetables and fruit if fun is involved. Make a colourful face on their plate. Count how many grapes or berries are in the bowl. Tell a story about Peter Pumpkin or Samantha Spinach.

• Experiment. Don't keep buying and cooking the same old things. This habit often ends up meaning reduced vegetable and fruit consumption. And don't just experiment with unfamiliar produce; prepare some of your old favourites in new ways or experiment with different ways of presenting them.

• Many people think vegetables take too long to prepare—but there are plenty of quick, simple dishes which can be whipped up in less time than it takes to order takeaway. You just need to get the right recipes.

• If you buy fresh produce when it is in season, it will be cheaper and taste better.

• The cost of vegetables and fruit is a major barrier for many families. Can you buy direct from the markets? Is there a local co-operative with discount prices? Could you join with other families and buy in bulk?

• If lack of time is stopping you from buying as much fresh produce as you would like, investigate other options: can you get home delivery, or order over the internet, or share the produce shopping with another family?

• Don't give up. If your children are eating some vegetables and fruit, that is better than if they are eating none. If they are eating more than they used to, that is a great step forward. Even better if you are eating more than before yourself.

What children say

Ask a bunch of 11-year-olds what they think about vegetables, and the message comes back loud and clear: they are good for you but they have a terrible image problem.

That was the firm opinion of one Year 6 class from Wilkins Public School at Marrickville in inner-western Sydney. The students, who generously donated an afternoon to share their thoughts with this book's readers, had plenty of nice things to say about fruit. But they felt vegetables were given a pretty raw deal; everything from TV programs to children's books portrayed them as unappealing.

'They just have a bad reputation,' said Eliza. 'Kids would say they hate brussel sprouts and they haven't even tried them. Even kids' books say brussel sprouts are gross. They don't taste gross; they just taste like cabbage. Vegies are advertised as something good for you, and a lot of kids don't care about that.'

Darcy agreed that vegies were poorly promoted. There were far more ads on TV for lollies and cars than vegies, she said. 'Some people think I am weird because I am a big fan of cabbage and artichokes and brussel sprouts,' she added. 'Seriously, I like the yucky vegies.'

Patrick felt that TV shows also contributed to vegies' bad reputation by implying that 'eating fruit and vegetables is punishment'.

When asked how they liked their vegies prepared, the general consensus from the class was that raw beats cooked hands down. 'I don't like the texture and taste of cooked vegies,' said Alice.

Tammy agreed with her classmates that vegies were treated unfairly. 'People don't think they taste nice but they are quite nice,' she said.

The message, for food producers, advertisers, parents and others who care for children, seems clear. Vegetables need a snappy PR agent—someone who can lift their profile and transform them from 'dull but worthy' to 'hip and happening'.

Sounds like a good creative project for some clever 11-year-olds...

The best way to lose weight— without even trying

Many women find they gain weight after having children. They are so busy they don't have much time for regular exercise or for looking after themselves.

But Jenni Adams shed several kilograms in the years following the births of her daughters, Sarah and Sophie, without even trying to lose weight.

The weight loss followed changes that Jenni made to her family's routines after being trained as a volunteer 'peer educator' to spread the word about the importance of good nutrition to other parents. Jenni, who lives in the small town of Penguin on the northwest coast of Tasmania, did the course after falling into some unhealthy habits when working long hours as a manager in the health sector. She often skipped meals and ate poorly.

After having her girls, now aged 6 and 4, she enrolled in the Family FoodPATCH project, which was funded through the Commonwealth Department of Health and Ageing, and run through the Child Health Association and Playgroup Tasmania. About 100 parents across Tasmania were trained as volunteer peer educators until the project ended in 2004.

Apart from sharing her new knowledge with other parents, Jenni made changes at home. 'I realised that a lot of things I thought were

OK, like cordial, white bread and full-fat milk, weren't good things,' she says. 'I had a daughter who would drink only cordial. So I got everyone drinking water and plain milk. I made other more gradual changes, using more whole grain products and having more vegetables and fruit.'

Now when Jenni goes to the supermarket, Sarah and Sophie choose the fruit and vegetables. 'They pick anything that's a baby,' says Jenni. 'We have baby corn, baby bok choy, baby anything. They're really open to trying stuff.' The girls also help with planning the week's menu and preparing meals. 'They have a lot more buy in,' says Jenni, 'so they are more prepared to try things.'

When giving talks to other parents, Jenni gives hints about how to 'hide' vegetables in sauces, muffins and cakes. She empathises when other mothers complain about a partner who refuses to change their eating habits.

'It's the husband factor,' says Jenni. 'It's a big issue. I'm prepared to make the changes in my diet to make a good example to the kids, but he prefers white bread, doesn't like cereals, wouldn't choose to eat fresh fruit, doesn't particularly like vegies, drinks soft drink, and snacks on salamis and cheeses.'

So what does she recommend to parents facing such a dilemma? There are no simple solutions, says Jenni, but her own approach has been to stick to her guns without resorting to food wars. 'I find that the biggest challenge is how to set the example, knowing that I'm only half of the example. All I can do is try and show that the right foods are the delicious foods.'

Jenni doesn't stress when her children have lollies or takeaways, so long as their diet balances out over the week. She has watched other parents' strictness result in children gorging themselves on junk at parties. 'I don't deprive my kids of those sorts of foods but they don't have a lot of them,' she says. 'At a birthday party they are more than likely to choose the strawberries and pineapple than the cakes and lollies.

'We don't talk about good foods and bad foods. We talk about things you have a little bit of and things you have a lot of. I don't talk of food as treats. If they want a treat or a surprise, it might be a book or a sticker or a new pair of undies.'

Jenni makes a point of not discussing her weight in front of the girls. When her weight loss attracts comment, she emphasises that she hasn't been dieting. 'I'm very conscious of saying "I'm just living a healthy life"', she says. 'I'm just more active and eating better.'

3. Hopping into breakfast

Only dull people are brilliant at breakfast, the Irish playwright Oscar Wilde once quipped. His remark captures many people's ambivalence about the morning meal, but does no justice to its significance. Breakfast is important for many reasons, not least that it really does encourage brilliance.

Breakfast is vital for refuelling the body and brain after the night's rest. Children who skip breakfast are more likely to have difficulty concentrating, learning and behaving appropriately in class. Breakfast is an important foundation of a healthy balanced diet; children who miss the morning meal are also likely to miss out on vital nutrients and to suffer constipation. People who skip breakfast are more likely to overcompensate later in the day by eating too many calories. Those who eat breakfast are less likely to gain weight and are also more likely to sustain weight loss.[12]

However, many parents feel too busy or too stretched to make breakfast a priority. Mornings might be difficult enough already. These are the reasons often given for allowing children free rein at breakfast time. As a result, too many children skip breakfast or have muesli bars or other concoctions of fat and sugar. One study of 5000 Australian schoolchildren found that 1 in 5 had nothing more than soft drink, cordial, tea, coffee or water for breakfast. Many children said they would not prepare breakfast themselves but would eat it if it was put in front of them or their parents reminded them to eat it.[13]

You don't have to be brilliant at making breakfast. The easier it is for everyone, the better. Here are some ideas that might help:

• Make breakfast a family habit—this means breakfast for everyone.

• Make time—you can make and drink a banana smoothie in a few minutes.

• Involve your children in selecting and preparing breakfast.

• Offer a variety of choices: cereal, fruit, toast, eggs, leftovers.

• Vary what is on offer—and eat according to what's in season.

• Have something special—maybe a picnic in the garden or the park—on weekends and other special occasions.

4. Shop smart

I have a theory about grocery shopping. As far as I know, it's never been tested by researchers, but it works for me. The theory is that the bigger the supermarket you visit, the more money you will spend and the more rubbish you will buy. That's certainly what happens with me. The more aisles containing junk food and processed food I have to push my trolley up and down, the more of these foods end up in my trolley. There must be some truth to the theory—otherwise why would supermarkets have turned into such super-sized monsters?

Conversely, if I start my weekly shop at the greengrocer, I end up with more vegetables and fruit, and less money and time for other foods. It's a sad sign of the times, however, that not everyone these days has access to a well-stocked and affordable greengrocer or a small supermarket.

Nutritionist Dr Rosemary Stanton has another approach. She sticks to the outside aisles of supermarkets, where the fresh produce tends to be displayed, and doesn't take her trolley down the inside aisles. Stanton has been told that one supermarket chain has 1765 snack foods on its shelves—those are exactly the shelves she advises avoiding.

Wherever you shop, keep in mind that mantra about making healthy choices the easy choices. What you buy determines how easy it is for your family to make healthy food choices—it's so much easier when there are no potato crisps or soft drink in the cupboard. Research shows that children are more likely to eat unhealthy snacks and to have soft drink if they are available at home. They are also more likely to eat fruit and vegetables if they are available at home.[14]

Stanton also advises being sceptical about foods that are promoted on the basis of health claims. Often these products will be more expensive but no better than foods which contain the same ingredients but do not make health claims. Stanton once did a quasi-experiment with a TV reporter in which they each took a trolley around the supermarket. The reporter filled his trolley with foods making a health claim and Stanton filled her trolley with equivalent foods of at least equal health value but that did not make any health claim on the packaging. Her bill at the checkout was significantly less than the reporter's.

In fact, it is advisable to have a healthy dose of scepticism whenever you see or hear claims made about the health benefits of foods, especially if they are processed goods. The food industry has a long history of engaging nutritionists and nutrition organisations in its marketing efforts. It does this by funding research, conferences and public relations and marketing campaigns. As US nutritionist Professor Marion Nestle points out in her book, *Food Politics* (2002), food companies are skilled at co-opting scientific and medical experts to support their marketing objectives, and they routinely place shareholders' needs over public health considerations. 'Food companies will make and market any product that sells, regardless of its nutritional value or its effect on health,' Nestle says.

Rather than relying on claims the food industry makes about its products, get to know the food pyramid endorsed by health authorities around the world. Try to make sure that your trolley includes different groups of food in the proportions of the pyramid.

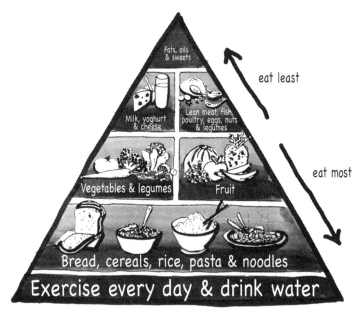

Food pyramid

Five practical strategies for eating well

Here are a few more tips for shopping well:

• Buy fresh produce that is in season. It will be cheaper and taste better, and you will also be doing the environment a favour—think how much energy is involved in transporting a punnet of strawberries halfway round the world.

• Plan ahead. Work out a menu for the week, and stick to your shopping list. Depending on their age, involve your children in planning and shopping. Get them to tell you the prices of different foods so they learn to work out value for money.

• Include a range of healthy snacks for after school on your shopping list. This is a key time of day when many children fill up on foods that are high in fat and sugar. Some research suggests that many children choose what to eat after school themselves, and that parents could play a greater role in ensuring healthy options are available.[15] If plenty of healthy snacks are available, it will be easier for children to choose well.

• Learn to read food labels and encourage the rest of your family to do the same. Be sceptical about health claims on food packaging—they are not always what they seem, and are often designed to confuse and mislead. When foods are described as 'lite/light', this may refer to the taste, texture, fat, salt or sugar content. Light products may not be lower in energy than other products. Reduced fat does not necessarily mean low fat, and these products often have so much sugar added that their calorie count is no less than the normal products. Reduced-salt products may still be high in salt even though they contain less salt than usual. Foods that contain toasted or oven-baked ingredients are likely to be high in fat. Foods that have 'no

199

added sugar' may contain other sources of sugar such as fruit sugars or milk sugars. Advertising such as '90 per cent fat free' sounds less enticing when you realise this means that fat makes up 10 per cent of the product. Sometimes labels give the amount of fat and calories per 100g when a typical serve is much more than 100g. Food Standards Australia has more information about food labels: http://www.foodstandards.gov.au/whatsinfood/foodlabelling.cfm.

• Don't go shopping on an empty stomach. Do not treat children with food when you go shopping. They will quickly learn to expect such treats, which will make shopping even more stressful than it need be. Find another way to treat them after shopping—perhaps a play on the swings or a visit to the library.

• Cost is a major issue for many families. However, there are lots of ideas for cheap healthy shopping and recipes around—see the Further Resources section of the Appendices lists. You can also save money by buying in bulk, buying bread when it's on special and freezing it, and making up large quantities of soup, stews, curries etc. and freezing them. Vegetables and fruit are often going at bargain prices if you go to markets late in the day. Dried beans, peas and lentils are cheap, nutritious and tasty. Staple foods such as rice and pasta are also relatively cheap and filling.

• Fresh fruit and vegetables may seem expensive, but they're not if you compare their cost on a dollar per kilogram basis with popular snacks such as muesli bars. Some popular snacks cost more than $30 per kilogram.

• Make a family policy on takeaways. This might mean setting a limit on how often you have takeaway—perhaps once a week or once a fortnight. It might also mean choosing healthier takeaways. When eating out, avoid the 'meal deals' and 'kids' menus', because these are often loaded with fat.

• If you eat out occasionally, make the most of it and don't worry about nutritional issues. But if eating out is a regular part of your routine, look for the healthy choices on the menu and be conscious of portion sizes.

Make the most of the season

Shopping in spring
Avocadoes, bananas, grapefruit, kiwi fruit, mangoes, oranges, rockmelon, strawberries, watermelon, pawpaw.

Asparagus, beans, beetroot, broccoli, cabbage, carrots, celery, lettuce, mushrooms, onions, peas, potato, pumpkin, silverbeet, spinach, zucchini.

Shopping in summer
Apricots, bananas, cherries, figs, grapes, mangoes, nectarines, oranges, passionfruit, peaches, pineapple, plums, rockmelon, rhubarb, strawberries, watermelon, pawpaw.

Beans, capsicum, celery, corn, cucumber, lettuce, mushrooms, onions, potato, pumpkin, tomato, zucchini.

Shopping in autumn
Apples, avocadoes, bananas, figs, grapes, oranges, passionfruit, pears, rockmelon, watermelon.

Beetroot, broccoli, capsicum, cauliflower, celery, corn, cucumber, eggplant, mushrooms, onions, potato, pumpkin, silverbeet, spinach, tomato, zucchini.

Shopping in winter

Apples, avocadoes, figs, grapefruit, kiwi fruit, lemons, mandarins, oranges, pears.

Beetroot, broccoli, brussel sprouts, cabbage, carrots, cauliflower, celery, corn, eggplant, mushrooms, onions, parsnip, potato, pumpkin, silverbeet, spinach.

Shopping for the environment

Many people feel they are doing their bit for the environment by using cloth shopping bags rather than disposable plastic bags. Buying fresh, unprocessed whole foods with a minimum of packaging is also doing a favour for the environment—as well as your health.

No less an authority than the National Health and Medical Research Council advises that we should consider more than the nutrient content when we go shopping for food. Dietary guidelines endorsed by the National Health and Medical Research Council state that eating in line with sustainable development includes avoiding overconsumption, eating food produced locally and in season, and eating less processed food.[16] Following these suggestions is likely to be good for your health as well as for the environment. As a general rule, the more highly packaged a food is, the more likely it is to be highly processed and energy dense.

Vast resources are used in the production of some highly processed foods, but some unprocessed foods can also take a heavy toll on the environment. For nutritionist Dr Rosemary Stanton, grain-fed meat production is a wasteful, inefficient exercise. It takes many kilograms of grain to produce 1 kilogram of meat, she says.

Five practical strategies for eating well

Liz Sanzaro, a food educator at Box Hill TAFE in Victoria, is deeply concerned at environmentally unfriendly practices in the production of many foods. As a general rule, she advises avoiding foods where the source is not clearly identifiable. 'You should be able to recognise what your food was 24 hours ago,' she says. 'If it wasn't picked off a tree, dug out of the ground or harvested from a bush or tree, or slaughtered or fished, it's a heavily manufactured product. When choosing cereals, can you recognise what sort of grass it was? If you can't recognise what plant it's come from, be highly suspicious of it.'

Sanzaro cites margarine as a prize example of a heavily manufactured food. She prefers to promote the use of butter—but in very small quantities. 'Environmentally I'm aghast at the trend to gobble up 15 kilos of vegetable and nut material (good foods in themselves) to extract 1 kilo of phytosterols so that this material can be incorporated into a plastic spreadable fat and marketed to consumers as an effective way to reduce cholesterol,' she wrote in a letter to the Food Chain newsletter.

The more manufactured a product is, the more complicated it is to work out its health benefits, says Sanzaro, whose motto is, 'Keep it simple.' She is a big fan of the Slow Food Movement, an international collaboration which encourages the consumption of locally grown produce that is in season (for more information, see http://www.slowfood.com).

Sanzaro's other staple advice is to focus on making small changes to the way you shop, cook and eat. When you feel overwhelmed by the prospect of making change, she suggests working on one small area at a time. For example, choose a couple of less processed foods at a time, and learn to prepare them and incorporate them into your regular diet; then take on another few. This helps keep it manageable.

'How do you eat an elephant?' asks Sanzaro. 'One bite at a time.'

Community Foodies

Many of the families who could most benefit from good nutrition advice are least likely to be able to get it. This might be because they are strapped for cash, or because they are busy with other issues—or just because of the stresses of everyday life.

Some people also find it confronting to deal with health professionals. Doctors and nutritionists can sound as if they are speaking a different language from the rest of us. Well-paid professionals can find it hard to understand what it is like to struggle to find enough money to pay the rent.

Community Foodies, an innovative program in South Australia, has been training 'peer educators' as a way of overcoming some of these barriers. The program is based on the principle that it is easier to learn from people of a similar age, background and socio-economic status as yourself.

The peer educators, or 'Community Foodies', are given training in basic nutrition, presentation and group skills. They give talks to schools, play groups, mothers' groups and other community organisations, and also work with community vegetable gardens, school canteens and breakfast clubs. They often become local advocates for improving nutrition choices in their area.

Community Foodies has had many benefits. Apart from helping improve people's skills and knowledge around food, it has helped boost the self-esteem and confidence of those involved and to build closer ties within communities and between community members and health services.

Here are the stories of three Community Foodies:

Better food, better life

Adelaide woman Sandy Tindall, 46, has had a tough life. She grew up in an abusive family situation and didn't have the opportunity to learn about cooking when she was young.

Five practical strategies for eating well

When Sandy had her own children, she didn't have the knowledge or skills to feel confident in the kitchen. She brought them up on a diet largely of takeaways, bread and chips.

When Sandy heard about the Community Foodies program, she was struggling to make ends meet on a pension. After paying her bills, some weeks there was just $10 left over for food.

Through the Community Foodies training program, she learnt how to stretch her food budget and to make cheap healthy meals using lots of vegetables. She then became involved in running groups to pass her new-found knowledge, skills and confidence on to other people. The groups included people recently released from jail, women facing domestic violence, and people struggling with drug and alcohol problems.

'Lots of the mums who come to my groups said their problem was how to get the kids to eat vegies,' says Sandy. 'So we learnt how to disguise vegies. We started making vegie hamburgers, dips and spring rolls.'

In the past few years, Sandy, has helped about 200 women learn how to feed their families better. She has also seen the benefits for her own family, especially her five young grandchildren. 'We have fun in the kitchen,' she says. 'They learn how to peel vegies.'

But one of the program's main benefits for Sandy has been the boost to her self-esteem and self-confidence. More than 30 years after dropping out of primary school, Sandy is now studying law at university. 'Doing Foodies really changed my life,' she says.

Delicious marketing

The Central Market in Adelaide is a famous tourist attraction, selling a dazzling array of produce. For Sharyn Spezzano, it has also become a classroom.

Since becoming a Community Foodie, Sharyn, 56, has taken groups on tours of the markets to introduce them to new fruits, vegetables and flavours, and the concept of shopping in season. She also takes groups on tours of supermarkets, teaching them to read labels and to get better value for their money, and pointing out the aisles to avoid.

The tours also take in the butcher and the fish shop, to give people the confidence to speak with the butcher and fishmonger, and to ask for advice on cooking and preparation. Sharyn also does demonstrations at community centres and other places, of how to prepare attractively presented, cheap and easy meals.

'People are under the misconception that "cheap" and "nutritional" can't be in the same sentence,' says Sharyn. 'I had someone asking me to write her a shopping list because she had only $20 a week to spend on food. You start with the basics: rice and pasta. If you have any sprouting onions or potatoes with eyes, you plant them. People don't think of things like that these days, because they think food is born in the supermarket.'

Sharyn has got tremendous satisfaction from being a Community Foodie. 'It's just wonderful to see people come out of their shells and say, "Hey I didn't think the family would eat vegies but when I gave them that dish, they came back for more". They come in beaming about how their family loved the food.'

Most people get their information about food and nutrition from family and friends, so it is not surprising that Sharyn has noticed a 'trickle-out' effect—family members, friends, friends of friends and neighbours have made changes to their shopping and cooking.

Eat well, feel better

Joanne Paynter, 40, has noticed an improvement in her family's physical and mental health since becoming a Community Foodie. She and her 18-year-old son are overweight and at high risk of type 2 diabetes because of a strong family history of it. But since making changes to their food habits—buying more vegetables and fruit and fewer foods high in salt, sugar and fat—Joanne has lost weight and discovered that she enjoys regular walks.

Joanne is a single mother living on a disability pension at Port Pirie, so she knows how difficult it can be to make the food budget work every week. 'It's not more expensive to eat healthily,' she says. 'It's just knowing how to do it. I go to the fruit and vegie place first, look for the specials, and try to go to the supermarket when they mark down the bread.'

Now she bakes and grills rather than frying, and is more likely to reach for fruit for a snack. Apart from the health benefits, she finds that she now enjoys food more. 'You just feel much better about yourself when you are eating well and exercising,' she says. 'My son is learning from my example.'

5. Eating together

Once it was just accepted that at the end of the day families sat down and broke bread together. These days so many forces have conspired to kill the family meal—television, parents' lack of time and energy, the proliferation of fast food and takeaways, the normalisation of 'eating on the run', longer and longer working hours...the list goes on.

On the other hand, there's also a long list of reasons why it is worth switching off the TV and resurrecting the family meal. Here are a few:

• Families that sit down together for meals tend to have healthier diets. They tend to have more vegetables and fruit and less fatty foods and soft drink. They are also less likely to be overweight.

• Children learn so much at the family dinner table. They learn about food and eating, as well as social skills such as table manners, sharing, and how to have a conversation with people. They learn to listen as well as to speak up.

• Family meals are a great opportunity for establishing healthy habits—such as having a glass of water or milk with the meal.

• They are also an important opportunity for parental role modelling, so be conscious of how you eat and behave as well.

• Conversations around the table help parents and children keep in touch with each other as well as with the day's events.

For many families, though, mealtimes are full of conflict and tension. Not every family can be The Brady Bunch (thank heavens). But everyone will benefit if the family mealtime is as stress-free and as pleasant as possible. Here are a few tips:

• Have structured, regular meals. If mealtimes are predictable, children will be more likely to arrive at the table with an appetite.

• They are also more likely to behave appropriately at the table if they know what is expected of them. Set some family rules for the meal table and apply them clearly and consistently. These might be as simple as saying 'thanks' and 'please' or not making rude comments about food.

• Ignore bad behaviour. Don't reward children for screaming or throwing food by giving them attention.

• Learn from McDonald's. One of the reasons children like going there (and to other similar places) is that the place is associated with pleasant family outings, with having a good time. People are more likely to behave nicely towards each other when they're out in public. See if you can apply the same standards at your home table. If an argument is brewing with your partner or another family member, try to resolve it away from the meal table.

• Encourage children to pay attention to what they are eating. Make sure the TV is off and there are no other distractions. Talk about what you are eating, where or how it was grown, how it tastes and smells, its texture. Cultivate the family's interest in food.

• Encourage children to eat slowly by eating slowly yourself. Eating slowly will help you and your children get back in touch with your internal signals of hunger and fullness. And remember, eating quickly is associated with being overweight.

• Stick to the division of responsibility rule. Parents are responsible for ensuring a variety of tasty, healthy foods are available at mealtimes. It will help if these are attractively presented. Children are responsible for deciding what they eat and how much. Don't make a fuss if they refuse food. No healthy child will starve themselves. Remove uneaten food calmly and without comment. Don't then offer a treat.

• Don't cook special meals for children.

• Family meals are an opportunity to support children as they learn to self-regulate how much they eat. Some experts recommend putting food in serving bowls on the table and letting everyone serve themselves; young children will of course need help with this. Research shows that preschoolers are less likely to overeat when they are allowed to help themselves to food.[17] If you are serving out food, remember that parents often expect children to eat more than they need. Don't dish out large portions. It is better to give small amounts and let them have extra if they want it.

A fussy eater

Julie Williams knew all the theory when she had children. She was a dietitian, so she was familiar with the research supporting the division of responsibility and the importance of remaining calm when children refuse food. But her first child, Reuben, was one of the most fussy eaters she had ever seen in her many years of working with families. He just did not want to try any new foods.

'I had all the theory, but putting it into practice was challenging,' says Julie, the Co-ordinator of Community Nutrition in the Tasmanian Department of Health and Human Services. 'I was really tested, but now I can talk with parents with a lot of empathy.'

She kept reassuring herself with the advice that she was used to telling other parents: no healthy child will starve. As Reuben grew, she learnt to relax and accept that he just did not need as much food as some other children. 'It was just a consistent, persistent effort,' she says.

It helped when her next child came along. Milla was an enthusiastic eater, and her example influenced Reuben, who has slowly become more adventurous.

Many parents, when faced with a fussy eater, find that it helps to have someone the child admires set an example. It might be a sibling, cousin, friend or grandparent.

Finding the pot of gold

Denise Greenaway became interested in nutrition when working as a school counsellor about 15 years ago. When girls came to her for help, whether about difficulties with their relationships, schoolwork or drugs, she noticed that they usually also had issues with food. Whether they were starving themselves or binge-eating, many girls' emotional and physical wellbeing was affected by their unhealthy eating patterns and relationship with food.

Greenaway, a psychologist based at Byron Bay on the north coast of New South Wales, now runs The Rainbow Food—Eating By Colour program, which aims to help young people develop more healthy relationships with food and their bodies. The program encourages children to think of food in colours and to eat as many natural colours as possible every day at every meal. The aim is to make eating a pleasurable, guilt-free experience.

She has become used to hearing gasps of delight when girls emerge from one of her workshops for morning tea. They find a huge table groaning with fruit and vegetables, beautifully arranged in all the colours of the rainbow, and with table decorations made from sculptured produce.

'You make food exciting by presenting it in a way that is visually pleasing,' says Greenaway. 'That's really important to girls. Fresh food, when it is presented well, is psychedelic.' The girls are asked to put something of every colour on their plates and to try at least one food they've never had before. They are told to eat as much as they want. 'The kids love it because they get to choose,' she says.

Greenaway says the rainbow is a fantastic device for engaging children with healthy food, because it is associated with magic and treasure.

The rainbow strategy is helpful for people of all ages. 'It's a wonderful way of reviewing your day, if you just write down how many colours you ate in a day,' she says.

When running workshops for boys, Greenaway takes a different approach to the stories of magic and fairies that she weaves for girls. Her goal with boys is to keep them physically active and engaged while she teaches them to cook porridge, pikelets and other simple meals.

Parents often are disbelieving when they hear what their children have eaten in Greenaway's workshops. 'I call Rainbow Food a taste recovery program,' she adds. 'Adults have this belief that their children won't eat anything healthy.'

Greenaway's experience suggests otherwise; you just have to make healthy food fun and enticing, she says. And a bit of magic helps too.

(For more information, go to http://www.rainbowfood.com.au, or http://www.mirrormirror.com.au.)

The voice of experience

Mary Mallett wants her four children to have more opportunities than she has had. When they grow up, she wants them to be able to run and play with their own children, and to be able to go to the beach or swimming pool without feeling painfully self-conscious.

Mary has been overweight since she was a child, and says it has had a huge impact on her life, affecting even her employment opportunities. She has also missed out on joining in many activities with her children. Weight is such a sensitive subject that Mary struggles to discuss it with even close friends. But recently she has found the courage to talk about her weight publicly, knowing that it lends extra impact to the advice she gives other parents.

Mary, 44, volunteers as a peer educator in Hobart for the Family FoodPATCH program, which aims to help improve families' knowledge and skills around nutrition and food. When she gives talks to parent and community groups, she describes the way her own experience of being overweight made her conscious of the importance of instilling healthy eating habits in young children.

Five practical strategies for eating well

'I know that it's so difficult to lose weight,' she says. 'It's better not to gain it.' She also knows from personal experience that food preferences which begin in childhood can be difficult to shake. 'I grew up in Ireland on a dairy farm,' she says, 'and I still love butter and cream.'

The most useful skill Mary has learnt as a peer educator is how to read food labels. As a result, she now rarely buys snacks that are high in fat and salt. The family has also changed its takeaway policy, preferring to buy noodle boxes instead of conventional fast foods.

She advises other parents how to deal with the soft drink issue. 'Once kids get used to drinking soft drinks and cordials, they will often refuse to drink water. But I know from experience that if you stop buying soft drinks and fruit juice and give them water consistently, eventually they are going to have to drink it.'

Mary also encourages parents to learn how to say no to their children, and to be consistent about it. 'Lots of parents of young children are really reluctant to say no to their children,' she says. She was shocked to discover, when giving a talk at a local private school, that only 1 out of 24 girls in the Year 3 class had a lunchbox that was completely healthy. It was probably no coincidence that this girl was the daughter of a dentist.

'It's just so difficult for parents,' says Mary. 'Modern Australian society makes it almost impossible for them to feed their children a healthy nutritious diet.'

9. Food and development

It starts from almost the moment they are born. *How much does she weigh? How much has he put on?* Parents—particularly mothers—often feel under intense pressure for their baby to conform to growth and weight expectations. This focus, dating back to the days when under-nutrition was much more common, can have unhealthy consequences today, when overconsumption has become the norm.

Julie Leask, a public health researcher in Sydney, is acutely conscious of the downside of such pressure. Her first child, Billy, 3, has inherited his father's thin build. Julie came to dread his regular weigh-ins at the baby health centre because he was always light for his age. 'Right from when they're born, the focus is on them conforming to this growth chart', she says. 'I felt tempted just to get weight on him, to give him chips rather than the fruit and vegetables that he loves, just to conform to this stupid curve on the chart.'

Julie is also conscious of subtle cultural and social pressures that can make parents' guilt even worse. 'It's as if his being thin is a reflection of my ability to nurture and provide for him,' she says, 'even though I know rationally that he's happy and he eats very healthily. There's unlikely to be anything wrong and I'm unlikely to be depriving him.'

Nutritionist Dr Rosemary Stanton is familiar with stories like Julie's, and she questions whether it is healthy to put so much emphasis on weighing well babies. 'It gives people the idea that big is good,' she says. 'The whole idea that the bigger and faster the baby grows the better it is may be from the days when wealthier people were bigger because they got fewer infections and had better living conditions. The mother is always made to feel there is something wrong with her if her baby isn't gaining weight at the rate someone else suggests. When I was first breastfeeding, in the late 1960s, I was told, "You will never ever be able to feed him with those small breasts."'

The pressure on mothers for their baby to conform to a growth chart can undermine their confidence in their ability to breastfeed, especially as the charts used to monitor growth were originally based largely on bottle-fed babies, who tend to gain weight more quickly than those fed at the breast. Some research suggests that infants who are exclusively breastfed to 6 months are on average 600–650g lighter at 12 months than bottlefed infants of the same height. New charts, based on the growth of breastfed infants, have only recently become available.

Wendy Burge, past president of the Australian Breastfeeding Association (ABA), believes too much emphasis is put on babies' weight. When she had her first baby, Kate, 20 years ago, she felt undermined by suggestions that her daughter wasn't gaining enough weight. It would have been easy for her to stop breastfeeding. 'It didn't stop me because I was fortunate to have enough support around me to keep going,' she says, 'but I can fully understand why women run away from it, because there is far too much pressure. You begin to doubt your own instincts. The ABA is constantly stressing to mothers not to get hung up on weight gain. If there is some weight gain and all the other signs say that your baby is doing well, you're OK.'

Breastfeeding matters

Breastfeeding is something of a holy cow. There's no doubt about its many likely benefits, for both mother and baby. But the mythology and mysticism that surround it can make it very difficult for women who find breastfeeding a struggle. They can feel like a failure if breastfeeding is not the joyous, natural experience they expect, and can find it hard to acknowledge that they are having problems and get help when they need it.

When the National Health and Medical Research Council published guidelines to promote breastfeeding, it included some personal reflections from a senior nutritionist which highlight some of these issues.[1] She wrote that breastfeeding is like holding down a full-time job—but more physically demanding than most.

'No one ever warned me just how hard it is to get breastfeeding established,' she wrote. 'In my mind I knew that this was the best food for my new baby and certainly the only option as far as convenience was concerned, but I found it quite frustrating (and painful) to learn this new skill at first. It was an eye opener when I realised that the 2 to 3 hours between feeds included the time you took feeding, which meant that sometimes there was a break of less than 1 hour between feeds to get anything else done. I relied a lot on the support and encouragement that I received from community nurses.'

Many couples—whether they are planning, expecting or

already caring for a baby—could benefit from reading these guidelines: they can be downloaded from the National Health and Medical Research Council website (http://www.nhmrc.gov.au). They have lots of tips for making breastfeeding easier for all concerned.

On top of all its other benefits, there is mounting evidence that breastfeeding reduces the risk of excessive weight gain during infancy and childhood. There is some evidence that the longer babies are breastfed, the less likely they are to gain too much weight in later years.[2] There is also some limited evidence that babies who start solid foods too early may be at risk of becoming overweight.

There are many theories about why this might be so. These include:

• Bottle feeding encourages parents to take control of how much and how often the baby eats. This may undermine the baby's natural ability to regulate their intake. Breastfeeding helps the baby learn to eat according to their appetite rather than according to external cues.[3]

• Breast milk exposes babies to the flavours of their mother's diet and may make it easier for them to accept a wider range of foods at weaning and as they get older.[4]

• Mothers of breastfed babies have a more relaxed attitude to their toddlers' intake of solid food and their toddlers consequently eat a wider range of solids and are taller and leaner than bottle-fed toddlers.[5]

• Some of the hormones and growth factors in breast milk may affect the body's mechanisms for governing appetite and fullness.

One review of the scientific evidence associating breastfeeding with a reduced risk of later obesity noted that research in the area is in its early stages.[6] It is possible that other factors at least partly explain the link: perhaps parents who are committed to breastfeeding are also more likely to regulate TV viewing and to encourage their children to be active, for instance. But many experts are convinced that the link is real and believe that supporting more women to breastfeed for a longer period may help reduce childhood and adolescent weight problems. It's even been proposed that the popularity of infant formula in the 1950s may have contributed to the weight gain occurring amongst many of those now in middle age.[7]

Of course there are plenty of other reasons, apart from weight control, to support breastfeeding. It has both short-term and long-term benefits for mother and baby.[8] It helps mothers bond with their baby and shed excess weight gained during pregnancy, and also may reduce their risk of breast and ovarian cancer. For the baby, it reduces the risk or severity of many health problems, including reflux, respiratory illness, asthma, gastrointestinal disease, inflammatory bowel disease, coeliac disease, type 1 diabetes, otitis media (a middle ear infection), urinary tract infections, bacterial meningitis, sudden infant death syndrome and some childhood cancers. It also helps intellectual development.

Reality check

What is recommended:

In an ideal world, all children would be exclusively breastfed until they are at least 6 months old. This means only breast milk, no solid foods and other liquids, until after 6 months. The National Health and Medical Research Council has set a breastfeeding goal: more than 90 per cent of babies should be breastfed, and 80 per cent should still be on the breast at 6 months.

What happens:

• A Queensland survey conducted in 2003 found that 57 per cent of infants were still being breastfed at 6 months.[9] Women who had made a commitment to breastfeed before having their baby were far more likely to do so. The survey also found that 18 per cent of children started solid food before they were 4 months old.

• A NSW study suggests that solids are being introduced too early into the diets of many babies. In 1995, 17 per cent of NSW infants were fully breastfed until 6 months of age (having only breast milk and no solid foods) but this figure had dropped to 5 per cent by 2001.[10] Public health nutritionist Dr Karen Webb says many women are discharged so soon after giving birth that they have not had a chance to learn the basic skills of breastfeeding. 'Support services for new mothers are very effective in extending the duration of breastfeeding, but there are simply not enough of these to help mothers with the steep learning curve they have as new parents,' she says.

• In 2004, a national study found that 37 per cent of babies had started regular solid foods by 4 months.[11] A national survey conducted in 2001 found that just over 50 per cent of babies were exclusively breastfed at 3 months and that only about a third were by 6 months.[12] In 1995 a national survey found that 57 per cent of babies were fully breastfed at 3 months. At 6 months, about 19 per cent were fully breastfed and about 46 per cent were fully or partially breastfed. Still, this is much better than in times past. When the Australian Breastfeeding Association first started in 1964 (when it was known as the Nursing Mothers' Association), only 23 per cent of mothers were breastfeeding on discharge from hospital.

None of this is meant to suggest that women should whip themselves if they struggle to meet the official recommendations on breastfeeding. It is a little like the obesity problem more generally, where it seems unfair to blame individuals for putting on weight when so many aspects of society encourage this. It is the same with breastfeeding: when employers, workplaces, health services and other powerful societal forces make it difficult for women to breastfeed, why should women be blamed? 'The mother shouldn't feel guilty if she can't manage to breastfeed,' says Wendy Burge. 'It's more likely the support and information that's failed her.'

One way women can make it easier on themselves is to get informed—the earlier the better. During pregnancy, many couples' focus is firmly on the birth and delivery, which is not surprising, considering it is such a momentous event. But pregnancy is also the ideal time for finding out about breastfeeding. And if both partners are involved in this, all the better—breastfeeding is more likely to be a success when the father is supportive. Have a look at the Australian Breastfeeding Association's website and get in touch with your local ABA support group. Read the National Health and Medical Research Council guidelines mentioned above. Find out if your hospital is accredited as Baby Friendly (this means you have a better chance of getting the support you need in those critical early days). Some employers are also accredited as being supportive of breastfeeding.

Chapter 15 includes a list of resources to help support breastfeeding. These are not only for women; they are also for their partners, families, health services and employers.

The pregnancy program

There is mounting evidence that babies' growth and nutrition before birth has a profound influence on their long-term health. Under-nutrition and over-nutrition during pregnancy may increase the risk of excessive weight gain in childhood and later life.

The Barker Hypothesis, named for the work of British researcher David Barker, has focused attention on the importance of nutrition during pregnancy. Barker and others believe that early influences on the developing foetus can produce life-long effects on organ structure and function. They argue that the origins of many adult diseases, including heart disease and non insulin-dependent diabetes, lie in this 'foetal programming'.[13]

Some of the evidence to support this hypothesis comes from the Dutch famine in the winter of 1944/45. The occupying German Army blockaded western Holland during the last 6 months of World War II, causing widespread famine. The official ration for pregnant women provided only about a third of the energy intake generally recommended. Studies following the health of babies born during the famine found that those who were undernourished in the first two trimesters of pregnancy were twice as likely to be obese at age 19 as those who received adequate nutrition during those stages of pregnancy.[14] One possible explanation is that nutritional deprivation during this crucial time influences the regulation of appetite and growth for life. This is supported by experiments showing that rats born to severely undernourished mothers are smaller at birth but have greater appetites than other rats, especially for energy-dense foods. They appear to have been programmed for a life of scarcity—to eat as if every meal was their last.

The other group influenced adversely by foetal programming appears to be bigger babies born to fatter mothers, or women who develop gestational diabetes during pregnancy. According to Ian Caterson, Professor of Human Nutrition at the University of Sydney, the intrauterine environment may affect their metabolic development in ways that predispose them to future weight gain and diabetes. This increased susceptibility may then be passed on to their own children, setting up a cycle in which future generations face an increased risk of weight-related problems. There is also some evidence that an adverse foetal environment—such as when the mother smokes during pregnancy—may also promote later obesity, independent of any effect on foetal growth.[15]

Caterson says research in the area of foetal nutrition and programming is still in its infancy, but it appears that babies who weigh less than 2.5kg or more than 4kg at birth may be at increased risk of weight gain and associated health problems in later life. While it is too early to make recommendations about how to best influence foetal nutrition and programming, he is in no doubt that pregnancy will prove to be a crucial period for intervention if obesity in childhood and adulthood is to be reduced.

He advises women to maintain fitness and a healthy weight before and during pregnancy. This is particularly important for those having difficulty conceiving; losing even a few kilograms may boost their chances of conception, he says. Smoking during pregnancy is, of course, never a good idea.

Different stages, different needs

Unlike adults, children need to take in more energy than they use in order to keep growing. But their needs around nutrition and feeding vary according to their developmental stage. Understanding how these things are connected will make it easier for you to help them establish healthy attitudes and habits. The early years are particularly important for this. There is some evidence that children's nutrition tends to worsen as they get older. One study, for example, found that 9-year-olds tend to have a poorer diet than 5-year-olds.[16] And anyone who knows anything about teenagers won't be surprised to hear that they are particularly likely to have poor nutrition.

1. Feeding babies (0–1 year)

The National Health and Medical Research Council recommends exclusive breastfeeding until about 6 months, then starting them on iron-enriched infant cereals. Vegetables, fruit, meat, chicken and fish can be added gradually. Babies often give clues when they are ready to start trying solid foods. They may watch and lean forward when food is around, put their fingers in their mouth, move their tongue up and down or reach out to grab food or spoons.

The first solids should be finely mashed and smooth, but you can soon move to coarser mashing. Nutritionist Dr Rosemary Stanton recommends avoiding sloppy baby foods— this can encourage lack of interest in any food that requires chewing. Even before their teeth emerge, a baby's gums can masticate food that has been mashed or blended. The infant should progress gradually to food chopped into small pieces. When infants begin to pick up everything and put it into their mouth, it is time to give them finger foods with texture. They may suck on them and make a mess, but they will gradually learn how to chew.

It is generally recommended that by the time babies turn 1, they should be eating much the same foods as the rest of the family.

Babies should not be given fruit juice before 6 months; between 6 months and 6 years they should have no more than about 150ml of fruit juice a day.

Your attitudes and behaviour around your baby's feeding may well influence their attitudes and behaviour around food for many years to come. So it is important to try to make the experience as enjoyable and relaxing as possible for all concerned. According to Ellyn Satter, your baby will feel about eating the same way you feel about feeding them. She compares good feeding with a nicely flowing non-verbal conversation. It is a two-way process where each of you responds to the other's cues. Your focus should not be on getting food into your baby but on observing what your baby wants and responding to those signals.

Children are more likely to eat according to their needs if they stay in control of the feeding process. This doesn't mean that you stop offering foods that they reject. 'I have learnt a lot about normal eating from babies', says Satter.[17] 'In fact I often teach my eating-disordered adolescents and adults about normal eating by talking about how babies do it. Older children are pretty good at eating normally, too, but since they have had time to learn strange ideas and habits from their elders, they aren't as good at it as babies.'

Remember that babies and children have an inbuilt survival mechanism based on rejecting new foods. They need to be exposed to new foods multiple times to learn that they are safe to eat. Some babies might try a new flavour the first or second time it is offered; others may need more than a dozen opportunities. Many parents are too quick to give up: one Australian study found that 53 per cent of those with children classified as fussy eaters gave up offering a new food if the child had not accepted it after two or three attempts.[18]

If you only give babies and children what you know they will eat straight away, they will not have the chance to learn to like a wide range of foods. But when you put a new food on their plate, don't make a big deal about it. Don't pressure them to try it until they are ready to do so.

Satter recommends sitting with your child at the family meal table and eating together—start as soon as they are able to sit up at the table in their highchair. This helps them learn by watching what everyone else does. It also helps cement the habit of family meals.

2. Feeding toddlers (1–2 years)

Few parents survive the toddler years without at least some food-related angst. It is much easier on all concerned if you can keep this to a minimum. It is easier to do this if you understand toddlers' take on food, life and the universe.

Toddlers are busy exploring their environment and asserting themselves and their independence—'no' becomes one of their favourite words and they continually test their parents' authority. They need a sense of security and routine. As Ellyn Satter says, toddlers are a little like a night watchman, 'checking all the doors but not really wanting to find any open'.[19] Toddlers can be easily upset and need help staying out of unnecessary struggles. Try not to let eating and mealtimes become a stage for struggles.

Food is of great interest to most toddlers—but not always for eating. They tend to be erratic and unpredictable eaters.

One day they might insist on feeding themselves; the next they will want to be fed. Or they might love a food one day and hate it the next. They might refuse a food at home but devour it when offered it somewhere else. Behaviour that can frustrate or worry a parent is often just normal for a toddler.

Toddlers have a limited attention span but they are very aware of those around them, and are great imitators. They are far more likely to accept and enjoy their food if others around them, whether children or adults, do the same.

Toddlers need room to express their autonomy but they also need structures and limits. 'If you treat him like you did when he was an infant, and simply accept and support his desires, you will fail him utterly,' says Ellyn Satter. 'He needs reasonable and firm limits in order to feel secure.' Toddlers need to know there will be three meals a day with regular snacks between meals. They also need to know how they are expected to behave at the table. This does not mean expecting them to clear their plate or eat tidily. It means offering them the same foods the rest of the family is eating and ensuring that, as much as possible, mealtimes are pleasant experiences. Parents who set limits, says Sattler, usually discover that once the toddler's initial storm is blown over, the child is happier and more settled.

In the second year of life, a child's nutrient needs are still high. It is particularly important to ensure toddlers are having plenty of foods rich in iron. Iron is essential for growth, and for motor and mental development, and the consequences of early iron deficiency may not be completely reversible. The best sources of iron are lean red meat such as beef, lamb, kangaroo or goat. White meats are also good sources, as are baked beans, wholegrain bread, some breakfast cereals and leafy green vegetables. Grains, dairy products and meats are important sources of the nutrients sometimes lacking in toddlers' diets.[20]

Restricting children's fat intake in their first few years of life is not a good idea; it may affect their growth and development. The National Health and Medical Research Council recommends that reduced-fat dairy products not be given to children younger than 2, and that skim milk not be given to children younger than 5.

3. Feeding preschoolers (3–5 years)

Preschoolers are very busy. They are learning new skills, striving for independence and have boundless energy and endless curiosity. 'Why?' is one of their favourite words. The preschool years are an ideal time for engaging children in the vegetable patch, in the kitchen and in food preparation. They are more likely to learn about food and to be interested in it if they have had a hand in growing or preparing it.

Food fads are common among preschoolers. They may insist on having a certain food prepared a particular way for several days. Then another food will come into vogue. Some parents might see this as a sign of fussiness, but really it is a common stage as children gradually expand their food range.

Preschoolers need routines—meals and snacks at regular times so they can eat small amounts regularly—but their appetite and intake will vary. Many prefer simply prepared foods that they can identify and manage themselves: vegetables or fruit cut into small pieces, for example. Make mealtime a pleasant and social occasion by including them in conversations and engaging them in meal rituals such as passing serving bowls. Using serving bowls helps children learn to regulate their eating. Remember not to pressure or reward them into eating.

Eating, as Ellyn Satter points out, involves a complex set of skills that are gradually acquired. Preschoolers are good eaters, she says, if they like eating and feel good about it, are interested in food, like being at the table, can wait a few minutes to eat when hungry, rely on internal cues of hunger and fullness to know how much to eat, enjoy many different foods, can learn to like new foods, can politely refuse foods they don't want, can be around new or strange food without getting upset, have reasonable table manners and can eat in places other than home.

Of course children's temperaments also vary. Some will adopt new foods enthusiastically, others will take a slow but steady approach and others will be late bloomers. Don't expect any child to fit neatly into any stereotype of what should happen at different developmental stages.

Fussy eaters

When children refuse food, it may be nothing to do with their view on the food itself—it may be their way of testing the effect of their response on people around them. If you assume that food is the real issue, you may end being caught up in an unwinnable game. The experts' advice for managing this sort of situation includes:

• Try to stay calm, and don't force your child to eat. Ignore behaviour you don't want to encourage. The more fuss you make, the greater your chances of entrenching your child's fussy behaviour.

• Allow your child some likes and dislikes.

• Start with a small serve and give more if your child is still hungry.

- If your child refuses to eat anything, let them sit quietly for a few minutes before leaving the table. Let them come to their next meal hungry.
- Do not bribe your child or prepare special food for them.
- Put the food in serving bowls on the table and let everyone help themselves. This way the child has to take responsibility for their choices. Coach other family members not to comment on the child's behaviour but to get on with enjoying their meal.

4. Feeding primary school children (6–12 years)

Children's first day at school is a huge milestone on their road to independence. School also often means the start of deterioration in children's eating. Parents have less control over what foods are available to their children, and schools don't always pull their weight in this area. Peer pressure also really starts to kick in.

But parents still have a great deal of influence. There are lots of ways you can affect your children's eating habits. Here are a few:

- Maintain the family habit of breakfast.
- Make sure your children (and their friends) have access to a wide range of healthy food at your home, especially for after-school snacks.
- Build relationships with other parents to try to counter the peer pressure problem. It is so much easier if your child's friends also have healthy snacks in their lunchbox and after school.
- Work with the school community on making healthy food choices available at school (see Chapter 15 for more on how to go about this).

Lunchboxes are often tricky. Children want whatever their friends are having, and often this means sugar and fat-laden snacks such as muesli bars and crisps. Some experts suggest making a list (help your child if they don't yet write) of all the things they are happy to have for lunch. You decide what is suitable, then try to come up with a list that you both agree on. Try to make sure the list includes plenty of variety.[21] And try to make sure that it does not include processed meats, chips, sweet biscuits, muesli and breakfast bars, fruit bars or straps, cordials, juices or soft drinks (see the Appendices for places to find ideas about making healthy, interesting and varied school lunchboxes; start by having a look at the Lunch Box World resources of the WA charity, Meerilinga, at http://www.meerilinga.org.au). And Choice magazine has an online, interactive tool to help with lunchboxes: http://www.choice.com.au

5. Feeding adolescents

It may seem narky to worry about what teenagers are eating when they have so many other issues to deal with—hormones and their emerging sexuality, annoying parents, irritating siblings, demanding teachers, stressful exams, drugs, alcohol, etc!

But food is a seriously important issue for teenagers. Adolescence is a high-risk period for nutrition. Teenagers have more money and opportunity to develop poor eating habits. Using alcohol and other drugs can also contribute to unhealthy eating patterns.

Good nutrition is critically important at this time, because teenage bodies are still growing and developing, and they need plenty of nutritious fuel. Adolescents are estimated to need about 1000 kilojoules more per day than adults.[22] The National

Food and development

Heath and Medical Research Council recommends that teenagers should have 3–4 serves of fruit and 4–9 serves of vegetables each day as well as 4–11 serves of cereal. Adolescence is an important period for calcium absorption and gaining bone density, especially for girls. A number of studies have raised concerns that many teenage girls may not be consuming enough dairy products for their long-term bone health.[23]

Adolescence is also a vulnerable time for putting on weight. Excess kilograms piled on at this stage have a nasty habit of lingering into adulthood. It is probably no coincidence that adolescence is also a time when stress levels in both parents and children rise. Parents' relationships are also particularly vulnerable to strain during children's adolescent years. According to one text, children's self-esteem often starts to fall from about age 11. By the time they turn 15, though, self-confidence starts to improve again.[24] A healthy diet and regular activity will help teenagers cope with their studies and the other stresses in their life.

Parents need to strike the delicate balance of being engaged and present in their teenagers' lives but not overly intrusive or critical. It is never a good idea to be critical of children's weight or body shape, and this is especially so during the adolescent years. Suggesting that adolescents join weight loss programs designed for adults is likely to be harmful—and ineffective.

In fact, you may need to actively discourage dieting. Many girls who have a healthy weight or are even underweight turn to dieting during adolescence. Disordered eating, whether it's binge eating, dieting or even fasting, is very common among teenagers. Studies of teenagers show that dieting is worryingly common, among boys as well as girls; dieting is so common among young women it is almost the norm.

Try not to do anything that will encourage your teenagers to follow fad diets or obsess about their weight and body shape. They need reassurance that weight gain, changes in body shape and increases in food intake are quite normal at this time. Discuss with them the downsides of dieting—including that it tends to lead to a vicious circle of food restriction and bingeing which ultimately leads to weight gain, not weight loss. Tell them that many women's lifelong battle with weight began with dieting in their adolescent years. If your teenagers are still not convinced, encourage them to see a health professional who can make sensible recommendations about changing eating habits and increasing activity—stay away from 'get thin quick' clinics.

If you are worried about your teenagers' eating habits, try not to just criticise them—it may make the situation worse. Some studies show that teenagers who are criticised about their eating skip more meals and have worse diets than those whose families are more supportive and accepting.[25] Rather than niggling at your teenagers, help make it easy for them to choose healthy foods. If the pantry and fridge are filled with a tempting range of tasty and nutritious snacks, there will be less room for the other sort. Research shows that teenagers are more likely to eat unhealthy foods and to drink soft drinks if that is what is available at home.[26] Equally, they are more likely to eat vegetables and fruit if these foods are readily available at home. Makes sense doesn't it?

If they complain that they're hungry, try buying healthy snacks with a low glycaemic index (GI) rating. Low GI foods take longer to be broken down and absorbed and may help ward off hunger pangs for longer. They tend to be less processed than high GI foods. But a word of caution: just because a food has a low GI does not make a food worth buying or eating. Nutritionist Dr Rosemary Stanton is concerned that the GI rating is sometimes used to promote foods that have dubious nutritional value. 'Chocolate has a low GI but that doesn't make it a useful food for people with diabetes or for those who need to lose weight,' she says.

She also advises giving teenagers more responsibility for buying food and preparing meals for the family. She suggests buying them a present of cooking lessons. Better still, suggest they do a cooking course with their friends.

10. Get moving

Remember how excited you were to see your child's first steps? Learning to walk is one of *the* significant milestones for both parent and child. It's pretty ironic that after we celebrate those first faltering steps, the adult world often then conspires to keep children sedentary. So many aspects of modern life—from concerns about safety to parents' busyness and the ever-increasing array of sedentary entertainment—reduce children's movement. In this chapter I hope to help counteract those forces: to give you some motivation and strategies for helping your children do what comes naturally for most—to enjoy being active.

The aim is not to try to turn every child into a sports star or athlete. That sort of approach immediately excludes those who are not interested in sports but who may well have the most to gain by being more physically active. Sport is an important part of many children's lives, but it is only one of the ways in which children can build skills and fitness. 'Team sport for kids who enjoy it is terrific,' says Associate Professor Melissa Wake, of the Murdoch Children's Research Institute in Melbourne. 'But one hour of sport on the weekend plus 80 hours of inactivity during the week doesn't add up to an active child. Children need to build activity into their everyday lives.'

Focusing on physical activity—which can be everything from playing a game to washing the car—rather than just on sport and exercise creates many more opportunities for children to burn off energy. It also means physical activity can be accumulated in short bursts throughout the day rather than in one long, hard slog. This is more in line with children's natural patterns of behaviour. It is not usual, for most children at least, to spend more than 20 minutes at a time in vigorous physical activity; the more usual pattern is to do short bursts, but lots of them. Taking a broad approach to physical activity also makes it easier to entrench it as part of your family's everyday routines. The goal is to develop the habit of being active every day, whether it is through enjoying a game of tennis or walking to the shop to buy the milk and the paper.

This is especially important because some research suggests that children's fitness is in decline because of falling levels of incidental activity, not because of falling levels of participation in sport or other organised activities. Many children play sport but don't get enough of other forms of activity, things like hanging out the washing, walking to school or playing in the backyard.

Even though this chapter's focus is on supporting and encouraging children being active, it is really adults who are the target. It is adults' attitudes and behaviours that need to change if children are to be given the opportunity to become more active. Research has shown that many parents think their children are more active than they really are, and that parents do not always place a high priority on their children being active.[1] Many factors influence how active children are: where they live, their genetic makeup (whether they are naturally energetic or lethargic, or have a calm or agitated personality, for example), and the school they go to. But many parents may not realise just how important they can be in influencing their children's activity levels. Parents can play a key role in helping their children develop the knowledge, attitudes, skills and behaviours that support an active lifestyle.

Activity matters

In recent years, health authorities in many countries have issued guidelines encouraging children and adolescents to be more physically active. This has been something of a challenge for the experts involved in developing these guidelines, because there has been surprisingly little research on the impact of physical activity during childhood to help them. The scientific evidence on the benefits of regular physical activity is clear for adults—it reduces the risk of many diseases and adds years to life (as well as life to years). But with children it is far more difficult to show such an impact, partly because serious diseases are rare in childhood. Few experts feel there is sufficient scientific evidence to make definitive pronouncements about the likely effects of any particular level of activity on children's current or future health.

However, common sense suggests that many children could benefit from being more active. One recent review noted the lack of studies documenting the effects of physical activity in childhood, but concluded:

> Considering the dramatic rise in the prevalence of
> overweight and obesity in Australian children and
> adolescents over the last decade and the importance of
> physical inactivity in the development and maintenance of

childhood and adolescent obesity, one could argue that it has never been more important to promote regular health-enhancing physical activity among our nation's youth.[2]

Here are some of the potential benefits of activity for children:

1. Healthy growth and development

Physical activity is important for the healthy growth and development of children's bones, muscles and cardiorespiratory system. Weight-bearing activities such as running and soccer are particularly important for developing bone density, which reduces the risk of osteoporosis in later life. Being active helps the development of flexibility, posture, balance, co-ordination and other skills. It also helps bring a good night's sleep and aids in regulating appetite.

2. Psychological and mental health

Active people are likely to feel more confident, happy and relaxed, and to have higher self-esteem. Physical activity can help ward off depression and relieve stress. Some studies suggest that adolescents who are active or play sport are less likely to smoke cigarettes, to drink alcohol or to use illicit drugs. The situation may change as they get older, however. Some research suggests that young adults may be more likely to drink if they are involved in sport. Perhaps this is connected to the alcohol industry's close association with sport.[3]

3. Social skills

Physical activity can promote the development of social skills and connections. Involvement in sport and other activities can help teach children about fair play, teamwork, discipline, competition and achievement. It can also help develop skills in goal setting, problem solving, conflict resolution, risk management and leadership. It may also help children learn to delay gratification and tolerate discomfort, which are helpful skills for dealing with the world at large.[4]

4. Potential academic benefits

Some studies suggest that increasing children's fitness boosts their academic achievement. However, not all experts are convinced; some argue that most of the evidence comes from small studies. Nonetheless, many people feel, through their own experience, that regular activity helps improve concentration, focus, thinking and energy.[5] At least one Australian study has shown that introducing compulsory daily physical education improved primary school children's behaviour in class.[6] 'Parents and teachers might say that cuts into the school day,' says Professor Terry Dwyer, one of the researchers involved in that study and now the director of the Murdoch Children's Research Institute in Melbourne. 'But our argument is that historically it's very unusual to have children sitting for 6 hours a day. It's not a natural state.'

5. Maintaining a healthy weight

Children are less likely to gain excess weight if they are physically active. And of course increasing activity levels is a key strategy for helping overweight and obese children reach a more healthy weight.

6. Reducing future disease risks

There is mixed evidence about whether active children are less likely to develop problems such as type 2 diabetes and heart disease in later life.[7] Some studies suggest that this might be the case; others do not. More conclusive answers will have to come from large, long-term studies. However, there are plenty of reasons why such studies might be expected to prove that there is a link. The process of atherosclerosis—the hardening of the arteries that can eventually lead to heart attacks and strokes— begins in childhood. Many risk factors for adult diseases, such as high blood pressure, high cholesterol, and insulin resistance, begin early in life. So it makes sense to assume that an active childhood may give some protection against later disease.

7. Influencing attitudes and habits

It is not certain whether children and teenagers who are fit and active are more likely to grow into fit, active adults.[8] Many other factors also influence adults' fitness and activity levels, and there are no doubt many middle-aged couch potatoes who were sports enthusiasts as kids. However, it seems sensible to assume that children who develop the habit, skills and confidence to be active will also have these resources at their disposal in later years.

8. Social benefits

Getting children and young people involved in enjoyable physical activity may also bring community benefits, including increased social cohesion.[9] Criminologists have long been interested in the possibility that participation in sport and activity might help prevent antisocial and criminal behaviour. A recent discussion paper by the Australian Institute of Criminology concludes that such programs may have an indirect effect on antisocial behaviour, by encouraging young people's personal and social development.[10] The paper says that sport and physical activity provide a socially acceptable outlet for tension and energy, and may help reduce behavioural risk factors for youth. 'The current consensus in the literature on boredom is that when youth have nothing else to occupy and sufficiently stimulate them they will seek out their own, often antisocial, amusement,' the paper says. 'Providing structured activities keeps young people occupied and out of harm's way.'

And some possible downsides...

Pushing children into sports or activities they do not enjoy or which are beyond their capabilities is not a smart move. It can lead to injuries or affect their self-esteem and confidence, and might even result in a lifelong aversion to physical activity. Encouraging children to be active in order to lose weight, or being overly controlling of their activity, may also be counterproductive. They are more likely to persist with an activity if they enjoy it for its own sake.

Injuries are relatively common with many popular sports. One NSW study found that 54 per cent of young people who play sport experienced some form of injury in a 6 month period. Rugby union, rugby league, netball, hockey, AFL, soccer and horse-riding produced the most injuries.[11]

But the risk can be minimised with a bit of forethought and preparation. Coaches, parents and others involved in supervising children's activities can help reduce the risk of injuries and accidents by making sure children have the right equipment, and use it correctly. Children should be encouraged to eat lightly about 2 hours before any vigorous activity, and to keep topped up with water before and during exercise. They shouldn't wait to feel thirsty before they take a drink of water.

The idea that doing some stretches before you exercise can help prevent injury is controversial, but many experts believe it is worth recommending. Stretching after exercise is certainly a good idea. So encouraging children to do some warm-up and warm-down exercises may help prevent injury, and will also cultivate an awareness of safety issues. Getting children in the habit of thinking about preparation and safety may have other long-term benefits too.

Some sports and activities which emphasise body image and leanness, such as ballet, aerobics and gymnastics, can lead to an unhealthy focus on weight and body image. They are also associated with a higher rate of inappropriate weight loss practices such as dieting. Such image-conscious activities can also affect some children's self-esteem.[12] The point is not to discourage children from being involved in these activities—just be aware of these issues and take steps to prevent or manage them.

Reality check

What is recommended:

• Children and young people should be physically active for at least 60 minutes (and up to several hours) every day, according to Australian Government recommendations for children aged 5 to 18. Activity does not need to happen all at once; it can accumulate during the day.

• The same guidelines recommend that children should not spend more than 2 hours a day using electronic media for entertainment (such as computer games, the internet, TV), particularly during daylight hours.

The big fat conspiracy

• In the United States, the National Association for Sport and Physical Education has made more specific recommendations for different age groups:

> • *Infants* should interact with parents and other carers in daily physical activities that help them explore their environment and facilitate their movement. They should be put in safe places that facilitate activity and do not restrict movement for prolonged periods of time.

> • *Toddlers* should spend at least 30 minutes each day in structured activity. This does not need to be all at once, but can accumulate during the day. They should also engage in at least 60 minutes and up to several hours of unstructured physical activity every day and should not be sedentary for more than 60 minutes at a time except when asleep. They should have safe indoor and outdoor areas where they can be active.

> • *Preschoolers* should accumulate at least 60 minutes of structured physical activity each day, and engage in at least 60 minutes and up to several hours of unstructured activity every day. They should not be sedentary for more than 60 minutes at a time except when sleeping, and should have safe indoor and outdoor areas where they can be active.

• Canada takes a slightly different angle. It advises all children to spend more time being active and less time being sedentary, and recommends taking a stepped approach, boosting activity levels gradually over a 5 month period. To start with, children should spend another 20 minutes each day on moderately energetic activities and another 10 minutes on vigorous activities. They should also start by reducing the amount of time they spend being sedentary by 30 minutes a day. By the end of 5 months, they should be accumulating at least 60 minutes of moderate physical activity each day and 30 minutes of vigorous activity. They should also have reduced sedentary time by 90 minutes.

What happens

There is not much reliable information about the physical activity levels of Australian children. Some studies examine only participation in sport or rely on children's or parents' reports rather than on an objective assessment.

The best national figures date back to 1985, when only 38–51 per cent of boys (depending on age) and 35–44 per cent of girls reported 3–4 bouts per week of sustained vigorous activity (defined as enough to make them 'huff and puff').

Other findings, from Australian Sports Commission publications, include that:

• About 62 per cent of children aged 5 to 14 participated in organised sport outside school hours in the 12 months before April 2003: swimming, outdoor soccer and netball were the most popular.

• During the same period, 62 per cent of children rode a bike (down from 64 per cent in 2000), and 23 per cent went skateboarding or rollerblading (down from 31 per cent in 2000).

• Almost a quarter of 15 to 24-year-olds reported doing no physical activity at all in the 2 weeks before a 1995 survey.

Associate Professor Tim Olds, a researcher at the University of South Australia, says children's fitness around the world generally improved between the end of World War II and about 1975. This reflected, among other things, improvements in child health due to reductions in diseases. But in developed countries like Australia, children's fitness has declined rapidly since then to levels that are now below pre-war levels. Professor Olds estimates that about half the fall-off in fitness is due to increases in fatness; falling activity levels also play a part.

Children today are generally less fit than children of similar weight and fatness 20 years ago, his research suggests. 'I am sure that most experts now accept that children's fitness is declining', Professor Olds says. 'Your kids are likely to be 10 to 15 per cent less fit than you were at the same age. It's pretty dramatic. It means they simply won't be able to do a lot of things. They will be excluded from a lot of life's experiences.'

Why parents are crucial

1. Rethinking some attitudes

If you can't get a park close to the shops or train station, do you moan and groan? Or do you welcome the opportunity to fit another 10 minute walk into your day? If it's raining, do you shelve plans for a walk—or do you grab the raincoat and brolly? At work or the shopping centre or the hotel, do you automatically take the lift, or do you look for the stairs first?

We have all become so used to labour-saving devices and clock-watching that many of us have been programmed into some unhealthy habits. Changing these habits means changing attitudes. Instead of seeing a longer walk to the carpark or a climb up the stairs as a waste of precious time, look at it as an opportunity to improve your precious health. Tweaking your attitudes like this may also help reduce stress levels. It's not only because exercise helps relieve stress or that the time spent walking is also time you can spend thinking, or problem solving, or daydreaming and losing sight of the clock. It's also because you have turned a negative into a positive. With this change of attitude, your day might well send you fewer annoyances.

The other important spin-off to changing your attitudes is that it is likely to rub off on the people around you. Children are more likely to create and enjoy opportunities for activity if you do too.

Many parents feel that they just don't have the time to be more active. What they really mean, according to Heart Foundation expert Trevor Shilton, is that being physically active is not a high priority for them. If it was, they would make time. Shilton points out that Prime Minister John Howard can find time to walk every day: 'I challenge anyone to say he's not busy.'

If parents make physical activity a high priority for themselves and their family, it is likely to result in all sorts of changes which will make it easier for children to be more active.

It could mean:

• changes to parents' working or transport arrangements;
• asking schools not only about their academic performance, but also about what they do to encourage students' activity;
• adding another dimension to discussions about where children should go to school, especially if one option involves a long drive and less opportunity for walking to school or playing with friends in the afternoon;
• changes to how your family travels on outings or what you do on weekends and during holidays;
• different types of presents at Christmas and birthdays— fewer computer games and more active games;
• changes to how you reward your children—perhaps taking them on a family bike ride rather than an outing to a fast food restaurant;

• changing the venue for children's birthday parties—instead of meeting at a fast food restaurant, meet at a park;
• turning off the TV and computer when your kids' friends come over to play; and
• something as simple as putting on some energetic music when you're all doing household chores, to get those bodies pumping.

Making physical activity a priority may also lead to a re-examination of adults' attitudes towards children's behaviour. So many aspects of society are geared towards immobilising children. TV screens have been introduced to cars and shopping centres because it is convenient for adults to keep children quiet and entertained. Are you in the habit of telling the kids to stop fidgeting, to stop running, to sit quietly? It's fair enough to not want them running amok through the house, or all the way to the other end of the shopping mall, but are there areas, inside and out, where they can run unrestrained and be boisterous?

For many parents, one of the most challenging areas for self-examination involves attitudes about children's safety. Today's parents are much more safety conscious and restrictive of their children's activities than previous generations were. It's not surprising considering the constant media diet of doom and gloom and the many groups that have an interest in making us anxious. One of the latest examples of how parental fears can be turned into profit is a new system allowing parents to track their children's whereabouts by mobile phone.[13] We are more aware of the risks in our lives than ever before, even though many of these risks are lower now than they used to be.

How you weigh up the pros and cons of various risks is a matter for your family. Everyone will have their own particular perceptions of risk, and their own list of how dangerous or safe various activities are. It can't be assumed that there is a 'right way' or a 'wrong way' here—people's perceptions vary according to their world view, their situation and their experience. But it's worth at least thinking through some of your attitudes and seeing if there is any room for movement. It might be as simple as rethinking your approach to a cold or drizzly day. Instead of seeing the weather as a reason to stay indoors, you might see it as a reason to rug up and enjoy a windswept walk along the beach or as a great opportunity to give your kids the pleasure of jumping in puddles or making mud pies.

When public health researcher Professor Boyd Swinburn moved to Australia from New Zealand several years ago, he noticed a greater tendency here to 'cotton wool' kids. He empathises with parents' concerns about risk but believes kids need to be allowed, up to some point at least, to follow their natural tendency to take risks. 'It's about how much you can hold your tongue and avoid saying no,' he says. Mothers, in particular, often find this difficult, he adds.

Girls are especially vulnerable to parents' concerns about risks, according to Geraldine Naughton, Associate Professor in Paediatric Exercise Science at the Australian Catholic University. Research has shown that gender differences in perceptions about risk are established as early as age 6, when girls are much more responsive than boys to parental concerns about hazards associated with play. Parents walk a fine line between exposing their children to unnecessary risks of injury and developing attitudes that constrain their children's activity.

Rethinking your attitudes to risk may bring other benefits for your children. Learning to negotiate risk is an important part of development. 'Every time you get a kid to take a healthy risk, you are giving them the opportunity to learn a little bit about themselves,' says Dr Michael Carr-Gregg.

2. Model that move

It's not only your attitudes that influence your children, of course. It's what you do, too. Children are more likely to be active if their parents are. They are also less likely to be overweight if their parents are active.[14] So it's worrying to see so many inactive adults. Estimates vary among studies, but it is likely that about half of all adults are not active enough to benefit their health.[15]

You can put this another way: many parents are not active enough to benefit their children's health. Parents can really help their children become more active if they build more activity into their own life. Even better if that activity also involves the children. Maybe you can walk to school together or, with older children, go to the gym or pool together. Or make it a regular weekend event to go on a family bike ride or bushwalk or roller skating or kite-flying. If you are going on a sedentary outing, such as a trip to the movies, can you incorporate some activity: walking to the bus or parking some distance away from the cinema?

Start the habit early. Take babies and toddlers for walks in their prams. That way they will be used to seeing you active from their earliest days. When they can manage, encourage them to walk part of the way. As they get older, get them to cycle while you walk or cycle.

Many people find it easier to be active if they've got

company. Having a friend to share your walk with is pleasant; it also makes it more difficult to skip that appointment with your runners. Similarly, it might help to find other families who also enjoy being active. Anything that makes activity more enjoyable for all concerned is a good idea.

It is not only parents who can be powerful role models: grandparents, aunts, uncles, neighbours, family friends, teachers, coaches and others who play a significant part in children's lives can also set active examples.

3. Psychological support

Children are more likely to participate in sport and other physical activities if they feel confident about their skills and abilities—if they believe they can do it. They are also more likely to be active if they think it will be a positive experience or bring benefits, such as having time with friends.[16]

Parents can help by encouraging children and praising their efforts. Young children, in particular, flourish in front of an audience. Watch them on the sports field or in the backyard, and be generous with your feedback. Children are more likely to be active if they think they are competent and if they believe their parents think they are competent.[17] Praise their efforts in games and sports, whether they win, lose or draw. If they are interested in a particular activity or sport, take them to a professional match or find a book about it.

Give them the opportunity to try a range of different activities, so they can find something they like. Make sure they are involved in activities appropriate to their age and ability. Pushing children beyond their abilities or into activities they do not enjoy is counterproductive. Some children thrive on competition, for instance, but many do not. Many will enjoy activity more if it does not involve competition and everyone has a chance to experience the buzz of success.

When children and adolescents are asked about what stops them being more active, they mention things like lack of time and energy, poor weather, homework, and lack of interest and motivation.[18] Parents can help children overcome these sorts of barriers, for example, by helping their children to manage their time better, so they can fit in both their homework and a game outside. Or kill a few birds with one stone—talk through homework or practise spelling while taking a walk together.

Girls may need different approaches from boys. One study of Year 6 children showed that boys were more likely to be active if they were involved in community-based organisations, but girls were more likely to be active if it had benefits such as spending more time with friends. The researchers emphasised the importance of providing opportunities that meet children's needs and interests.[19] Research has also suggested that boys are more active than girls because they are more confident in their ability to overcome barriers to physical activity. The researchers speculated that girls may be less active because they are not given the same encouragement and support as boys. They may also need to learn the behavioural skills that will let them overcome the everyday barriers to participation in physical activity. The researchers suggested that girls should be given plenty of opportunity to participate in non-competitive activities they can enjoy throughout their lives, such as walking, callisthenics/resistance training and aerobic dance.[20]

Special care may be needed when children are overweight. They tend to be less confident of their ability to be physically active. They may need more support and encouragement than other children—but it is important that it is not coercive. One study concluded that the best way to encourage obese children to be more active is to provide enjoyable, developmentally appropriate activities that let them experience success with a minimum of anxiety. It also found that obese children are encouraged to get moving by watching influential others—parents or peers—being active.[21] Generally speaking, children should not be made to feel that the goal of activity is weight loss; they should be encouraged to be active because it is fun and it will help them feel good.

4. Practical support

Many studies have shown that children are more likely to be physically active if their parents give them practical support.[22] This support can take many forms:

• Ensure there are safe places, whether inside or outside, at home or elsewhere, for activity.

• Provide appropriate equipment. This might be as simple as a ball. Or it might mean installing a trampoline or basketball hoop in the backyard. Some families find it useful to store balls and other games equipment in the car so they can be ready for action whenever an opportunity arises. The more items of sporting equipment a family has, the more likely the child is to be active.

• Do what is needed so that your children can participate in sports and other activities—drive them to weekend games, pay their registration fees, make sure they have the correct equipment and uniforms.

• Make sure that when they meet up with friends, they have opportunities to be active.

• Have a stock of suggestions ready for when you hear, 'I'm bored.'

• Plan ahead. Identify events which might be of interest to the children and incorporate them into the family schedule. If your children are passionate about a particular sport or activity, take them to professional games or performances or buy them books or magazines about that activity.

5. Authority figures

Parents can help children be active by setting some rules, and not just about the amount of time spent in front of a screen. Many studies have shown that children who spend more time outdoors are more active. It's so much easier to be sedentary indoors. Sending children outside to play is a very simple way to get them moving. There are other good reasons to encourage kids to explore the great outdoors; it is thought that the increasing incidence of allergic diseases may be due to the sterilisation of childhood—children being kept indoors and having minimal exposure to the germs that help their immune systems to develop.

Setting some rules to encourage outdoor time is a good idea. Make it a habit, for example, for the family to spend at least one weekend day or half day outdoors. Involve the children in household chores such as gardening, sweeping or walking the dog. And don't forget the sun protection.

Rethinking home

People use many criteria when they choose where to live—how close it is to the train station or school or family, or how much it costs could be on that list.

Another issue you should perhaps consider is whether your home will make it easy for you and your children to be active. If it is a house, does it have a backyard? Research shows a correlation between the size of a backyard and a child's level of activity: the bigger it is, the more active the child is likely to be.[23]

If you are considering moving to a unit, is there a courtyard where the children can play?

Can they walk to school? Does the local neighbourhood encourage activity—can you walk to the shops or the library or the doctor's surgery? Are there cycle ways?

Even the way the streets are laid out can influence your family's ability to be active. A grid network makes it easier to walk to the shops or other destinations; cul de sacs can discourage this. On the other hand, some families prefer to live on a cul de sac because they feel it makes it safer for children to play on the street. Denser development can create a residential area which also supports shops, cafés and other services that are walkable destinations.

Is there a park nearby? A Perth study found that people were more likely to be active if they had access to large, attractive public open spaces. This was particularly so if such spaces were designed for a range of uses—walking, cycling, dog-walking, picnicking and games, for example. It found that people who used public open spaces were nearly three times as likely as other residents to achieve recommended levels of activity.[24] Another Australian study found that people were more likely to use parks, and to use them more often, if they lived within 500 metres of one.

Of course affordability is a key criterion for most families when selecting where to live. But Associate Professor Billie Giles-Corti, a public health researcher at the University of Western Australia, believes that if more attention were paid to the factors that influence physical activity, many parents might see their options quite differently. Choosing an activity-friendly place to live will not necessarily cost more, she says.

Balancing risks

As a public health professional, Glenn Austin is familiar with the idea of weighing up benefits and risks. Rationally, he knows that public fears about 'stranger danger' are sometimes exaggerated and often lead to restrictions on children's ability to be active. But now that he has three young daughters, he has quite a different perspective on the issue. No matter how small the actual risk is of his girls being abducted or injured if they play in the streets, it is not one he wishes to take.

However, Glenn, a former teacher who now works in health promotion in the central Queensland city of Rockhampton, is also determined not to expose his children to the risk of inactivity. His solution has been a backyard landscaped to provide plenty of interesting play areas, including a bicycle track and a cubby house. There's also an outdoor entertaining area to make it easier for adults to keep an eye on the kids.

Not everyone has the space or the money to create a backyard fun park. But even simple measures—like turning part of the lounge room or the spare room into an activity den for vigorous play or sharing supervision at the park with other parents—can help protect children from the often under-appreciated risk of inactivity.

Rethinking cars

Here's another one of those paradoxes: you might have to slow down to get you and your family moving faster. Cars are so much part of the Australian way of life that we tend to take them, and their impact on our children and cities, for granted.

Taking some time out to reconsider your transport needs and arrangements could pay large dividends if it leads to less car use and greater reliance on active forms of transport, such as cycling and walking. Most people, even those who identify as environmentally conscious, don't base their transport decisions on health or environmental considerations. Research shows that time constraints, habit and practical issues are the major influences.

If you want to make some changes to how often you use the car, maybe you could start by trying to think of strategies that might help make active travel more practical and efficient for your family. You need to be realistic about your goals and how to achieve them.

You might also be surprised by how easy it is to make changes. When Perth researchers conducted a study, simply telling residents in one suburb about the active transport options that were available to them, there was a significant drop in car travel and an increase in walking, cycling and use of public transport. The changes were sustained over two years.[25] Similar results have been achieved with Travel Smart programs elsewhere. So it is not impossible to make changes to how you travel. A little bit of information and planning may be all you need.

It might also help to work out how much your car/s cost, taking into account much more than the price at the bowser. Many people overestimate the advantages of car use and underestimate the disadvantages.[26] Some researchers use the concept of 'effective speed' to capture the true cost of cars to motorists. While most people probably think of speed as the distance travelled divided by the time taken, the notion of effective speed also incorporates into this equation the time taken to earn the money to pay all the costs associated with car travel. Taking this approach can throw a whole new light on the benefits of car travel.

One study compared the effective speeds for one person driving a car, travelling by bus, cycling or walking in Canberra. The effective speed ranged from 14.6km/h for a Monaro to 12.8km/h for a

Landcruiser Sahara, 23.1km/h for a Hyundai Getz, 21.3km/h for a bus, 18.1km/h for a bicycle, 37.1km/h for a train (using Perth data for comparison) and 6km/h for walking. The study was based on 2004 data and included only the costs to the individual of each form of transport—it didn't take account of other costs such as greenhouse emissions or pollution.[27] 'The most important thing we need to do in changing our culture is to slow down and to realise the absolute futility of trying to save time with cars,' says one of the study's authors, Dr Paul Tranter, a senior lecturer in geography at the Australian Defence Force Academy in Canberra. For most car drivers, how fast they drive makes little difference to their effective speed because they spend so much time earning money to pay for all the costs of their transport. However, for people using a bus, train or car, any increase in trip speed is reflected in a significant increase in effective speed.

Many adults also fail to consider the effect of their car use on children—whether their own family or others—in making roads and neighbourhoods unsafe for children. In Canada, researchers showed that parents became more open to reducing car use when told about the impact of cars on children.[28] Questioning your car use may help children in many ways. If you start to look for other forms of transport, especially on those short trips when cars are so often used, your children may be less likely to grow up thinking that cars are the only way to travel. If they get in the habit of walking to the shops or school with you, they will also have the chance to learn much more about their environment.

Tranter and his colleagues argue that being able to play in the streets has many benefits for children.[29] They cite Denmark, which has recognised the importance of having streets available for children to play in and designated some as 'rest and play' streets. In Munich, some streets have signs saying 'children can play in this street' and require cars to travel very slowly. 'If children are allowed to play on the streets, walk around their own neighbourhood, get to know their own city and community, then when they do become adults, they may be less inclined to defend the levels of motorised traffic which are limiting children's access to their environment,' say the researchers. 'If we can encourage more people to use residential streets for walking, cycling, social interaction and playing, then cities will become more sociable, more liveable places for all city residents.'

A Brisbane inventor, David Engwicht, has developed some ideas for making the streets safer, which at first might sound counterintuitive. In his book *Mental Speed Bumps: The smarter way to tame traffic* (2005), he recounts noticing that a child playing on the footpath could be more effective than a speed bump at slowing traffic. Intrigued, he investigated further and concluded that the speed of traffic on residential streets is governed, to a large extent, by the degree to which residents have psychologically retreated from their street. Simply reversing this retreat creates what Engwicht calls 'mental speed bumps'. His book also describes how a traffic engineer working in Holland, Hans Monderman, made a similar discovery at the same time. Monderman found that removing all traffic signs, speed humps, line markings and traffic lights dramatically reduced traffic speeds and actually made streets safer. The lack of signs and traffic control devices created a mental speed bump that slowed motorists, without their even being aware that they had slowed down. This new approach to street design has been applied in over 30 cities and villages in Europe.

Even if you do not have control over the design of your street or neighbourhood, you may be able to help make it safer by encouraging street life. Hold a street party, or leave the car at home on your next outing.

Some state, local and territory governments have Travel Smart programs which offer advice to help you plan car-free journeys (see

Appendices for contact details). The active marketing of such programs in a variety of suburbs and towns has led to reductions in car use and increases in walking and cycling.

Some schools and organisations run courses to help parents and children become more confident with cycling. Your local cycling organisation may be able to help with details of these.

Dr Chris Rissel, a cycling enthusiast and public health expert at the Sydney South West Area Health Service, advises parents to start off with recreational cycling—taking the kids somewhere safe to build up their skills and confidence.

Even in a city like Sydney, which is notorious for being car-centred, a little bit of research will turn up many routes offering opportunities for safe cycling, says Rissel.

Trapping an expert[30]

Dr Paul Tranter, senior lecturer in geography at the Australian Defence Force Academy in Canberra, is passionate about the harm being done by society's unquestioning reliance on cars. In his research and his lectures to students, he unpicks the many hidden costs of car ownership and usage.

But he knows how easy it is to fall into the car trap. He almost did it himself a few years ago, when he started a new job which involved an hour-long commute (each way) by bicycle or bus. He and his wife considered buying a second car so he could squeeze more work into his day.

'While we were looking for a car I recalled a lecture I had given to my transport geography students...and I reflected on just how little time, if any, I would save by getting a second car, and about how I might be able to use my time in a bus, and decided I could save more time by continuing to bus it to work and paying for an occasional taxi when I needed to get home quickly in the evenings.'

He also thought about how the bus allowed him some time for work as well as some exercise (walking to the bus stop). 'As a bus commuter I lose less "effective time" than I do as a car driver,' he says. 'I also arrive at work less stressed than the driver who has dealt with peak hour traffic. Leaving aside the environmental and social arguments in favour of public transport, I can now see that catching the bus gives me more time to complete the tasks I need to do.'

If you do these sorts of sums on your car habits, you too might discover some downsides that you hadn't previously seen, as well as some benefits to other forms of travel that you hadn't previously thought about.

Play on

When children play, they are having fun. But they are also learning—about themselves and their world—and developing their physical, intellectual, emotional and social skills.

And they are burning up energy. Many experts believe that giving children plenty of opportunity for spontaneous play is one of the keys to making sure they are active enough to prevent weight problems emerging. Some research suggests that children use up more energy in active free play or unstructured play outdoors than they do in other kinds of physical activity.[31] One US study, for example, found that preschool children were more active in their free play than in structured activities.

Play is particularly important in the first 10 years of a child's life, when they are too young for sport, according to Associate

Professor Beth Hands, a human movement expert at the University of Notre Dame in Western Australia. Pushing children into sport before about age 10 can be counterproductive, she says, because they often don't have the skills or confidence to cope with the challenges involved, and the experience can put them off. 'So many children are burning out from starting sport too early,' Hands says. 'They start playing football at 6, and by 9 or 10 they are burnt out.'

Hands also cautions parents against filling up every minute of their children's day with activities. It's better, she says, to just make sure children have the time and opportunity to develop their skills and to entertain themselves with physical play.

However, many children do not get to do this. One study of Year 5 students in western Sydney in 2003 found that about a quarter of the children reported having no or a minimal amount of time for free play after school during the 3 days of the study.[32] Only about half the children spent more than an average of 30 minutes a day in free play. They were otherwise occupied—with homework, structured activities and the mesmerising screen.

After school and weekends are critical times for children's play, and variety in venue and activity are also important. Dr Paul Tranter has studied how different environments influence children's play, and says that many parks, playgrounds and school yards serve children poorly.[33] Rather than neatly manicured lawns and gardens, children need a range of environments, so that they get involved in a range of activities. They need access to spaces where they can be with friends, solitary places where they can be alone, and wild places where they can get dirty, whether by digging holes or making hideaways.

Apart from ensuring that children have time and space for play, one of parents' most important jobs is to play with their children, especially in those formative years. A parent's praise and approval has almost magical properties for young children. Children are more likely to be active if their parents play with them regularly.[34]

The National Association for Prevention of Child Abuse and Neglect offers the following tips to help parents be good playmates:

• Play at the right level for your child. Play that is too easy might bore your child, and play that is too hard may frustrate them.

• Let your child lead the play. Don't take over.

• Make sure the play is safe.

• Ask your children what they would like you to do as part of the play.

• Allow enough time for play.

• Don't compete with young children.

• Be patient if your child wants to repeat the same play over and over. New skills require lots of practice. Stay enthusiastic.

• Appreciate and encourage their efforts.

Associate Professor Geraldine Naughton, an expert in children's exercise science at the Australian Catholic University in Sydney, says that the parents' role as partners in their child's activities gets smaller as the child gets older and more independent. 'But the role of the parent as a facilitator of activity never stops,' she adds.

One of the easiest ways to get young children moving is to have their friends over to play.

Developing skills

Like most people, children are more likely to do activities they enjoy. They are more likely to enjoy an activity if they feel competent at it. So helping children develop the skills to master activities is an important part of helping them to be active.

When young children play, they are also developing the fundamental movement skills that will let them play sport and do other activities later.

Parents have an important role in supporting children's acquisition and development of these skills. This is especially so during the preschool and primary school years, when children are very open to learning new skills, have not yet developed bad habits, are not very self-conscious, and are not as worried as they will be later about being injured or teased by their peers.

Taking time to help children develop their skills and confidence in things like running, jumping, throwing a ball and using a bat may pay long-term dividends. Some researchers believe being confident with these skills plays an important role in preventing unhealthy weight gain among children and youth.

Children who master these skills early are more likely to be active throughout childhood and into adolescence, research shows. They are also more likely to be fit and less likely to carry excess weight.[35] Conversely, those who lack fundamental movement skills are more likely to become frustrated and have difficulty learning more advanced skills. They also are less likely to be fit and active, and more likely to be overweight. They are also more likely to suffer the consequences of public failure, including ridicule and humiliation, which may also discourage their future involvement in physical activity.[36] 'Humans don't do things they are not successful at,' says Jeff Walkley, Associate Professor in the School of Medical Sciences at RMIT in Melbourne. 'They tend to prove their competence in an area and stick with it, and avoid and reject activities which lead to failure and frustration.'

It can become a vicious circle. Poor skills may lead to low levels of activity, which lead to weight gain, which discourages activity, which reduces the opportunity to improve skill levels. Studies suggest that many Australian children are trapped in this unhealthy cycle.[37] A 1997 study of NSW primary and high school students found that, with the exception of one skill, no more than 40 per cent of students were proficient in all aspects of any of the skills that were assessed. Boys generally performed better than girls.

Girls may benefit if they get some extra attention from parents, coaches or teachers on their skills and confidence.[38] Such help might be particularly useful for adolescent girls. 'Even small increases in skill proficiency could increase adolescent girls' participation in organised physical activity,' says Dr Tony Okley, from the University of Wollongong, who is an expert on the link between fundamental movement skills and health.

Once again, parents who force or push their children into learning and practising skills may do more harm than good. Learning how to throw or kick a ball should happen naturally, as part of fun and play.

It is especially important for children who are overweight or unconfident of their physical prowess that this kind of learning happens in a relaxed and encouraging way. One study showing that overweight children were quite aware of their lower levels of movement skills concluded that they need opportunities to learn and master such skills in a supportive environment where parents, teachers and coaches gave them positive and specific feedback and modelling.[39] Making a child learn or practise such skills 'because it will help them lose weight' could just make things worse—by turning activity into an unpleasant chore.

Walking to school

Once upon a time, children walked to school and nobody thought anything of it. These days it takes a great deal of energy, organisation and commitment to arrange it. That, at least, has been the experience of many of those involved in walking school buses, where adults acting as bus drivers and conductors collect children along agreed walking routes to and from school.

The concept has many pluses. It gives parents and children the chance to do some physical activity and to get to know their neighbours and neighbourhood, and it helps build a sense of community. Children learn about road safety and spend some out of school time with friends. Rather than being strapped into a vehicle and removed from the world, they get some adventure and interaction with the environment. They are less likely to observe and absorb their parents' irritability with the traffic or, in extreme cases, road rage. Teachers often say that children who arrive on the walking bus are in a better mood and more ready to concentrate in class than those who have come by car. Some schools notice a reduction in absenteeism and late arrivals.[40]

Walking school buses reduce traffic congestion around schools and can help parents, in the words of researcher Dr

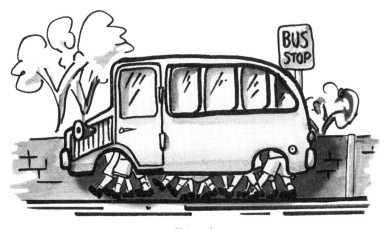

Walking bus

Paul Tranter, escape the 'social traps' that push them into driving children to school to protect them from the traffic dangers created by parents who drive their children to school. They may contribute to safer, more child-friendly neighbourhoods. In the City of Port Phillip in Victoria, the walking school bus led to a pedestrian safety research project after bus volunteers reported that pedestrian lights did not give the walking bus enough time to cross the road.[41]

Those are some of the pluses. On the other hand, many communities have found it difficult to sustain walking school buses. They rely on the motivation and availability of volunteers, and not all schools, local governments or state governments have done enough to support them. Some attempts to establish walking school buses have been stymied by red tape and concerns about liability and safety issues. As well, some researchers criticise the concept, saying it encourages parental paranoia about their children's' safety.[42]

In 2002 and 2003, Associate Professor Jeff Walkley was part of a team which worked hard to establish walking school buses at several primary schools in the City of Whittlesea in Melbourne's northern suburbs. Only about 65 children, out of a possible 4200 children, joined the buses. The project had trouble getting volunteers to run the buses because most parents were working or couldn't spare the time. Many were also concerned about their children's safety. The layout of local streets may have been a deterrent, Walkley says, because parents couldn't keep children in their line of sight from when they left home until the 'bus stop'. However, those children who joined the buses became enthusiasts and reported many benefits.

A study of New Zealand's experience with walking school buses suggests they are most likely to succeed in well-to-do areas. They are least likely to survive in poorer areas, which also tend to have the most to gain from reducing traffic because of their higher rates of child pedestrian injuries. The researchers concluded that walking school buses have limited ability to solve the public health problems arising in car-dominated cities.[43] As ever, there is unlikely to be a single or simple solution for complex problems, like children's inactivity. 'Walking school buses are not for every community,' adds Associate Professor Melissa Wake at the Murdoch Children's Research Institute in Melbourne. 'But where you have the community behind them, it's terrific.'

A number of resources are available to help parents, schools and community organisations establish walking school buses (see Useful Resources). Many models have been developed, for a range of communities and needs.

If you think a walking bus is more than your community could do, you might want to consider setting up occasional or weekly walk-to-school days. Perhaps you could join the International Walk to School Week. In 2004, more than

3 million children, parents and community leaders from 36 countries joined in this project. For more information, go to http://www.iwalktoschool.org.

Several years ago, a health promotion team from the Sydney South West Area Health Service began working with Forest Lodge Primary School in inner-western Sydney, and the local council, Leichhardt Council. At that time, 80 per cent of the school's students lived within 1 kilometre of the school, but 60 per cent were driven to school. Parents told researchers they were reluctant to let their children walk because of safety issues, including footpaths being blocked by cars. The council made changes that reduced such hazards, and within a year, more children were walking to school.

The project has been expanded, and it now incorporates a controlled trial involving 24 primary schools in Sydney's inner west. Half the schools are getting interventions designed to promote walking to school. These include classroom activities mapping where students live and where they can walk, newsletters to parents, and travel access guides showing families how to get to school without a car. A safety audit is also conducted around each school to identify and fix hazards that stop parents letting their children walk to school.

It is too early yet to know the project's impact on the rates of children walking to school, but it gives some hints about what might be useful for parents and schools in other areas. 'All the things we've done could be picked up for use elsewhere,' says Dr Chris Rissel, director of health promotion for the area health service. 'They're all sensible things that can help families and schools, especially the idea of helping parents with travel management. If parents knew how to use public transport themselves, they could teach the kids how to use it.'

The big fat conspiracy

Some schools have found other transport solutions, including an early release from class for children who walk or cycle to school. This gives them 5 to 10 minutes to make a safe getaway and avoid the car crush.

Now that's an incentive for taking an active approach to school.

One school's lesson

A few years ago, Graeme Brims became increasingly concerned by what he was reading, in almost every publication he picked up, about the sedentary lives of modern children. He decided to do something about it. As the principal of a primary school in a disadvantaged part of southwestern Sydney, he felt he had a special responsibility to take action.

At Carramar Public School at Villawood, there are students from more than 40 nationalities, and most come from families where there is no spare cash for extracurricular sport or other such activities.

After consulting with colleagues and parents, Graeme oversaw the introduction of a regular fitness program, in addition to the existing Friday sports afternoon. From 9am until 9.30am every Monday, Tuesday and Wednesday, all students from Kindergarten to Year 6 are involved in activities aimed at getting their bodies pumping. They might do aerobics, dance or a fun run.

Graeme's main motivation was to improve the children's learning rather than their physical fitness. 'There's a lot of research to show that healthy, fit kids learn better,' he says. 'They're much more attentive in class and their concentration spans are longer.'

The school also introduced classroom sessions on healthy eating.

Graeme has noticed an improvement in students' performance—both in sporting competitions and the classroom—and is quick to recommend the program to other school communities. 'I would say it's made a difference,' he says. 'I'm really, really happy with it and so are the parents, teachers and kids. We try and make it fun. It's not like a chore. The kids understand the links between fitness and learning.'

Critical times for encouraging activity

Adolescence

Whether you're talking about dogs, children or horses, the same thing happens when young animals grow up. They become less playful, so they become less active and burn up less energy.

According to Associate Professor Tim Olds, this makes perfect sense when you consider that young animals play in order to develop skills and knowledge of their environment. When they are young, the benefits of play generally outweigh any associated risks, such as predators, injury or straying too far from a protective parent. 'As young animals learn more, they gain less from play but the risk remains the same,' Dr Olds says. 'They reach a tipping point around puberty, where it becomes more sensible, from an evolutionary point of view, to conserve energy.'

Keep that in mind next time you're tempted to label your teenager a sloth. They are just doing what comes naturally at their time of life—sleeping, eating and conserving their energy. Other factors may also be involved, of course—puberty often coincides with the transition to high school and increased demands on children's time, as well as broader attitudinal changes. Running around the school yard is just not cool after a certain age.

Whatever the reason, however, puberty often means the start of inactivity. One Victorian study, which used an instrument to assess activity levels in 5 to 6-year-olds and 10 to 12-year-olds, found a striking difference between the two groups. The younger children spent about 200 minutes a day in moderate activity, including walking, and about 30 minutes in vigorous activity. The older children spent only 100 minutes a day in moderate physical activity, and 20 minutes in vigorous activity.[44]

Other research has reported a 50 per cent decline in physical activity levels between the ages of 6 and 16.[45]

Many parents feel, wrongly, that they have little influence over teenagers, so they shrug their shoulders and give up instead of working out ways to help adolescents develop and maintain active habits. 'Parents harbour a view that what they say doesn't matter to adolescents,' says Trevor Shilton, a physical activity expert at the Heart Foundation. 'That flies in the face of research. What you say as a parent and your permissiveness on issues is absolutely central. The popular image is that peer pressure is a key driver of smoking in adolescence, for instance. It is important, but the most important influence on whether a child smokes is whether their parent smokes, not whether their friends smoke.'

Parents can make a difference by being active themselves and supporting their teenagers to follow suit. But they need to try to see the world from their teenager's viewpoint. Associate Professor Geraldine Naughton is only partly joking when she says that the ideal solution to adolescent inactivity would be a phone that works only when they are walking. Her serious point is that parents need to be creative and responsive to teenagers' interests. She cites the example of a high school which offers girls the opportunity to 'power shop' rather than doing sport. They probably use up more energy walking to the shops, talking and laughing, than they would standing unenthusiastically on a sports field. Asking teenage girls to exercise for hours at a stretch would probably just get groans. But many will happily dance for that long without even looking at their watch.

An Australian study which asked 213 children aged 7 to 17 to rank the benefits of physical activity, provides some useful hints for helping to motivate teenagers. At the top of their lists were the social benefits, including the opportunity to socialise with friends, teamwork and the impact of fitness on other areas of life, including coping and life skills and parents' approval. They also appreciated the sense of achievement, pride, self-esteem, confidence, discipline, enjoyment of challenges and excitement. And they liked how it made them feel physically, including improved strength, sleep and energy levels, and less fatigue. Lastly, they mentioned their improved sport performance and fitness and cognitive benefits, including stress relief, relaxation and having an outlet for aggression, frustration and anger.[46]

All the age groups in the study said they would like to do outdoor games and activities with their parents, and for their parents to encourage them to become involved in physical activities. The teenagers told the researchers that existing PE programs were often boring. They wanted to try new things, such as aerobics, martial arts, yoga, archery, hiking and rock climbing. The girls said they would like female-oriented sports and activities taught by female teachers in private facilities. They suggested having doors on the school showers and changing rooms, and wanted to be able to select the type of sports uniform they wore.

Teenage girls may be particularly vulnerable to inactivity because they are self-conscious about their bodies. Mothers can be particularly influential on the activity levels of teenage girls—research suggests they are important role models in this area. In one study, sporty teenage girls said they were inspired by their mothers being active, and being generally interested in and supportive of activity.[47] Other research suggests that high school girls are more likely than boys to give up activity during winter, which means we need to focus on what they might be interested in doing, physically, during the colder months.[48] Girls from Mediterranean, Asian and Middle Eastern backgrounds may need more—and more carefully targeted—support to be active, as research shows they are more inactive than other teenage girls.[49]

Teenagers in country areas also need special attention. A South Australian study conducted in 1997 found that rural children aged 9 to 12 were significantly fitter than their city counterparts, perhaps because they were more likely to participate in club sport and school PE.[50] These findings contrast with another South Australian study showing that adults living in country areas tended to be heavier than those living in Adelaide. If you put these two sets of results together, it seems that adolescence is a critical time for those living in the country, and they may need extra help to make a healthy transition from childhood to adulthood.

Get with the VERB™

In the United States, health authorities decided to learn from the marketing experts when putting together a campaign to encourage activity in the so-called tweens set (kids aged about 9 to 13). They knew that this was the time when children began to be more influenced by ideas about what was cool (or not), and were at risk of becoming set in sedentary ways.

The result was VERB, a national campaign, co-ordinated by the Centers for Disease Control and Prevention, that used advertising and social marketing strategies to persuade tweens that it is both fun and cool to be active. Just like product marketers, the campaign's organisers did market research when developing their 'brand'. This found that tweens would respond positively to messages encouraging them to explore and discover physical activities that are fun, occur in a socially inclusive environment, and that emphasise self-esteem and belonging to their peer group.

The campaign, based on the active properties of verbs, included resources and hints for parents, teachers and relevant organisations. Tweens also have their own website with cool active characters and games. Here are some of VERB's tips for teachers:

• Have students name a VERB or action they would like to try for the first time, and help them develop a plan to make it happen.

• Ask students to get into groups and invent a new game by combining aspects of different sports, dances, or games. Then have each group teach the class how to do the new activity.

• At the start of class have students take a quick stretch break or do a VERB or action. The break helps rejuvenate the students and is a great opportunity to learn about different muscles—and VERBs.

• Set a project researching how different cultural groups play games or sports, and

- Have the class draw up a map of free or affordable activities in the area to share with the students' families.

Sadly, it seems unlikely that VERB will be extended beyond its first five years, and experts have bemoaned the likely demise of a 'well-designed and effective program'.[51] Unfortunately this is a familiar story the world over. Just because a program is effective, doesn't mean it will last. But you can still get plenty of tips from the VERB websites:
http://www.VERBnow.com, or
http://www.cdc.gov/youthcampaign/

After school

If you want a quick test for whether a child is being active enough, find out how they spend the time between finishing school and dinner. If they're slumped in front of the TV or computer, the odds are not in their favour.

Many experts say the after-school hours are a critical window of opportunity for influencing children's activity. 'What they do then is one of the distinguishing features between the active and inactive kids,' says Boyd Swinburn, Professor of Population Health at Deakin University in Victoria. The Australian Sports Commission says 3pm to 6pm is 'perhaps the single most important time' for increasing movement and stopping sedentary behaviour.

Of course this presents a dilemma for the many working parents who can't be at home to influence their children's behaviour during these hours. And for all the other parents who are flat out with chores such as looking after younger children or preparing dinner, and also can't help their kids make the most of this time.

But even some simple strategies might help:

• If you are home after school, prompt the kids to be active: make sure the TV is kept switched off, or pull out the games box, or invite friends over to play, for example. One study, of Year 5 students in western Sydney, found that about 40 per cent did not receive any prompt to be active after school.[52]

• Set up a roster with other parents to give children the opportunity for supervised play, whether at a park or at each other's places.

• Consider enrolling your child in after school care.

• Encourage after school care services to provide plenty of opportunities for active play if they are not already doing so.

• Some parents may be able to arrange greater flexibility in their working arrangements so that one parent can be home some days after school for at least some days of the week.

Children's best friend

Some people say there are just three types of people in the world: dog people, cat people and the rest. Dog people know there are just two types: themselves and those sad others.

So I'd better declare my interest here. Every morning, two sets of beautiful brown eyes fix themselves firmly upon me and do not let up until they've got what they want: their morning walk. Who needs a personal trainer when dogs will do the job just fine?

Of course dogs are not for everyone, but there are plenty of public health experts ready to sing their praises. Several years ago, an authoritative publication known as *The Medical Journal of Australia* published a study suggesting that a campaign to encourage dog owners to walk their dogs more often could save millions of dollars in health care costs by reducing the need for heart disease treatment.

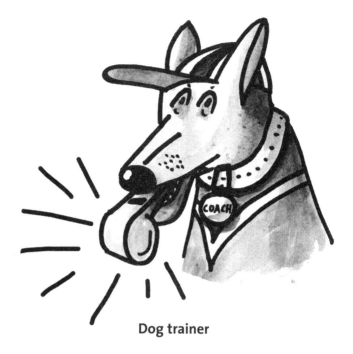

Dog trainer

The most unusual aspect of the study—apart from the proliferation of puns such as 'this report cuts to the bone and unleashes an incisive public health argument for increasing dog walking'—was the species of one of its authors. Shroeder J. Russell, a 'canine walking advocate', was listed as the second author on the paper, after his owner, public health expert Professor Adrian Bauman.[53] 'It's one of my most cited papers,' says Bauman, who now has two Jack Russells. They ensure that he rarely misses his daily walk.

Bauman, like many other public health experts, believes dogs can play an important role in encouraging families and children to be more active. It is his top suggestion for parents wondering how to bring more activity into their family's lives. 'Walking is an adult thing that bores kids,' he says, 'but walking the dog is a family thing.'

Dogs make walking a more interesting experience for young children and have also been shown to encourage teenage girls to walk more, he says. Victorian research shows that 10 to 12-year-old girls were more likely to be active if they had a dog, perhaps because it helped alleviate safety concerns about them walking the streets.[54]

'People often ring the Heart Foundation and ask me what kind of exercise equipment I recommend,' says Trevor Shilton. 'Exercise equipment is probably the leading item in people's garage sales. You get it and use it for a week and never use it again. I always say "Do you have a dog?" Second question, "Does it have a leash?"'

'It's funny how people will always take their dog for a walk because it's good for the dog, and they don't fully appreciate how good it is for them and their family.'

Walking the dog is not only good for physical health; it can also have social and psychological benefits. A Perth study found that pet owners were more likely to interact with neighbours, to be involved in their local community and to describe their neighbourhood as friendly. They were also more likely to rate their health as excellent or very good and less likely to feel lonely.[55]

Children learn about responsibility and nurturing when caring for animals. Pets also give them companionship, affection and a playmate.[56] One study of primary school children found many ranked their relationships with pets as more important than some of their relationships with humans.[57]

Even devotees admit that dogs are no miracle solution. They involve care and commitment. Some breeds are more demanding than others. Not all dogs and breeds make suitable family pets, and far too many children are injured by dogs each year.

And there's nothing sadder than a pooch deprived of regular exercise. Adrian Bauman's study found that 59 per cent of dog owners did not walk their mutts. There's no point contemplating a dog for the family unless you're prepared to walk the walk.

Nor are dogs' many merits universally appreciated. Virginia Jackson, a town planner at the Melbourne firm of Harlock Jackson, believes local government and planning authorities need to do more to create dog-friendly neighbourhoods. Many new housing developments make it almost impossible for dogs (and therefore also their owners) to be active, she says. She cites one new, fast-growing development in outer Melbourne which does not have a single off-lead area for dogs. 'We can't even get it right when we are building new suburbs on the urban fringe,' says Jackson. 'Dog owners are not regarded as legitimate users of open spaces. Town planners just don't seem to think that planning for dogs is an issue anyone needs to think about.'

But Jackson is doing her bit to make cities and suburbs more dog-friendly. She is writing animal management stratcgies for councils, and has developed pet-friendly urban design guidelines (available at http://www.petnet.com.au) as well as some guidelines to promote the integration of dogs into public open space. She knows from her own personal experience just how helpful a dog can be to a family's health. 'With all the concerns about stranger danger, parents might actually be happier letting their kids play or walk outside if they have a dog with them,' she says. 'I am starting to let my 10-year-old walk half a kilometre to the milk bar, but I insist she takes my mobile phone and the dog with her.'

Did I mention the other reason dogs are so much better than your average walking machine? They don't just motivate you to walk every day; they also reward you with love and laughs.

Learning from Australia's beef capital

The bull statues dotted around Rockhampton are symbolic, and not only because the central Queensland town likes to be known as the beef capital of Australia. Many locals are themselves, to put it bluntly, a bit beefy—carrying more weight than is good for their health. But in public health circles, Rockhampton has recently developed quite another sort of reputation. It is now rather famous as the setting for a large-scale experiment—using the entire town as a laboratory—which tested the power of the pedometer.

Vets, hairdressers, community groups, employers, GPs and other health professionals and local media outlets and identities were enlisted in the campaign to encourage locals to take 10,000 steps each day. This is equivalent to about 8 kilometres or 100 minutes of walking—and it's about 30 minutes more walking than most people do each day—and is considered the level of activity needed to reap health benefits.

Hundreds of pedometers, which are small devices attached to a belt to count the number of steps you take, were distributed to help motivate locals as well as to monitor their progress, while a media campaign helped raise awareness about the health benefits of physical activity. The project—funded by the Queensland Government and carried out by researchers at the University of Queensland and Central Queensland University—also involved environmental changes, such as improvements to footpaths, to make walking more appealing.

An evaluation of the 2 year project compared trends in activity levels between 2001 and 2003 in Rockhampton and Mackay, the city used as a control.[58] It identified some measurable benefits, especially for women:

• In 2001, 48.3 per cent of residents in Mackay were physically active, compared with 41.9 per cent in Rockhampton. Two years later, 41.9 per cent of Mackay residents were active, compared with 42.8 per cent of Rockhampton people. The campaign appears to have stopped the fall in activity levels which happened elsewhere.

• Between 2001 and 2003, the proportion of women in Rockhampton who were active rose from 35.8 per cent to 40.8 per cent, while in Mackay the proportion of women who were active fell from 47.1 per cent to 43.1 per cent. The increase in women's activity in Rockhampton was not quite statistically significant so it may have been a chance finding or statistical aberration. However, the study's other findings suggest that it was a real increase.

• Between 2001 and 2003, the proportion of men who were active in Mackay fell from 49.6 per cent to 40.7 per cent. The decline was smaller in Rockhampton: from 49 per cent to 44.8 per cent.

• In 2003, 18 per cent of the Rockhampton residents who were surveyed said they had used a pedometer in the last 18 months, compared with 5.6 per cent of those in Mackay.

For all the effort involved, the changes may seem modest. But they sound more impressive when you consider all the forces encouraging people to be sedentary—and remember that the study was able to achieve increases, for women at least, at a time when activity levels across Australia were declining.

Wendy Brown, Professor of Physical Activity and Health at the University of Queensland and chief investigator on the Rocky project, also cites research showing that every 1 per cent increase in physical activity is estimated to prevent 122 deaths from heart disease, non insulin-dependent diabetes and colon cancer each year—and save about $3.6 million in direct health care costs.

The Rockhampton experience suggests that pedometers can be useful for getting people walking. Even some of the athletic types involved in running the project were shocked when they put on a pedometer and discovered how few steps they did some days.

Many schools and families everywhere have found pedometers a fun tool for motivating and monitoring activity. Recommendations for how many steps children should do each day vary. One guide says that children aged 8 to 10 should aim for 12,000 to 16,000 steps and that adolescents and healthy young adults should walk between 7000 and 13,000 steps each day. Others believe that rather than making a blanket set of recommendations for all children, it is more helpful for each child to set an individual goal.

Pedometers have also been used successfully to boost activity among obese children and adults. In one study, young people in Brisbane were given a pedometer to evaluate their baseline levels of activity and were then were helped to set a goal of increasing their steps over the following fortnight. Their parents were also given pedometers and encouraged to do the same. During the 10 weeks of the program, the children increased their daily step count by an average of 36 per cent. The researchers concluded that a home-based activity program incorporating positive reinforcement, parental support, problem solving and self-monitoring via a pedometer could increase physical activity among obese youth.

Pedometers are now widely available and are relatively inexpensive. Another option when you're looking for an active gift, perhaps? If they help keep children moving in the years after those celebrated first steps, they might be worth a try.

11. How to tell if your child is overweight... and what to do about it

How does your child measure up?

Parents often find it hard to acknowledge that their child is overweight. This has been found in many studies. In one case, Australian researchers found that about half the parents of obese children thought their children were of a normal weight or even underweight.[1] Parents may be in denial, perhaps conscious of their own weight or lifestyle issues. They might think their son or daughter must be OK because they are about the same size as their friends. They may be concerned, quite rightly, that making children weight-conscious is not a good idea. Or they might think a bit of puppy fat is just a passing phase and nothing to worry about. That might have been the case in generations past, when chubby children probably had a much greater chance of growing out of their plumpness. But these days, the big fat conspiracy ensures that many overweight children will grow into overweight adults, with all the risks that brings for their health and wellbeing.

It can be difficult to tell whether or not someone is at a healthy weight. Adults are not good at judging themselves either, and sometimes think they are closer to a healthy weight than they really are. Overweight men are particularly likely to do this. Indeed, one Australian study found that 43 per cent of overweight or obese male university students were satisfied with their body size; some even wanted to be bigger. The same study also found that most underweight women were either satisfied with their body size or wanted to be even slimmer.[2]

It is even more difficult to judge weight in children, whose bodies grow and change rapidly. It is not always easy to distinguish between weight gain that accompanies normal growth and weight gain that should be cause for concern. Dr Michele Campbell, a paediatrician and researcher at the Murdoch Children's Research Institute at the Royal Children's Hospital in Victoria, says even paediatricians, nurses and obesity researchers like herself can get it wrong when they simply 'eyeball' a child to judge their weight. Parents also interpret their children's weight differently according to gender; Dr Campbell's research shows parents are more likely to be concerned if a daughter is overweight. It is sometimes seen as an advantage for a boy to be big.

This chapter gives some pointers on how to tell the difference between weight gain that is healthy and weight gain that may be a health risk. It also offers some suggestions about what to do if the warning bells are ringing.

Understanding normal growth and development

We come in different shapes and sizes. Thank goodness. What a boring world it would be if we didn't. Our aim should not be to strive for some ideal body but to respect and celebrate individual differences. A whole range of shapes and sizes fall within the range of healthy growth and development. Some children will be tall and wiry; others will not. And girls and boys, it need hardly be said, follow different paths along the growth track.

Infants

Fat cells can be found in the developing foetus from about the 14th week of gestation. In a newborn, fat accounts for about 13 per cent of the baby's body mass. It is perfectly normal for babies to look chubby. By the end of their first year, babies are typically about 28 per cent fat.[3] About the time of weaning they begin a trend towards leanness.

Early childhood

In the 3–5 years following a baby's first birthday, the proportion of body fat declines.[4] Dr Michele Campbell says many parents become anxious at this stage, worried that their child might not be eating enough. 'It's important for parents to know that slimming down in preschool is normal,' she says.

Between the ages of about 4 and 6, children reach what is known as 'adiposity rebound', a point where growth patterns switch. 'Adipose' is a medical term for fat. At adiposity rebound, children typically move from getting thinner into a stage of getting fatter again. This stage usually lasts until around puberty. If a child's body mass index (BMI: see below for more on this) is regularly charted, it will typically show a dip around the time of starting school. The point where the BMI bottoms out and then starts to steadily increase again is the point of adiposity rebound.

A number of studies have shown that children who reach adiposity rebound early (younger than other children) are more likely to become obese in later childhood and adolescence—regardless of whether they were lean or fat before that point. It is not clear why this might be so and it may not be a simple matter of cause and effect. It might reflect another one of those circular chains: that children who are genetically predisposed to obesity mature earlier as a result of being heavier and then go on to be fatter in adolescence. Alternatively, some experts believe the association might indicate that the effects of behaviours learnt earlier in childhood—around eating and activity, for example—are becoming apparent at about the time of adiposity rebound. Some research also suggests that an early adipose rebound may be more likely in children exposed to the effects of their mother's gestational diabetes while still in the womb.[5]

The difference between the genders begins well before puberty. Girls as young as 4 tend to have a higher proportion of body fat than boys, even when you are comparing boys and girls of similar age, height weight and BMI.[6]

Puberty and adolescence

After growing steadily through their primary school years, children usually hit a growth spurt about the time of puberty. This is associated with significant changes in body composition. The adolescent growth spurt typically begins around age 10 or 11 for girls and 12 to 13 in boys. During this stage, boys gain an average of 20 centimetres in height and 20 kilograms in weight, and girls typically gain around 16 centimetres in height and 16 kilograms.[7]

Girls are reaching menarche (their first period) at younger and younger ages. This is probably due to improvements in living standards, and it is thought to be an important factor contributing to overweight—the younger girls are at menarche, the greater their risk of being overweight later on. By the time of menarche, girls are already about 95 per cent of their height.

The difference between girls' and boys' bodies really becomes obvious during adolescence. Girls are programmed for curves; boys are more linear. In girls, body fat typically accounts for about 17 per cent of body mass at the start of adolescence and about 24 per cent by its end. Boys tend to put on weight later in puberty and it mainly reflects an increase in their lean body mass.[8] While boys' body fat typically declines during adolescence, it tends to become more concentrated around their middle.[9]

Adolescence is one of the periods when people are most likely to gain excess weight that they then can't lose.[10] One review estimated that almost a third of obese adults became obese during adolescence.[11]

The body mass index (BMI)

It's not surprising that parents have such difficulty knowing when children are overweight or obese—the experts have trouble drawing that line themselves. As mentioned in Chapter 4, the BMI is generally accepted as the best tool for assessing overweight and obesity. It is calculated by dividing weight (kg) by height squared (m^2). BMI charts for children use cut-off scores that take stages of growth and development into account.

But it's always sensible to be cautious about what a test result actually means, and this is especially the case with using BMI charts for children.

In adults, studies have helped establish when a BMI is likely to signal an increased risk of health problems. An adult with a BMI of 25 to 30 is overweight, and a BMI of above 30 signals obesity. The same degree of precision cannot be used for children because there are no large, long-term studies that establish what level of BMI in what age child signals an increased risk of health problems in later life. As you might imagine, these studies would be expensive and take decades. So the BMI cut-offs used to signal overweight and obesity in children are rather arbitrary. They are based on experts' best guesses about what is appropriate rather than on hard evidence.

As well, the BMI reflects a person's weight rather than their degree of fatness; two children with the same BMI may have quite different levels of fatness. One may be tubby around the tummy (which is of particular concern) and the other may be solidly muscular. Using the BMI charts may result in some overweight children being wrongly classified as of normal weight, but very few children would be classified as overweight if they were not.[12] BMI charts may be less reliable in children or adolescents who are particularly short or tall for their age or whose body fat is distributed unusually.

And then there's the fact that the BMI charts recommended for use in Australia are not based on studies of Australian children. They were developed by the Centers for Disease Control in the United States. If there are any significant differences between the growth trends of Australian and North American children, they will not be reflected in the charts.

This may be an issue for Aboriginal and Torres Strait Islander children, whose growth patterns have not been clearly defined by research. The BMI charts may also be less relevant for children with Asian, Pacific Islander and other non-Caucasian backgrounds.

Having said all that, the BMI charts are the best available tool for monitoring children's growth and weight gain (an on-line calculator for determining children's BMI has been developed by NSW Health at: http://www.health.nsw.gov.au/obesity/youth/bmi.html). Children's waist size is another good indicator, especially because fat around the middle seems to carry more of a health risk than fat elsewhere. Again, however, there are not reliable figures to indicate which waist size should trigger alarm bells.

The National Health and Medical Research Council has recommended that children's height and weight should be measured at least twice a year as part of routine care by their family doctor[13]. This is important for plotting trends and for detecting any sudden upswings in BMI.

In practice, however, you can't assume that this will automatically happen. Researchers have found that few GPs routinely weigh and measure the children they see in their practice or calculate their BMI.[14] Many do not even have the equipment to precisely chart changes in a child's BMI over time. The researchers concluded that this National Health and Medical Research Council recommendation seems to be a 'pipe dream' at the moment. And not all experts are convinced it is a good idea anyway, given uncertainty about the impact of this sort of clinical focus on overweight children. 'There is no evidence yet to support the idea that intervening with these kids clinically does more good than harm,' says Dr Melissa

Wake, of the Murdoch Children's Research Institute in Melbourne.

If parents are concerned about their children's weight, they may need to raise the issue themselves with their family doctor. It is best to do this in a way that does not make your child self-conscious about their weight—perhaps discuss it with the doctor before bringing your child to the surgery.

Of course a BMI is easy enough to calculate yourself, but whether parents should monitor their children's BMI is a vexed question. Certainly they should understand the BMI and have an idea where their child fits on the charts. But some experts worry that encouraging parents to monitor children's BMI at home might foster an unhealthy focus on weight which could, in the long term, be counterproductive. Children who worry about their weight and diet or restrict their food intake are more likely to end up with weight problems. 'I don't want parents measuring and plotting the child on the charts,' says Sydney specialist Professor Louise Baur. 'That is a recipe for encouraging labelling of children as overweight.'

Warning signs and children at increased risk

The best way to understand a child's BMI is generally to look at several measurements over time rather than one measurement. This lets you monitor how the child's growth and development is going, in comparison with what might be expected.

How you interpret a child's BMI depends on many things. A BMI suggesting obesity is, of course, of greater concern than a BMI suggesting overweight. And a child who is overweight but whose BMI is consistent over time is less cause for concern than an overweight child whose BMI shows a marked increase.

Excess weight in a preschooler is generally less worrying than excess weight in a teenager. Then again, a young child who is overweight and whose parents are obese and have family histories of diabetes may arouse more concerns than an overweight teenager who is fit and whose parents are both active and healthy.

So many factors have to be weighed up. Here are some:

Family history

Children are more likely to carry too much weight if their parents or siblings do. Obesity is more likely to present health problems for children if there is a family history of type 2 diabetes or heart disease.

Some ethnic groups

Aboriginal and Torres Strait Islander children, and those from Middle Eastern and Mediterranean backgrounds, are more likely to develop excess weight.

Preschool years

Children typically lose fat in the years before the adiposity rebound (which is usually sometime between 4 and 6). Children who become fatter in the years before adiposity rebound are probably at increased risk of significant and persistent obesity.[15]

Early developers

Children who reach adiposity rebound early, or who reach puberty early, are at greater risk of significant weight gain. Because overweight children are often tall for their age, it can be difficult to determine their degree of fatness by just looking at them.[16] Studies of children who became overweight have found that they tended to grow upwards at about the same time as they grew outwards.[17]

Adolescence

Adolescents who carry too much weight are at risk of becoming overweight or obese adults.[18]

When overweight is a sign of an underlying medical problem

These days, most children who gain excess weight are simply responding naturally to the obesogenic environment. For a small proportion, however, it can be a sign of an underlying medical issue:

• A number of medications have weight gain as a side effect. These include glucocorticosteroids, which are used to treat kidney disorders, juvenile rheumatoid arthritis, inflammatory bowel disease, chronic severe asthma and other inflammatory diseases. Some drugs used to treat psychiatric disorders and epilepsy can also cause weight gain, as can treatment for acute lymphatic leukaemia.[19]

• Adolescents with type 1 diabetes often gain weight, especially if their diabetes is not well controlled and they have unstable blood glucose and use high doses of insulin.

• Children with physical disabilities or mild learning difficulties may be more susceptible to weight gain.

• A number of endocrine disorders are associated with childhood obesity. They include hypothyroidism associated with thyroid enlargement, Cushing's disease and Cushing's syndrome, growth hormone deficiency, growth hormone resistance and some forms of rickets.[20]

• The National Health and Medical Research Council says obesity features in a number of rare congenital syndromes. It recommends that children who are obese, intellectually disabled and who have multiple physical abnormalities should be assessed by a paediatrician, an endocrinologist and/or a geneticist. Children with the Prader-Wili syndrome, which is caused by a chromosomal abnormality, have an insatiable appetite which is extremely difficult for clinicians and families to manage.[21]

...and what to do about it

When and where to get help

This is truly a tricky issue, for several reasons. With any intervention—no matter how well meaning—there is always the potential to do harm as well as good. When to seek professional help depends to a large extent on a child's age and situation. If other family members are obese or suffer problems such as diabetes, that's a good indication that it might be worth seeking professional help sooner rather than later.

The National Health and Medical Research Council recommends that children and adolescents with a BMI showing they are overweight or obese should be considered for intervention, especially if they are suffering from problems related to their weight. If their BMI is borderline, they should be reviewed over a 6 month period before any decision is made about intervening.

But intervention must be carefully managed; it can make a child self-conscious, which can be counterproductive at a number of levels. It would be particularly worrying if it made them feel rotten about themselves or led to rigid dietary controls—these could send the child into the vicious circle of disordered eating habits, and could also harm their growth and development.[22]

And it must also be remembered that not all overweight children become overweight adults. Seeking professional help for every overweight child would result in an unnecessary focus on some children who will simply grow into a healthy weight as they get older. On the other hand, there is some evidence that weight management is more successful in children than in adults, so it makes sense to tackle the problem early in the children who are most likely to benefit. Some experts also argue that early intervention is most likely to be effective because the family has greater influence over the child's behaviour in the years before adolescence.[23] 'The beauty of working with children is that you can usually change their trajectory to overweight a lot more easily than [you can] with adults,' says Dr Zoe McCallum, a paediatrician at the Centre for Community Child Health at the Royal Children's Hospital in Melbourne. 'We're all set in our ways as we get older, but certainly if you work with a family with children at a preschool age, you can really change some behaviour patterns.'

Again it comes back to assessing an individual child's risk. The authors of one US study cautioned against intervening with obese children under the age of 3 if their parents were not obese, because these children were not at high risk of being obese later on. By contrast, the study found that 1 and 2-year-olds who were obese were also more likely to be obese as young adults if they had at least one obese parent.[24]

Many studies have shown that health professionals, like other people, often have negative attitudes towards people who are overweight or obese.[25] Dr Zoe McCallum says it is probably no coincidence that obese adults with the lowest self-esteem have often had the most interaction with the health system. 'Health professionals often don't do this very well, particularly if they come from what I call "the skinny person bias",' she says. 'In other words, they lack comprehension and empathy about how difficult it is to remain at a healthy weight in this environment.'

When you seek professional help, you and your family are entitled to feel comfortable and supported. The process may involve some challenging moments—including some re-examination of family attitudes and behaviours—but you have a right to be treated with respect and compassion. If you do not feel this is happening, find another health professional or service. Just don't let one bad experience stop you trying to make changes or find help.

With young children, it is generally agreed that the best approach is to work through the parents. Apart from regularly assessing the child, the most benefit comes from engaging parents in therapy aimed at changing the family's lifestyle and environment. Engaging young children in treatment may simply make them anxious. The situation is a little different for adolescents. The National Health and Medical Research Council recommends that both they and their parents be involved in treatment. Parents and adolescents should attend consultations together and separately. Dr Zoe McCallum says taking a 'solution-focused approach' can work well. This involves the therapist talking through (with the parents or the adolescent) what changes they think might work, as well as what hasn't worked in the past. This is a meaningful conversation, and is more productive than the health professional simply giving instructions about what the client should do, she says.

It's important to be realistic about what treatment can achieve, too. Many children who are moderately overweight will be able to grow into their weight with only minor modifications to the family lifestyle. Keeping these children at the same weight while they grow taller will lead to reductions in their BMI. But for more serious weight problems, quick solutions are unlikely. If that is what is promised, you are unlikely to be disappointed. Managing obesity usually requires a long-term commitment and has been shown to bring 'modest success' for children and adolescents in the medium to long term.[26] For some children and adolescents, the goal of treatment will be to relieve any associated symptoms and to ensure the best quality of life possible. Many obese children and adolescents never reach an optimum BMI; they can be helped, however, to have a healthy and active lifestyle and to feel good about themselves. The National Health and Medical Research Council guidelines note that fat loss is not the only goal of treatment—it is also important to monitor children's emotional and psychological wellbeing.

The main tools of treatment are those described in Chapters 5 to 9. These include changing the family's behaviours and environment so it is easy for all family members to be active each day (including decreasing sedentary activities such as TV watching) and enjoying a healthy diet. Many medical reviews have noted the lack of evidence about which of these approaches is the most effective for managing overweight in children and adolescents.[27] It also depends on the individual family's situation: some may find it easier to alter their diet; others may find it easier to build more physical activity into their life. Professor Louise Baur says it is important that the approach is appropriate for the age of the child. 'We would deal with a 4-year-old very differently from a teenager,' she says.

Finding ways to increase activity levels in seriously overweight children can be a challenge, particularly because of the discomfort—chafing, sweating, heat rashes and breathlessness—that they often experience with exercise. It is particularly important with these children to find activities that they enjoy and can sustain. They may need extra help as they build the skills and confidence to participate. Be patient; this may take time. The National Health and Medical Research Council guidelines say overweight children and adolescents are more likely to continue with lifestyle exercises (such as games, swimming, dance and cycling) than with programmed aerobic exercise. Competitive sport may be inappropriate and may only exacerbate any psychological or social problems. Children should be given positive reinforcement for participating in physical activities. But try not to measure their success according to whether they have lost weight. Instead, praise their improved skills or acknowledge their changes in behaviour.

In extreme cases, where a child's health is seriously compromised by their weight, more extreme approaches to treatment may be needed, including very low energy diets. The National Health and Medical Research Council says this should only be attempted in a tertiary institution and under the care of a specialist multidisciplinary team. For adolescents in this situation, the Council says drug therapy or surgery may be worth considering. However, such treatments should be used only as a last resort and with great caution.

Another reason why the treatment issue is so tricky is the desperate shortage of services available to help the families of overweight children. In an ideal world, families would have an expert medical assessment followed by numerous consultations with a dietitian, psychologist and exercise physiologist, as needed, to provide ongoing advice and support, says Professor Louise Baur. In the real world, most families do not have access to this range of services. And even if they were available where and when families needed them, the cost would probably be prohibitive.

This lack of appropriate treatment services is yet another reason why prevention is by far the best approach. For many families, though, the horse has already bolted; they need help to try to stop it becoming even more of a problem.

Finding the most appropriate source of help for your family may take some research and effort. If at first you don't succeed, don't give up. Don't be tempted to try clinics offering quick fixes (more of that in the section on 'dieting dangers'). Here are some ideas for where to find help:

General practitioners (GPs)

GPs are often described as the cornerstone of the health system, because they are in a unique position to assess patients' needs, to provide ongoing primary care and to refer them to other services where necessary. Many obesity experts believe GPs are ideally placed to act as the frontline troops in managing and preventing childhood weight problems. They also have an important role in managing medical problems associated with obesity, such as checking for early warning signs of diabetes. The National Health and Medical Research Council has published guidelines to support GPs in managing obesity in children and adolescents. These are freely available on the internet and provide useful advice for families as well.

Many GPs, however, have not been trained in how to manage weight problems generally, let alone in children. Many do not feel confident about their skills in this area and are unsure of whether or how to raise the issue with patients. Some, no doubt, don't particularly want to get involved. They can find it confronting, time consuming and frustrating. Many GPs already feel overburdened with all the other problems they are expected to manage, and have little time or energy to be proactive about children's weight.

Dr Louise Roufeil, program director with the NSW Central West Division of General Practice, has conducted research asking people in her region about what they would do if their child was obese. Many do not even think of seeing their GP; they see weight as a problem which they have to solve themselves. 'My concern is that people don't see a role for health professionals, and that dovetails with what we know about health professionals not feeling comfortable to intervene,' Dr Roufeil says.

But many people will find it difficult to make the necessary changes without professional support. Try to find a GP who is willing and able to engage with you and your family. If weight is a family problem, you may also need help from allied health professionals such as a dietitian, psychologist or exercise physiologist. Ideally, your GP should be linked into these networks so they can all work together to support your family in making change.

If you have trouble finding a suitable GP, ask around. Specialist childhood obesity clinics at children's hospitals or your local Division of General Practice may be able to give you some recommendations. So might dietitians or other allied health professionals.

Step by step[28]

The National Health and Medical Research Council recommends that GPs take a step-by-step approach to assessing and managing weight problems in children. The steps include:

1. Assess extent of overweight or obesity in the child or adolescent relative to their stage of development. Measure their height, weight and waist circumference and pubertal stage.

2. Assess health complications associated with weight and treat these independently where appropriate.

3. Assess why and how energy imbalance has occurred.

4. Determine the level of clinical intervention required.

5. Devise treatment strategy with the patient and family.

6. Devise treatment goals, including ones unrelated to weight.

7. Review and provide regular assistance for weight management and maintenance of weight change.

8. Change program as required.

Dietitians

Dietitians can identify problems in the family's shopping and eating habits, and help you work out some strategies to fix them. However, it can be difficult to access dietitians. Those in public health services are often overloaded and have long waiting lists. Some families may not be able to afford those in the private sector. And private dietitians are scarce in some areas. In New South Wales, for instance, two-thirds of the dietitians who specialise in weight management are in northern, central or southeastern Sydney[29]. People living in outer suburban, rural, remote or regional areas may have to travel to find help.

For help in finding a dietitian, contact the Dietitians Association of Australia or ask your local GP or Division of General Practice for a recommendation.

Psychologists and other behavioural therapists

Changing entrenched patterns of behaviour and dealing with complex issues of family dynamics can be extremely challenging. Working with a professional can be confronting, but it can also help make the change process easier and more effective. There are many techniques, including cognitive behavioural therapy and solution-focused coaching. Again, cost is sometimes an issue, because most people will not be able to access these sorts of services through the public system.

Contact the Australian Psychological Society if you need help finding an appropriate therapist. Or ask your GP or local Division of General Practice for a recommendation.

Specialist weight management clinics for children and adolescents

These services are usually based in children's hospitals or other teaching hospitals. They are in short supply and great demand, and it is not uncommon for families to wait more than a year to be seen.

These clinics have the great advantage of involving a multidisciplinary team. But if you do not live close to such a service and are put off by the long wait, ask your GP if there are any other options available. Your GP or the Paediatrics Division of the Royal Australasian College of Physicians may know of other specialists who could help.

The National Health and Medical Research Council recommends that children with severe and early onset obesity should be referred for specialist assessment. Children whose obesity is suspected to be the result of a medical problem should also see a specialist.

Community health centres

Community health centres provide another option for treatment, but not every area has one. Your state or territory Department of Health or local Division of General Practice should know what services are available in your area.

Universities and researchers

Another way to get help might be through a study or trial testing various treatment approaches. Check with local universities and hospitals; you may be able to leave your details for future reference if nothing is immediately available.

By now something important has no doubt become obvious: despite all the political and professional rhetoric about the perils of childhood obesity, there is remarkably little support available to help families grappling with these issues. Perhaps Dr Louise Roufeil's finding—that parents believe they have to find the solutions themselves—is not so surprising after all. One way parents could help themselves (and others) is by becoming advocates and lobbying politicians and bureaucrats for better services. More on that in Chapter 13.

Mind your focus
Focus on the family, not the child

Weight management is far more likely to be effective if the whole family is involved. The family environment has a powerful influence on a child's weight.

Singling out the overweight or obese child is a recipe for trouble. First, children have little control over their environment. It is unfair and unproductive to expect an individual child to change their ways when the rest of the family is not. 'How can you expect a child to enjoy their vegies if Mum and Dad don't enjoy theirs?' says Dr Janet Warren, Senior Research Dietitian at the University of Newcastle in New South Wales. 'How can you expect a child to be physically active when they get home if the rest of the family sits around watching TV?' Professor Louise Baur says every family member who buys and prepares food, including grandparents or other carers, needs to be involved in the change process.

Making the individual child the focus of attention also risks making them self-conscious and resentful. It can encourage victim-blaming attitudes in the family.

Adolescents can take more responsibility for their environment and behaviour. But they too may be more likely to respond positively to change if everyone in the family is doing it. They may also be more likely to participate if they've had a hand in working out some of the solutions and feel that their concerns are being taken seriously and dealt with. Most people don't like being told what to do; teenagers, like the rest of us, are more likely to do something if they feel some ownership of what's being done.

Focus on healthy eating and activity, not on weight

The overriding goal is for children to be healthy and happy. This is most likely to happen if their family and broader environment make them feel valued and supported and make it easy for them to eat well and be physically active.

Making children and adolescents self-conscious about their weight is a recipe for trouble. It may send their self-esteem plummeting and encourage unhealthy eating patterns which set them up for a lifelong battle with food and weight.

Doctors who specialise in treating obese children often hear parents use negative language, which only compounds their children's problems. Telling children they are 'bad eaters' or 'lazy' won't do anything except make them feel miserable.

When you are making changes to family routines, try not to raise the weight issue. Instead, talk about healthy eating and activity making everyone feel better.

If you focus on healthy eating and activity, everyone benefits. Many family members who do not have a weight problem could also benefit from eating better and moving more.

Dangerous dieting

Now, where shall we start? There are so many reasons to steer clear of dieting. And that's if you're a grown-up. For children and teenagers, dieting is even worse:

• Restricting children's energy intake when their bodies are still growing can adversely affect their growth and development.

• Dieting encourages an unhealthy focus on food and promotes disordered eating patterns. It helps people lose touch with their internal cues for hunger and fullness.

• Dieting often starts a vicious cycle of food restriction and bingeing, which leads to weight gain. Binge eating is implicated in many cases of obesity.[30] It typically begins in late adolescence and is associated with body image dissatisfaction and regular dieting.

• Diets are impossible to sustain—particularly today in Australia, where food is abundant, readily available and relatively affordable.

• Dieting makes eating a painful rather than a pleasurable experience. It makes people feel deprived and miserable. Rather than feeling rotten about eating less, it's far better to focus on eating differently—and enjoying it.

• Parents who diet are encouraging unhealthy eating patterns in their children.

• Dieting reinforces unhealthy concerns about body image.

• Dieting is bad for self-esteem and mental health. When it doesn't work, as always happens, dieters often blame themselves for 'failing' when it is actually the diet that failed them.

• Dieting often restricts the range of foods people eat, making it more difficult to get the full range of nutrients needed for good health.

• And last, but not least, dieting doesn't work. If anything, it is likely to lead to weight gain. If your body feels it is being starved, it will use every physiological trick at its disposal to make the most of the food you do eat. The best way to lose weight and to keep it off is to make permanent changes to your lifestyle. Move more, eat better.

It's no wonder that weight loss guru Garry Egger describes television current affairs shows as 'the most fattening thing in Australia'. 'They are always selling stupid diets,' he says.

Ellyn Satter says diets or restrictive feeding practices for children are, quite simply, a disaster:

I can think of no better way to get a family to fight, or to make a child a scapegoat, than by imposing a weight-reduction diet on a child. We have to reconcile ourselves to children not necessarily being at the weight we might like…We have to stop making kids feel like they will lose all their excess weight if they will only try hard enough. Being so unrealistic with them about their chances of being thinner is not motivating—it is just setting them up again and again for failure. The popular perception that anyone can get thinner if they only want it badly enough and are willing to work on it hard enough is simply not true.[31]

Caveat: Very low energy diets may be helpful for some children and adults with serious obesity. But the National Health and Medical Research Council guidelines stress that these should be administered only under specialist care and supervision. This is a medical treatment—far removed from the 'quick-fix' diets often promoted in the media.

The no-diets doctor

When Rick Kausman graduated from medical school in the late 1980s, he landed a job in a general practice in Melbourne that specialised in weight management. Patients were put on strict diets, told to take appetite suppressants and given long lists of forbidden foods.

It's an approach which is a million miles from how Dr Kausman now works. Over the last 20-odd years, he has listened closely to his patients' stories and learnt from them about what helps and what doesn't.

An advocate of the non-dieting approach to healthy weight management, Dr Kausman says that helping people reach a healthy weight is like trying to put a challenging jigsaw together. 'No two puzzles are exactly the same, but there are common themes,' he says.

Many people make the mistake of trying to complete the puzzle using just two pieces: nutrition and exercise. However, they are only part of a much more complex picture, Dr Kausman says. Other important pieces are people's attitudes to food, themselves and their bodies.

'Eating more slowly is a very important piece of the puzzle,' says Dr Kausman. 'You have to help people understand why they were eating quickly in the first place. One of the reasons is often because they feel guilty—if they feel a food is bad or wrong. There's much more to being a healthy weight than exercising more and eating less. We're at the same place where depression was 15 years ago—where there was this simplistic idea that people should just try harder and think happy thoughts.'

Dr Kausman emphasises the need for families to try changes that are realistic, empowering and sustainable. He jokes: 'I can guarantee to you that I can make you fitter—but it means you are never allowed to go in a car or public transport ever again. You must walk everywhere!

'In theory you might be able to get fitter in this way, but it wouldn't be compatible with normal living. We have to give people ideas and strategies that are possible to manage and achieve in the long term.'

Surgery?

Many people are disturbed by the idea of subjecting young people to surgery as a treatment for obesity. It seems such a drastic measure. Professor Paul O'Brien, Director of the Centre for Obesity Research and Education at Monash University, Victoria, understands such concerns—and in fact shares them.

But he believes that surgery is a valuable option for the small proportion of adolescents who are so severely obese that their health is in serious jeopardy.

For young people with severe obesity, O'Brien says lifestyle modification and drug therapy are rarely effective in the long term. He cites research suggesting that severe obesity at the age of 20 is associated with a 12-year reduction in life expectancy.

'People who get upset when we talk about surgery often don't recognise that severe obesity is such a serious health problem,' says O'Brien.

O'Brien specialises in a gastric banding procedure that involves placing an adjustable silicone band around the top part of the stomach, causing a feeling of fullness. Generally this is done using a minimally invasive surgical technique known as laparoscopy; there is no need for large surgical incisions. The procedure is reversible.

O'Brien has performed the procedure on about 1800 patients, including about 30 people under the age of 20. He is now involved in a randomised controlled trial, together with the Royal Children's Hospital in Melbourne, which aims to evaluate the procedure in adolescents aged 14 to 18.

One half of the group are being randomly allocated to have surgery plus a lifestyle modification program; those in the control group are having only the lifestyle modification program. The study will examine the impact of surgery on the teenagers' weight and quality of life, as well as the costs involved.

O'Brien expects the results will help define the role of surgery in treating obesity in young people. Australia's growing weight problem is already escalating demand for gastric banding surgery, but O'Brien expects adolescents will only ever account for 1–2 per cent of the total caseload.

The National Health and Medical Research Council guidelines say surgery for obesity should be the 'last possible' option for severely obese adolescents with health problems, and undertaken only in an experienced centre after extensive consultation, assessment and education. After the operation, continuing care should be provided by an experienced weight management service.

Handling children's concerns

Children are bombarded by conflicting media messages about their bodies. On the one hand, huge headlines sound the alarm about childhood obesity. On the other hand, so much media imagery promotes the virtue of unrealistically thin figures. It would be surprising if children weren't weight conscious, especially as so many of their parents are also caught in this trap.

All children, overweight or not, can benefit from understanding the role of the media and marketing in promoting unrealistic body images. This may be a fruitful topic for family discussions, which can become more complex as children grow older.

For children who are overweight, the best way to handle their concerns will depend on their age and individual situation. The issue probably does not need to be raised with young children. Studies show that preschoolers are not usually conscious of weight as an issue. Being overweight doesn't seem to affect their self-esteem.

But as children get older, parents need to work out ways to handle weight and related self-esteem issues. Older children and teenagers, particularly girls, are more likely to suffer self-esteem problems related to overweight.

Doctors and others who specialise in treating obese children hear lots of horror stories of bullying. This is likely to be an extreme end of the spectrum: children who end up in treatment may be more likely than the many children who do not end up in treatment to have suffered such problems. Jane Cleary, a clinical dietitian at Wollongong Hospital in New South Wales, says families often seek help for social reasons—because their children are being bullied—rather than for health reasons.

Parents may not always know if their children are being picked on. Weight management experts often hear of children who haven't told their parents about the harassment they suffer. Professor Louise Baur advises parents to talk to their kids about bullying, to explain that some people bully others to make themselves feel better. Help them work on problem-solving skills to deal with bullying. Professor Baur also cautions parents to be aware that it is not only children who may make disparaging comments; it can also be adults. She says this is a reflection of the deeply moralistic views about overweight that are entrenched in our society.

If children have a serious weight problem, parents can help by disentangling the disorder from the child, Professor Baur says. Children who have been labelled as fat may have trouble seeing themselves as anything else. Parents can help them see all their positive characteristics by praising these things. They might be good at art, or good friends. Parents can help create new, more positive labels for their children, Professor Baur says. Parents may be able to help older children develop some problem-solving skills in this area too. Reading this book, for instance, might help them understand the power of the big fat conspiracy and so make it easier for them to deal positively with their situation, rather than sinking into self-blame and destructive behaviour.

Getting adolescents involved in the change process may also help them feel better about themselves. If they are involved in first identifying changes the family could make and then in helping to make these changes happen, they may gain a greater sense of control. And they may also be more motivated to make the changes themselves.

Dr Zoe McCallum says adults are often reluctant to raise the subject of weight with overweight children, though older children will almost certainly be aware of it. 'I've never had a consultation with a teenager who didn't acknowledge they were concerned about the issue themselves and were happy to have it followed up,' she says.

How you handle your children's concerns about their weight will also depend on your relationship. If you are in the habit of discussing big issues openly and frankly, you'll probably be OK. If your relationship is difficult at the best of times, it could be worth trying to enlist the help of some other influential adults, such as grandparents or neighbours.

Be careful with the language you use: it could make all the difference to how children respond. Careless or critical language may only make them more worried. One medical text recommends talking about weight rather than 'fatness' or 'obesity'—these words may be upsetting or offensive.[32] You may also need to examine your own attitudes. Some parents, perhaps without even realising it, express society's negative attitudes towards overweight. Jane Cleary says parents need to make sure that bullying and teasing do not happen in the home. 'The home needs to provide a supportive environment; it needs to be a safe haven for the child,' she says.

Ellyn Satter says that obesity can in many ways be viewed as a handicapping condition. 'However, unlike other handicapping conditions, it is blamed on the sufferer,' she says. 'It is hard to raise an emotionally healthy obese child in today's weight-prejudiced society.'[33]

Of course one of the best ways for parents to help children deal with their concerns about body image and weight is to lead by example. If you are confident and happy about your own body and look after yourself, it will be easier for your children to do the same.

Children and teenagers may be concerned about their weight or body image even if they are not overweight. These concerns can be self-fulfilling if they lead to dieting and other unhealthy eating patterns. As well, concerns about body image can discourage girls, particularly teenagers, from participating in physical activity. All children, from an early age, need to be supported in being confident about their body and their physical abilities.

Ellyn Satter has some more sensible advice on this subject: 'We can help preserve children's ability to eat in a positive and healthful way, we can help preserve their joy in moving their bodies, we can love them without reservation or criticism, and we can thereby support them in feeling good about themselves. But we can't make them thin.'

Thinness most definitely should not be the goal. As much as the glossy magazines would have us believe that thin is beautiful, children will be better off if they grow up knowing that true beauty lies in feeling healthy, strong, confident and happy.

Disconnection

'I really like your yellow dress,' Dr Tony Grant tells me over coffee one day. It makes me feel really uncomfortable. We are sitting at a café at the University of Sydney, where he heads a coaching psychology unit. Whenever I try to change the tack of the conversation, Grant comes back to my yellow dress. Actually I am wearing black trousers and a black top patterned with pink and red hearts.

Grant is trying to help me understand what it feels like to have someone completely disregard your understanding of reality. It's such a simple experiment, but it had a powerful effect; I didn't trust what Grant was saying, but I also began to doubt myself. Maybe I really was wearing yellow...

I had asked Grant for his advice about what parents should say to an overweight child who raises the issue of their weight.

On the one hand, you don't want to exacerbate or reinforce their anxiety.

On the other hand, little white lies—'You're not fat, darling'—are not helpful either, says Grant. They can undermine children's confidence in their own understanding of themselves and the world.

'Kids realise there is a split between what mummy says and what other kids say,' he says. 'They think, *If I am wrong about this, then maybe I am wrong about other stuff*'.

How one family changed

When one family decided to seek help for their young daughter's weight problem, it led to many small changes to their daily routines which added up to a significantly more healthy lifestyle for everyone. David and Kim Aislabie, from Newcastle in New South Wales, were already concerned about 8-year-old Katelyn's obesity when they read about a new program to combat childhood obesity.

It was being offered as part of a study by the University of Newcastle and the University of Wollongong known as HIKCUPS (the Hunter and Illawarra Kids Challenge Using Parent Support). The 10-week program provided education to parents and enjoyable physical activities for the children.

As a result, the Aislabie family now spend less time in front of the TV. Most nights they now have dinner at the table, and they spend more time on their meals than when they ate in front of the box. It's not just because they're eating more slowly; they're also chatting more.

The family is now less likely to eat out, and is more careful about reading the food labels when shopping. David also spends more time going on walks or bike rides with Katelyn. 'For me, it's been a re-education process,' he says. 'Even with portion sizes—we used to give her an adult portion. Because she could eat it doesn't mean we should have given her that much.'

David and Kim have tried not to focus on Katelyn's weight, but are pleased that she has trimmed down. More importantly, within several weeks of starting the program, Katelyn was participating in PE at school for the first time. David says they have noticed 'major, major changes' in their daughter. 'She is absolutely more confident with physical activity and her co-ordination skills have improved out of sight,' he says.

David says the lifestyle changes have been good for everyone in the family, including Katelyn's two young brothers. 'I see other kids who could benefit, but it's a really hard thing to broach with other parents,' he says.

Dr Janet Warren, Senior Research Dietitian at the University of Newcastle, says feedback about the study has been extremely positive. 'Parents and teachers have commented that the children are showing a new enthusiasm for physical activity as their skills and confidence levels increase,' she says.

'By providing practical support programs on fitness and nutrition for overweight children, we can break the cycle of childhood obesity progressing to adulthood.'

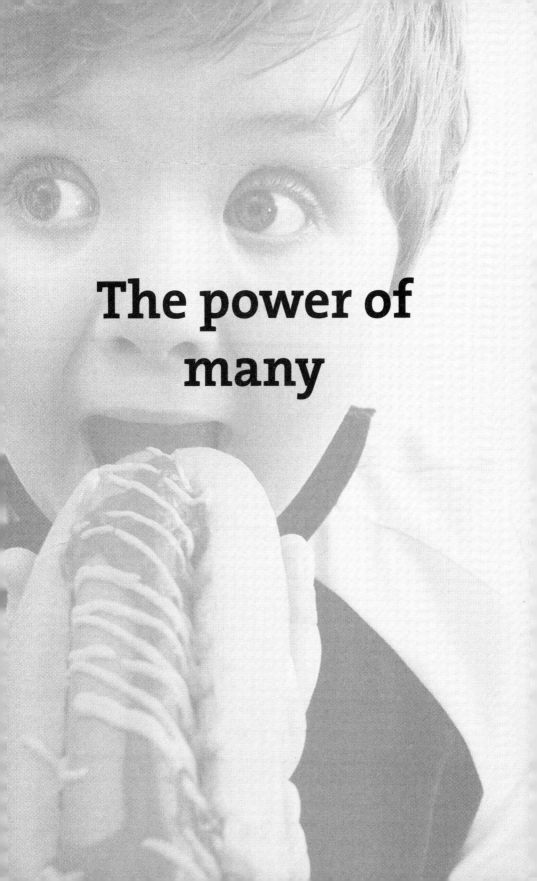

The power of many

12. The bigger picture

So far, we've mainly looked at the steps parents can take to make it easier for their family to enjoy a healthy diet and an active lifestyle. But it's not fair to lay the burden solely on parents. We all are products of our environment and culture, and it is also the broader society that needs to change if children are to be given the opportunity for a healthy future. Creating an environment which is more supportive of children's health will aid others too. Many adults could benefit from help to eat better and move more. And, of course, parents wear many hats. They are also teachers, council workers, employers, town planners, farmers, nurses, builders, politicians...some are in a position to influence the lives of many children and families.

These last two chapters offer a smorgasbord of ideas and practical examples of how schools, employers, local government, childcare services and other sectors can make positive changes for children's health. The number of examples given in these chapters may give a misleading impression that all is well. And it does seem that the constant barrage of newspaper headlines about childhood obesity may be having

316

an effect. There are signs that something of a sea change may be occurring among business, political and community leaders. No less a heavyweight than former US president Bill Clinton, who once was probably the world's best known junk food junkie, has thrown his considerable clout behind efforts to reduce school children's soft drink consumption.

And it is true that many teachers, schools and community groups are doing wonderful work. But often this reflects the drive and passion of individuals, and results in one-off or short-term success rather than any far-reaching changes that will have lasting effects on all children—not only those who are lucky enough to go to a school that makes its students' health a priority.

That is why these chapters also offer some suggestions for exercising parent power. Parents may not always appreciate the influence they can wield as advocates, both in their local community and more broadly. Just writing a letter or picking up the phone and contacting a newspaper, business or school principal can have a significant effect. Surely there's a car sticker in it: parents vote too.

Schools

Schools can promote children's health in many ways. Here are a few:

Schools' physical environment

Do the school grounds invite children to run and play? Are there areas where children can explore nature and interact with their environment? Are there areas that can be used as outdoor classrooms so that physical activity can be built into learning activities?

Are there areas that cater for the needs of children at different ages and stages? Girls and boys will often have different requirements. Not all children will want to run around on sports grounds or play ball games. Is there a range of equipment, games and venues to cope with children's different interests and abilities?

Are the sports facilities and venues and equipment well maintained? Do they cater for a variety of interests or are they narrowly focused on a few dominant sports? Is there shade? Do students have easy access to drinking water throughout the school grounds? Does the school identify itself as a healthy learning environment by promoting healthy eating and activity? Are there, for example, signs to encourage children to drink water rather than soft drink?

Promoting physical activity

Physical education needs to be an important and valued part of the school curriculum. This is not simply a matter for PE teachers; school leaders have a responsibility to foster a culture that places a high priority on children's health. In the past, PE had a low status compared with all the other issues vying for teachers' and students' attention. This is often still the case, despite the immense public focus on children's weight and health; a recent NSW study found that about 50 per cent of primary schools do not allocate the recommended amount of time (120 minutes per week) to physical activity.[1]

PE should help children develop skills, be as enjoyable as possible for all children, and cater for a range of interests and abilities. It should not focus on just a few sports. Teachers need to be well trained and resourced to teach PE, and may need support, such as backing from the school hierarchy, and opportunities for professional development When their teachers enjoy and feel confident about teaching PE, children are more likely to enjoy and feel confident about being physically active. In the United States, many schools see PE as a way of encouraging children's interest in a range of activities they can pursue throughout their life. This is reflected in the name of one school's PE policy: 'Fit for the Future'.[2]

PE classes are only one of the places where schools can promote physical activity. The broader school curriculum can also encourage kids to be active. Many schools are getting children moving in science, maths or other subject lessons.

Promoting healthy eating

The whole school community needs to be engaged. There's little point teaching children in class about the benefits of eating well if the school canteen is stocked with foods full of fat, salt and sugar. Or if the school's fundraising efforts rely on selling chocolates or sweets. Or if parents (or children) pack school lunchboxes with muesli bars and chips. Or if pies and soft drink are the standard fare at sports days, camps and other school functions.

Similarly, it is much easier to encourage children to drink the water they need if it is freely and easily available and soft drinks are not. It also helps if teachers and parents set a healthy example with their own water consumption and lunchboxes and if teachers do not use sweets as rewards and treats in the classroom or elsewhere.

According to Deakin University academics Dr Colin Bell and Professor Boyd Swinburn, children get only about 16 per cent of their total energy intake from the food they eat at school, with probably less than 3 per cent coming from school canteens. But even if school canteens are providing a relatively small proportion of kids' food, their symbolism is big. Too often they have helped reinforce the message of so much food advertising: that foods high in salt, fat and sugar are for eating every day rather than occasionally.[3]

The Apple Slinky sensation

A few years ago, some bright sparks at a Sydney school stumbled across a clever little device which transforms apples into a single, long piece of the fruit, or 'slinky'. The Apple Slinky Machine, which cores, peels and slices, was at that time sold mainly as an aid for drying apples.

But after one school realised its potential for making apples more child-friendly, the Slinky found a whole new market and set of fans. Word spread quickly, and thousands of schools have now bought the device, and use it in canteens, at fundraisers and at school fêtes and other such functions. In Queensland, schools can also buy the Slinky through the Queensland Association of School Tuckshops.

'Schools have just latched onto them,' says a spokeswoman for the Adelaide-based Hillmark company, which distributes the device. 'You hear stories every week of school canteens going from selling one apple a day to 60 kilograms a week. Sales have grown astronomically; last year we sold nearly 8000 units around Australia. But the big winner is the fact that kids are eating fruit.'

Trent Ballard, a dietitian at the Queensland Association of School Tuckshops, describes the Apple Slinky as a 'whizz-bang little machine' and a 'fantastic success story'. 'The kids get such a buzz out of it,' he says.

Healthy profits

School fundraising has traditionally relied on sausage sizzles, chocolate drives and other similar activities, all of which tend to undermine healthy messages. Some schools seem oblivious to the contradiction of running a chocolate drive in order to buy sporting equipment. As well, some companies have seen a market opportunity in the funding squeeze facing many schools: they've been prepared to provide funds or equipment in return for access to young customers, or, as they describe it, the opportunity to 'build relationships' with their customers of the future.

However, concerns about children's health are now leading many schools and parents to rethink their approaches to fundraising. Several organisations have developed resources to help with this. These resources include not only ideas for healthy fundraising, but also some detailed strategies for how to market them. This is important at a few levels: members of the school community such as P&C committee members may need to be persuaded of the merits of changing their fundraising ways, and effective marketing plays a huge role in ensuring healthy profits. Here are two good resources:

• In Queensland, the Fresh Ideas for Fundraising project has plenty of ideas for healthy fundraising and how to promote such ventures (see http://www.qast.org.au/).

• In Tasmania, the Fruitful Fundraising Directory is also chock full of ideas, many of which also support Tasmanian growers and other local businesses (see http://www.parentsandfriendstasmania.asn.au).

Parent power

If ever you doubt that a single person can make a difference, think of Liz Broad, a mother of five from Hobart.

A few years ago, Liz decided to become a peer educator, volunteering to teach others in her community about healthy eating. She'd been out of nursing for more than a decade, bringing up her children, and was looking for an activity which would use her passion for health and help build her confidence to rejoin the workforce.

After doing some training through the Family FoodPATCH program, Liz teamed up with a nearby early childhood teacher to give talks to new mums' groups. They also began working with St John's Primary School in Richmond on a whole-of-school approach to promoting healthy eating and activity.

This led to Year 6 students developing a nutrition policy for the school, which includes making special time in class to have fruit and water. The school also introduced a 20 minute activity session to the start of each day, which is run by Year 6 students. The project was such a success that it is now being implemented across Tasmania.

Liz says the changes at St John's made it easier for her family to follow some of the suggestions of the Family FoodPATCH project. 'It shows the need for a whole of school community approach,' she says. 'When the whole school switched to having water, my kids weren't the odd ones out. Before that, they were starting to say, "I wish you hadn't done this course." They initially saw it as a negative thing not being able to drink cordial, but once the school changed, they started to see it as a positive thing.'

Similarly, Liz's children were not so worried about the absence of muesli bars and other such snacks from their lunchboxes once other children were also having healthier lunches.

As for Liz, she is now working part-time in a doctor's surgery, which gives her plenty of opportunity to continue raising the community's awareness of the benefits of healthy eating and activity. 'I started that project after having lost a lot of confidence, having been home for a decade,' she says. 'It helped put me into networks to access skills and resources that I didn't have and to develop skills for myself that have really helped my confidence and made me much more employable. It's been a win–win situation.'

Promoting active transport

Schools can encourage children to walk or cycle to school by: promoting the benefits of active transport to parents and families; providing secure facilities for bicycles; and working with local government and health authorities to develop and promote safe routes for walking or cycling to school.

Teachers and other school leaders can also set an example themselves, and foster a supportive school culture.

Collaborating with other groups

Schools can work with other organisations to help make the environment, both within the school and the community, more healthy for children. Many schools are already working with local public health units, councils, Lions Clubs, sporting and recreation organisations, youth groups and others. Experts believe that many schools could do more to open up their grounds and facilities to the broader community outside school hours to promote physical activity.[4] Some schools have done this.

One fine example of collaboration comes from the small town of Warialda in northern NSW where the local school, council, businesses, and other organisations formed a partnership to improve training opportunities for young people in the region. As one offshoot of this, a gym has been opened to enable local high school students to train in physical education. It's been a boost to the young peoples' self esteem and confidence, and has also proven popular with the public, says the Warialda Mayor, Mark Coultan. The council also subsidises staff to attend the gym, and local doctors are referring some patients to the gym, particularly if they've got diabetes or weight problems. 'We've had some quite significant achievements with people losing weight,' says Coultan.

Collaborating

• Schools on the central coast of New South Wales have been working with local health promotion experts on ways to improve students' health. Tens of thousands of primary and secondary school children have participated in Q4 Live Outside the Box, a project encouraging children to eat more vegetables and fruit, and to spend less time in front of screens. It involves children keeping a diary of their food and activity habits over a fortnight, as a technique for raising awareness of their current habits and stimulating changes. Parents are also involved.

'It's a way of engaging families through their kids,' says Doug Tutt, director of health promotion at the Northern Sydney and Central Coast Area Health Service. Preliminary findings from the project suggest that many children find it easier to change what they eat than to reduce their TV and computer time.

Tutt and his colleagues have also been helping primary school teachers improve their practical skills in simple playground games, and are developing resources to help parents provide healthier lunchboxes. Tutt says many of their programs may be useful for schools in other areas (see http://www.healthpromotion.com.au).

The bigger picture

• In Western Australia, public health and nutrition experts have been helping schools, parents and students make healthy changes. Nadine Paull, Nutrition Co-ordinator at the Wheatbelt Public Health Unit in Northam, has several key projects:

CaterWise is aimed at schools that don't have canteens and rely instead on commercial outlets such as roadhouses to provide children's lunches. It involves a workshop presented to school principals, teachers, parents, P&C members, and the food outlet. The aim is to help the school and food outlet come to an agreement about what foods can and can't be served. The project also involves students. At one school, students had a 'design a sandwich day'—they made their favourite sandwiches and then voted for which ones should be included on the lunch menu.

The Bibbulmun Track, one of the world's great long-distance walking trails, stretches nearly 1000km from the hills near Perth to Albany on the south coast, and meanders through stunning scenery. It is named after an Aboriginal language group who inhabited some of the areas the track passes through.

Many primary school students in Western Australia's wheatbelt have managed to walk the track without leaving their classroom as part of the Bibbulmun Track School Challenge. Year 4 and 5 students are given a map of the track and do daily exercise sessions which take them along the route on the map, learning about the places they 'pass' on the way. It's a great way to combine learning with physical activity and fun, says Paull.

The north of Western Australia boasts one of the world's toughest and most remote tracks, the Canning Stock Route. The 1781 km track runs from Halls Creek to Wiluna, and these days is usually travelled by well-equipped four-wheel drive vehicles. However, many primary school students in the Kimberley region have 'travelled' the track as part of the Canning Stock Route

Challenge, a project which aims to engage schools in preventing type 2 diabetes. Developed by public health experts, the project involves students in physical activities and in learning about diabetes and the importance of a healthy lifestyle (see http://www.community.wa.gov.au/Communities/Indigenous/PSIC/The_Canning_Stock_Route_Challenge.htm).

Paull's unit also makes small grants to schools to support activities during the annual Fruit and Vegetable Month. Paull has prepared many articles on nutrition and health which are freely available for use in school newsletters and other such publications (see http://www.wheatbelthealth.org.au/html/populationHealth/popHealthDocuments.htm).

The birth of a big idea

When parents enrol their children at Parklands, an independent primary school at Albany on the south coast of Western Australia, they are asked to send them to school with healthy lunchboxes. The school also has a water-only policy: fruit juices, flavoured milks and soft drinks are not allowed. Each day begins with 20 minutes of skipping, games or other activity, and after lunch, children in the older grades have a piece of fruit and some water in class while they work.

The principal, Ruth Vertigan, says the fruit and water break helps the children's concentration at a time of day when they might otherwise start to flag. 'We've had parents say their children have never had water,' she says. 'The odd kid says they don't like water, but if that's all there is, they do have it. It's been an education for parents.'

Ruth has noticed that starting the day with physical activity helps some of the students, especially the boys, settle down better and

The bigger picture

therefore concentrate better on their lessons. Parklands is only a small school, but the policies it has introduced over the past several years have had a far-reaching impact. One of the school's parents is Kate Hawkings, a public health nutritionist in the Great Southern Public Health Service. She has helped support the evolution of the fruit and water program at Parklands into the Crunch & Sip™ program, which is now operating in schools across Western Australia. Kate helped put together booklets and information to help other schools set up the water and fruit break. 'We've had inquiries from all around Australia,' she says.

Fruit and water breaks are becoming part of the daily routine for increasing numbers of schoolchildren. When primary schools in disadvantaged areas of Melbourne's inner west introduced them as part of the Fresh Kids program, it had a huge impact, according to community dietitian Sharon Laurence.

'It was so effective because kids got excited about the fact that they could eat in class,' she says. 'It created a positive context for eating fruit and a positive form of peer pressure, because all the other kids were participating. Kids were going home and saying, "Mum I've got to have a piece of fruit for school". It created a daily routine and became part of the culture of the school. After a while the kids were reminding the teachers, "It's time for fruit break." It just became a habit to eat fruit every day.'

Sharon and her colleagues at the Western Region Health Centre also worked with a local disability agency and fruit and vegetable wholesalers to organise Seasonal Fruit Weeks where fresh fruit and vegetables were delivered to participating schools, giving children the opportunity to taste a wide variety of produce in season. Every school term the teachers linked nutrition education activities in the classroom to the fruit weeks, which were also an important part of reinforcing the fruit and water break program.

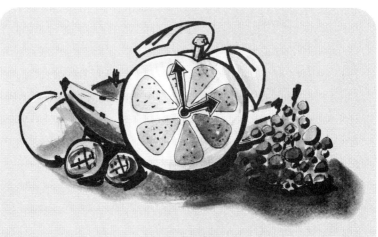

Time for fruit

Sharon says one of the reasons for the success of Fresh Kids, which has expanded to include more than 30 primary schools, was that schools were not expected to do everything by themselves. It helped to have a health professional who could drive the project, negotiate with local businesses, and be an advocate in the school community.

'Schools have an enormous number of social issues to contend with—they are overwhelmed,' says Sharon. 'You need to work with schools if you want something to be on their agenda. You need an advocate at a local level. Just providing a manual won't work.'

A holistic approach

Several years ago, teachers at one Melbourne primary school began to notice that students were not only putting on weight, but also seemed less active and energetic. They often complained of tiredness and their concentration in class was suffering.

Since then, the teachers, parents and students of Tucker Road Primary School at Bentleigh have developed a whole-of-school program to improve students' fitness and wellbeing.

The bigger picture

Its components include:

• Raising the entire school community's awareness of the importance of eating well and being active. Fruit platters are offered when parents and children meet with teachers at the start of the preparatory year. For principal Stan Oakley, this is an important way to show that the school supports healthy eating habits. 'We promote ourselves as a healthy, active school,' he says.

• Introducing a fruit/vegetable break in the classroom. The Parents' Club takes fruit platters into classrooms several times a year for tastings, to encourage children to try new fruit.

• The parents have built and manage a vegetable patch. Students help grow and cook its produce.

• A fruit market makes an annual presentation to students about the benefits of fruit and vegetables and gives students samples to take home.

• A nutritionist takes occasional classes. An information evening helps parents with ideas for preparing healthy, interesting lunchboxes. Parents are encouraged not to send junk food to school and lunchboxes are regularly checked.

• The school canteen's menu has been revised, and healthy choices are vigorously marketed.

• An all-weather running/walking/cycling track has been built, and it is available to families on weekends. Students are encouraged to use it during their breaks.

• A PE teacher was employed. This teacher, among other things, measures each child's fitness level at the beginning, midpoint and end of each year and sets individual improvement goals. Some overweight children are given extra support to improve their fitness.

The school has been careful to avoid focusing on weight, and has kept the emphasis firmly on improving children's health, but Stan says there has been an obvious reduction in the proportion who are overweight.

Teachers say the improvement in students' fitness and health has been noticeable. Their concentration in class has improved, as has the school's performance at swimming and athletics carnivals. Staff are also more health-conscious and are eating better, says Stan.

The school grounds have also benefited. John Allin, who was heavily involved in introducing the changes when he was president of the School Council, says the changes led to less litter: 'Instead of there being wrappers from pies or lollies, the banana skins were being tossed into our new compost bins.'

Stan says the school succeeded in implementing changes because everyone—staff, parents and children—was involved. 'Change can be generated, but you have to bring people on board fairly slowly,' he says. 'You can't just go in and wave a wand. You have to show parents the need for change. Children will go along with it, so long as everyone else is.'

It's Your Move

Students have taken the lead in a health-promoting project involving five high schools in the Geelong East and Bellarine region of Victoria. They have designed an action plan to promote healthy eating and activity, a logo and the project's name: It's Your Move.

The project aims to promote healthy eating, regular physical activity and healthy bodies among adolescents, and to improve the capacity of families, schools and community organisations to support adolescents in making healthy choices. It also highlights the importance of accepting all body shapes and sizes.

Each school has a project officer who oversees the project. Lyndal Taylor, the project officer at one of the schools involved, Catholic Regional College, says the lunchtime walking group has been a resounding success. It has been particularly effective at engaging inactive children and encouraging them to socialise. 'Rain, hail or sunshine they turn up for their walk,' she says. 'They enjoy getting out of school and doing something different at lunchtime. They chatter away to one another and have improved their social networks.'

Lyndal also organised 'tasters' of yoga classes, self-defence lessons, aerobics lessons and other activities. 'We're trying to give the kids a broad range of activities to do at lunchtime,' she says. They might find something they really enjoy that they can take up and do on an ongoing basis. We want to improve the environment and culture of young people to springboard them into a healthy adulthood.'

It's Your Move is primarily funded by the Victorian Department of Human Services, and its impact on students' health is being evaluated.

Childcare services

There are so many issues when it comes to childcare. Does it provide a safe, supportive and friendly environment? Are the staff caring and well trained? For many parents, access and affordability are key issues. Many do not have the luxury of choosing the service that best reflects their particular needs and priorities; they simply have to take what is available. In this environment, it's easy to see how children's needs for activity and healthy food might not have the priority they should have. As well, many services are, understandably, risk-averse. This can have a downside if it means using videos and other screen-based entertainment to keep children quiet and out of harm's way. Similarly, an emphasis on food hygiene can mean providing processed, packaged foods rather than fresh food. Some services, overwhelmed by the costs and demands of meeting food hygiene requirements, have stopped providing food altogether, leaving this responsibility to parents.

There are several resources and initiatives to help childcare services be more proactive in promoting children's activity and healthy eating, including:

• The Start Right–Eat Right Award Scheme, which offers resources and training to promote healthy eating in childcare services. To achieve the award, services must have staff who have completed recognised nutrition training, suitable menus and nutrition policy—and then be assessed. The scheme was developed in Western Australia, and is now also used in Tasmania, Victoria and South Australia as well.

• The Queensland Branch of Nutrition Australia runs a Child Care Advisory Service which gives childcare workers current information on food issues via a quarterly newsletter and telephone enquiry service. Its staff also do menu assessments and food safety audits to help centres get accreditation. The service also runs nutrition and food handling courses for childcare workers.

• New South Wales and Queensland have developed a physical activity training package for staff in out-of-school-hours (OOSH) care centres, and Victoria has funded the *Kids—Go for Your Life* initiative. The Australian Government is also funding physical activity programs for OOSH care.

• The Heart Foundation has developed a comprehensive manual to give services that provide OOSH care ideas on promoting activity and healthy eating. Called *Eat Smart, Play Smart*, it contains over 100 recipes, from afternoon tea ideas to breakfast dishes and kids' cooking activities. Parents might also find many of its suggestions helpful for around the home. The manual can be ordered from the Heart Foundation's Heartline 1300 36 27 87, or at http://www.heartfoundation.com.au.

• Kindergartens, parents and others involved in caring for young children are the target of *Romp and Chomp*, a social marketing campaign aiming to encourage active play, water, fruit and vegetable consumption and less screen time for children up to the age of 5. It has been developed for use in the Victorian city of Geelong. For more details, go to http://www.deakin.edu.au/hbs/who-obesity/ssop/ssop.php.

Communities

It surely is no coincidence that in this era dominated by globalisation, the mass media and multinationals, many people feel a longing for connection to community. They lament that in the global village, many people no longer know their neighbours. Some have voted with their feet and become part of the downshifting movement, changing their priorities or moving to smaller communities where they hope to have a better quality of life with more time for their family. One national survey found that almost a quarter of adults in their thirties, forties or fifties had downshifted during the previous decade, and that about a quarter of them wanted a healthier lifestyle.[5]

A community can take many forms. It might be the people in your street, your social group, other parents at your children's school or childcare centre, or people who share a similar cultural background, political concerns or hobby. People who feel connected to a community generally have better mental health than those who do not. Being part of a community has other benefits, too—it's a case of the whole being greater than the sum of the parts. If a neighbourhood's residents push for better walking facilities, they are more likely than a single walking enthusiast to be successful. Holding a community working bee to install new playground equipment will do more than get the equipment set up. By bringing people together and forging connections and relationships, it may also make the local community healthier for children. When neighbours know each other, they may be more confident about letting their children play in the park down the road or walk to school.

Dr Helen Berry, a researcher at the National Centre for Epidemiology and Population Health at the Australian National University in Canberra, says that obesity should be seen as a problem for communities rather than for individuals and their families. Solutions will come from communities mobilising, she says. 'It's not just about changing the school canteen, although that is important,' she says. When parents take children to sport or other activities or get involved in local volunteering or charity work, they are building connections that can help lead to healthier neighbourhoods. In the United States, the Department of Agriculture employs community nutrition workers who help communities identify their concerns and issues and then learn the skills they need to solve their problems.

And making changes to a community's services and facilities can make it easier for individuals and their families to have healthier lifestyles.

It's not surprising that many people feel overwhelmed by the force of the big fat conspiracy. 'You don't want to be at constant war with your child,' says a friend whose 3-year-old recently said she needs a computer in her bedroom so she can play computer games. 'You want to feel that the community and the society around you are supporting you in making healthy choices, and that it's not you against the supermarkets, or you against the big food companies, or you against the advertising industry.'

It can be a lonely fight for any one parent. But when people come together, in a community of whatever sort, they can be a powerful force: when one hundred or one thousand people say no, it is a lot louder than one parent saying no.

How can your community get involved in the fight against the big fat conspiracy?

A special delivery

In some parts of northern Australia, a special delivery follows the arrival of a newborn. New mothers in Arnhem Land are handed a basket of fruit as part of a push to improve their community's nutrition. The program is the brainchild of the Arnhem Land Progress Association (ALPA), which runs retail stores in the communities of Minjilang, Milingimbi, Ramingining, Galiwin'ku and Gapuwiyak.

Poor nutrition has been a major cause of health problems in remote indigenous communities, where fruit and vegetables have often been prohibitively expensive, in limited supply and of poor quality. Foods high in fat, sugar and salt have often been far more accessible and affordable.

ALPA has been working with public health experts and commercial suppliers to promote the availability, appeal and affordability of fresh produce in these communities. It subsidises the total cost of the freight on fresh fruit and vegetables and gives away tonnes of fresh produce to schools, and at sporting and other community events. ALPA is also training peer educators—the Good Food People—to spread the word in local language about the importance of healthy eating. The Good Food Person conducts instore promotions and is the person who presents new mums with their fruit basket. 'The whole idea is to give the new mother a taste of some fruits she may not have had previously and to benefit the baby during breastfeeding,' says ALPA's health and nutrition manager, John Given.

ALPA has also begun selling and promoting indigenous foods as a way of boosting both nutrition and activity levels. 'In most communities we are the only show in town, and we have a responsibility,' says ALPA general manager, Alastair King. 'I often say to our store managers, "You don't have a clear understanding of your power in this community. You decide what people eat or don't eat by stocking it or not and by having it on show.".

'We will never say to people, "You can't have chips, hot dogs, hamburgers or Coke", because what right do we have to make those choices? But we will be proactive in putting the better stuff right in front of their faces. By doing that, slowly but surely we will change people's eating habits.'

It's a reminder of what can be achieved when community leaders make health a priority.

A living laboratory

Colac, a town of 11,000 people in a fertile volcanic plain in Victoria's picturesque southwest, has traditionally been known for its abundant agricultural produce and the recreational opportunities offered by the large lake nearby. But in recent years, Colac and the surrounding South Barwon region have hit the spotlight as the setting for a large, community-based experiment aimed at determining whether a raft of changes to local facilities and services can halt the increase in childhood obesity.

The *Be Active, Eat Well* project, with its theme of 'making healthy options the easy options', involves many different programs aimed at improving the health and wellbeing of children and at strengthening the local community. It is a collaborative effort of the Victorian Department of Human Services, local health services, the local council and community leaders, and academics at Deakin University. According to Dr Colin Bell, a senior research fellow in the university's School of Exercise and Nutrition Sciences, the project has included:

• A training workshop for people working in local government, schools, day care facilities and local health services to raise their awareness and understanding about the obesity epidemic and the importance of healthy eating and activity. This was run by Deakin University staff, and led to the development of a local action plan. The academics also trained local leaders in social marketing techniques—for raising the community's awareness of the benefits of making changes;

• A Choice Chips campaign to reduce the amount of fat in hot chips. This followed a survey showing that hot chips sold at local outlets were 10.4–18.5 per cent fat, when 8.4 per cent is the maximum level recommended by health authorities. The campaign worked with 7 out of the 13 local outlets and led to a significant reduction in the fat content of their chips;

• Challenging local sports clubs to think beyond their traditional competitive focus, to the broader role they could play in promoting physical activity. This resulted in an after-school activity program. Over eight weeks, children paid $2 per session to try four different sports, including croquet and tai kwon do. Where possible, schools allowed the sports clubs to run the sessions in their grounds, so children didn't need to travel. The program resulted in significant increases in local sports club membership—and to the number of children who are active after school;

• A walking school bus. This was established after a survey showing that more than half the children living within walking distance of their school were driven there. However, the walking school bus ran into difficulties because of red tape and the struggle to attract parents to run it. In retrospect, says Bell, it might have been better to get other volunteers to do the walking school bus, such as grandparents, police officers or retirees;

• Changes to school canteens, including the launch of *Be Active Lunch Pack*. These are brightly coloured cardboard boxes that contain a pita salad wrap and a fruit salad tub. They are also being sold in local milk bars; and

• *Powerdown Week*. This was a campaign to raise families' awareness of the benefits of reducing screen time.

At the start of the project, in 2003, 28 per cent of children in the South Barwon region were overweight or obese. It is too early to know the project's impact on children's health and weight, but a preliminary evaluation suggests that some families have made important changes to their lifestyle. Bell says a survey found that in response to the program, 68 per cent of families reported limiting consumption of sweet drinks, 68 per cent reported participating in the after-school activity program, and 57 per cent were providing healthier lunchbox foods. However, only about 4 per cent said they changed their choice of takeaway foods, and 32 per cent said they had made no changes because they believed their family was healthy already.

Bell says an important goal was to ensure that the local community felt they owned the project, and developed the skills to keep it running. 'Universities have a bad habit of coming in and running projects and then disappearing and taking the data away and leaving nothing much behind,' he says. 'We've purposely designed this so that the skills and the expertise are left in the community.'

For communities wishing to introduce similar projects, Bell has this advice:

> One of the key things I've learnt is that to get people involved, you need to demonstrate to them the benefits of participating. The benefit to local sports clubs of participating in the after-school care program is that kids are introduced to their sport and many go on to take up membership with their club. Parents love it because it's a 'taste and see' for their kids. They can introduce their kids to tennis without having to buy all the gear.

He advises communities to be realistic about what is possible with the resources they have:

> If I'm a mum and want the canteen to start selling healthier food options, I have to ask myself, 'What is my capacity to make that change?' Sometimes people's enthusiasm outweighs their ability to make change, which leads to frustration and burnout. One solution can be to link up with other people and groups who are also keen to make change.

Growing up in New Zealand, Colin Bell was inspired to study nutrition after seeing a World Vision advertisement showing how an inexpensive, simple feeding program could restore life to severely malnourished children. But as his career progressed, it became clear that overconsumption was also a major health problem for many of the world's children, even in developing countries. He has since worked on projects to improve the nutrition of Pacific Islanders living in New

Zealand, and on documenting the impact of urbanisation and the rise of the motor car on health in China.

When he moved to Australia to help oversee the Colac project, Dr Bell wanted to live somewhere that made it easy for his own young children to be active and healthy. His family built a small home on a big block near Geelong to maximise the space available for play. It is in stark contrast to many of the other homes nearby, where large buildings leave little space for children to run. As a result, the local kids tend to congregate at the Bells', because there they have room to play.

Community gardens

To the uninitiated, gardens are simply places where plants grow and die. To those who know otherwise, gardening is good medicine—and not only because it gets you moving and can help your diet be lean and green. Gardening also helps mental health and wellbeing. It is relaxing, and promotes creativity and connection with nature. And it is a fine teacher, providing endless opportunities for learning, whether about the seasons, the environment, or design. It also instructs in philosophy and the nature of life and death. Gardeners learn patience and acceptance, and to cope with loss and frustration as well as joy and success. Gardening can also be a social facilitator—by connecting neighbours who share excess produce or cuttings, for example.

For children, gardens are particularly important as places for play, fantasy and exercise. Involving children in gardening can encourage their taste for fresh produce and their interest in food and its preparation.

Not everyone can have their own backyard garden. However, the concept of community gardens is gaining increasing popularity, and it is estimated that there are now more than 280 around Australia.

Establishing and running a community garden can be challenging, because there can be many practical and financial barriers. Conflict can also arise. Cultivating Community, an organisation which supports community gardens on more than 15 public housing estates in Melbourne, has developed a resource kit to help people establish gardens and deal with some of these issues.

The *Community Garden Good Practice Guide* is available at: http://www.communitybuilders.nsw.gov.au/building_stronger /safer/commgard.html.

The Australian City Farms and Community Gardens Network also offers plenty of helpful information and links: http://www.communitygarden.org.au.

Growing a community

When members of a community come together to make a garden, they do more than grow plants. They also grow themselves. That, at least, has been the experience of a community garden at Ravenswood, a disadvantaged suburb on the northeastern fringes of Launceston in Tasmania.

The garden has had its share of ups and downs since it began in 1996, but locals' perseverance and passion have paid off. Their efforts—in creating a beautiful, productive patch which has brought many rewards for local children, unemployed people and other community members—were recognised recently when the garden won the inaugural Community Garden Excellence Award.

'We haven't used the garden just for growing; we've used it to change the social fabric of our community,' says the garden's coordinator, horticulturalist Tamara Johnston. 'Because everybody works on it together, there's a growing together.'

The garden, which measures 200 metres by 200 metres and boasts 130 beds, attracts about 150 volunteers each week, who take produce home in return for their labour. The garden also involves local schoolchildren and teachers. Apart from developing practical and social skills in the garden, the students make good use of the garden's kitchen. And they take home fruit, vegetables and recipes.

A special program is run for children who are struggling at school or who have been excluded from classes because of behavioural problems. 'We often find we are the only contact they have with education,' says Tamara. 'The kids say, "We're only here because we're the shit kids." I say, "That's OK because we use a lot of that on the garden."' More seriously, she adds that working in the garden has boosted these students' self-esteem and confidence. 'They've got this status they've never had before,' she says. 'We've had kids coming in during their school holidays who want to work.' At least one has gone onto a horticultural traineeship as a result.

The project relies mainly on government grants but also sells produce at local farmers' markets. For Tamara, it represents a holistic approach to improving a community's health:

Ravenswood Community Garden is not a picture perfect or a totally wonderful example of a permaculture environment, not even of the best garden practices—but we are making a difference for groups that are not being supported anywhere else.

We are sowing the seeds of change and of a future for groups that struggle to see that they can make change happen, or that there is a future. We grow not because we are organic or environmentally friendly—though these make the journey more meaningful—we grow because we value all who come into the garden. We believe that everyone can succeed but understand that success for each person is very different. We work to develop pathways for reconnecting people to their communities and allow the garden to have successes and failures.

Farmers' markets

In 1997, Jane Adams went to a food and wine festival in Melbourne and heard a provocative speech asking why Australia, with all its fantastic fresh produce, lacked farmers' markets.

The question struck a chord. Jane, a Sydney-based food writer and marketing consultant, had enjoyed shopping at farmers' markets throughout Europe and thought them a wonderful vehicle for connecting farmers with their customers. Some time later she found herself on a six-week fellowship, investigating how farmers' markets were run in the United States. As she spoke to town planners, food policy experts, nutritionists, market managers, farmers and others involved in the markets, she began to realise their potential for Australia.

When she returned home, Jane set up workshops, offering communities throughout Australia and New Zealand advice on how to establish farmers' markets. Since her first session in the New South Wales town of Orange in 1999, she has delivered dozens of such workshops. Australia is now thought to have about 100 farmers' markets.

Some health authorities promote farmers' markets as an effective way to increase fruit and vegetable consumption, and recommend providing financial incentives for them to run in needy communities.[6] Indeed, one large medical centre in California opened an onsite farmers' market in 2003 so that patients, staff and local residents could have easy access to fresh produce, and has plans to expand the initiative elsewhere.[7] Some public health experts also see farmers' markets as a tool for improving mental health: by promoting community networks and social contacts, they build resilience and the ability of individuals and communities to withstand stresses. Jane also sees the benefits broadly. She has watched farmers' confidence, skills and productivity flourish as a result of having direct contact with their customers. Jane has also observed the environmental benefit of produce being sold locally rather than being transported vast distances for sale— or even in some cases being transported back to its area of origin.

But most of all, she is passionate about how the markets help reconnect people with the environment and the sources of their food, at a time when many people do not know whether their strawberries come from the other side of the world or the other side of town. For Jane, farmers' markets are a political statement which help honour and sustain farmers. 'I don't think people go to farmers' markets to make a political statement, but they discover it's a much more pleasurable way of getting food than a supermarket. At a farmers' market you have conversations with the people who grew your food.'

When working with a community to establish a farmers' market, Jane does the following:
• She runs a workshop for the local community, taking care to invite a broad spectrum of stakeholders and even potential competitors, such as supermarkets. This is an opportunity to

discuss the potential benefits to the community as well as to identify any potential hurdles. For example, she reassures shop owners who may be concerned about competition that farmers' markets generally boost everyone's business by bringing more customers to the area.

• She holds a meeting for the local primary producers, and stresses the importance of having a diverse range of local produce. Ideally, shoppers should be able to put together a meal from a farmers' market. Jane compiles a list of what produce is grown locally or within the region, to identify gaps that may need filling. Sometimes this leads to new local businesses being established to fill the gap.

• She suggests guidelines for how the market will be run. Usually they are held on a Saturday or Sunday morning. Ideally they should be held weekly, so people can get into the habit of shopping there. Choosing an appropriate site is critical. It needs to be prominently located, flat, have some form of shelter and good access to parking. It also needs to be big enough to cope with expansion.

• She helps work out a publicity and marketing strategy. Farmers' markets must provide a positive experience if they are to be successful. Customers need to feel they have got a 'good deal', because of price or because of getting something special, such as first season produce. 'You have to come away with a reward that you wouldn't have had access to in conventional food systems. It may be that you are taking home a story, such as the name of the chook who laid the eggs that you bought.'

Jane, who is city born and bred, has been transformed by her own involvement in farmers' markets. She has given much of her time freely but has also gained plenty from the experience and from her many new contacts around the country. 'It gives me a great deal of faith in human nature and in the power of individuals to create change,' she says. 'I get a lot of satisfaction from knowing that I have contributed to what now appears to be lasting social change. It's nice to have made a little toeprint on the earth.'

Keeping it local

When Pam Lincoln moved to Albany on the south coast of Western Australia more than a decade ago, she was shocked by what she saw. Much of the region's wonderful fresh produce was transported 400 kilometres to Perth before being sent back to Albany for sale. Not surprisingly, its quality often left much to be desired by the time it finally reached shoppers.

Pam, a dietitian who had moved to Albany to set up a vineyard and enjoy a sea change, joined forces with two other friends and enlisted the help of Jane Adams to set up a local farmers' market. They almost had to beg producers to attend the first one. Several years later, the market is a local fixture. More than 1000 people visit it every Saturday, buying tonnes of fruit and vegetables, and also snapping up free range pork, and organic beef, lamb and chicken. The market has helped many local producers' sustainability. 'The feedback has been really, really positive,' says Pam. 'You can see that it's really created a sense of community. Neighbours speak to each other at farmers' markets.'

Kate Hawkings, a public health nutritionist who helped establish the market, says it's also had a noticeable impact on the vitality of the CBD. 'There's much more activity in town on a Saturday morning,' she says. 'It's had a flow-on benefit to other traders, some of whom were quite reluctant initially.' Kate has no doubt that the market has helped boost local consumption of fruit and vegetables. You know what they say about fresh tasting best.

Jane Adams also contributed to the success of another market, thousands of kilometres to the north of Albany. Traditionally much of the horticultural produce from the Gascoyne region was also carted to Perth, leaving many locals and visitors with limited access to fresh fruit and vegetables.

The Gascoyne Growers' Market, held every Saturday in Carnarvon from May to November, was established as a joint partnership between health, agriculture, primary producers and local government in 2001. It has been extremely popular, and now attracts up to 2,000 customers each week—equivalent to about a third of the region's population.

Research conducted in 2005 found that the markets have brought significant health, economic and social benefits. More than two-thirds of shoppers report eating more fruit and vegetables, and many stallholders said their businesses had benefited. They also took great satisfaction from the direct interaction with their customers, felt proud of their contribution to the local community and had improved their marketing skills. 'I love selling to people who like my produce,' one stallholder said.

The evaluation concluded that the market 'provides a model for other rural towns to harness local resources and build on assets to deliver practical benefits, increase the local economy and build community pride'.[8]

13. The picture gets bigger

Local government

We tend to look to our state, territory and national governments to provide leadership on health issues because of their role in funding health services and setting health policy. The impact of local government on our health is often overlooked and under-appreciated. Yet local government can play an important role in creating environments that make it easier for us to make healthy choices. They are major providers of sport, recreational and physical activity infrastructure. Their decisions often shape the development and nature of our community, and can also have a powerful influence on the local food supply. They can be powerful advocates for their areas. There are many examples of local government taking strong action to support communities' health, but no doubt many could also do much more in this area. Most of us can only dream of having the facilities that the City of Chicago provides to support cycling commuters: a bicycle transit station that includes free indoor parking for 300 bikes, showers, lockers, bicycle rental and repair, and a café.[1]

In Western Australia, the Premier's Physical Activity Taskforce has produced a guide for how local government can promote walking, with plenty of practical advice for how to set up walking groups, pedometer challenges and loan schemes, community walking events, walking maps and trails.[2] Here are some other suggestions for how local government can help support health:[3]

• Make it easier, safer and more appealing for people to walk and cycle for recreation and transport, especially to schools and other community centres and facilities—by providing secure bicycle parking and seating at shopping centres, bus stops and train stations, for example.

• Develop safe walking and cycling routes to schools in conjunction with local students, teachers and parents.

• Help make it easy for people to use public transport.

• Ensure that new developments have pedestrian and cycling links to nearby areas and destinations. Encourage the use of stairs and walkways in commercial and residential developments. The simple measure of putting up a sign that says, *please use the stairs*, has been shown to make a difference.

• Provide street lighting, shading and signposting on pedestrian and cycling routes.

• Increase residential density through development of existing community centres, in order to help neighbourhoods retain or attract shops and community facilities. People are more likely to walk or cycle to shops and other facilities if they are nearby.

- Help and encourage residents to care for street trees.
- Provide street furniture and shelter/shade at activity centres to make it easier and more comfortable to sit, meet and talk.
- Design parklands and ovals to provide a variety of opportunities for physical activities in addition to sport—for example, have shaded walking paths, water features, gardens, play facilities, marked walking tracks. Something as simple as erecting a sign saying '2 km walking track' will get more people walking.
- Set up a pedometer loan scheme at libraries.
- Incorporate physical activity into community festivals and events. For example, include games that get children moving.
- Support community groups and businesses that promote physical activity and healthy lifestyles. Acknowledge their efforts publicly.
- Involve children and youth in recreation and community planning. They are more likely to become involved in activities they've had a hand in planning.
- Ensure council childcare programs provide healthy food and plenty of opportunity for children to be physically active.
- Use child health centres to recruit parents, particularly mothers, into physical activity programs.
- Provide and maintain hygienic and safe rest rooms, water fountains and recreation facilities for outdoor environments.
- Preserve market gardens and other local food supplies.
- Support community gardens.

Professor Billie Giles-Corti believes municipal councils could also learn from the experience of Glasgow, where swimming pools in some disadvantaged areas are free to children during school holidays. Apart from the physical benefits, Giles-Corti says the move has also helped reduce antisocial behaviour. 'Kids are less likely to get into trouble if they've got things to do,' she says. More generally, Giles-Corti argues that local government could do much more to overcome the financial barriers that prevent many children from being involved in sport and other physical activities.

Back to the source

Efforts to improve people's nutrition often focus on the demand side of the equation—trying to influence consumers' food choices—rather than on the supply side, such as farmers and other food producers. This probably reflects our tendency to put the blame for poor nutrition and other health problems onto the individual: 'If you don't eat properly, it is your fault.' This approach overlooks the fact that many aspects of our society make it difficult for people to eat well, particularly if they live in disadvantaged or recently developed areas that are not well served by affordable fresh produce and other healthy foods. And of course it is far easier to blame the individual than to attempt the complex, difficult task of changing the underlying societal and structural factors that contribute to their problems.

In the early 1990s, Dr Karen Webb, a public health nutritionist at the University of Sydney, and her colleagues decided it was time to change focus. She wanted to develop a project that would influence the food supply in a way that made it easier for people to eat well. She knew such projects had been successful overseas—there is a famous one from the Knoxville City Council in Tennessee, which has made major gains from working on local food supply and distribution networks.

Webb's sights settled on Penrith, at that time a fast growing area in western Sydney with many young families and more takeaway outlets than food shops. Penrith was on the doorstep of many of the farms supplying food to the Sydney region, but had fewer food shops than most other places in Sydney. Residents in one particularly disadvantaged suburb had to travel 16km to the nearest fruit and vegetable shop. Many suburbs had no supermarket or fruit and vegetable supplier, although most had butchers and all had several takeaway and liquor shops. Not surprisingly, the people of Penrith were more likely than other New South Wales residents to suffer health problems related to poor nutrition.[4]

Webb and her colleagues from the university and the local area health service's health promotion unit had an enthusiastic response from the Penrith City Council, which established a Food Policy Committee in 1993. This provided a mechanism for a variety of interests, including Webb and other academics and nutritionists, health services, businesses and other local stakeholders, to work together. The committee's initial goals were to: improve access to food outlets and related transport services; expand the availability of healthy choices in food outlets; increase community facilities and support for breastfeeding; promote local agriculture; and increase the safety of the food being sold. Its achievements have included:

• Establishing an open farm day to support local farmers and develop greater awareness of their importance in terms of a healthy local food supply.

• Establishing local farm sales, which also helped stimulate locals' interest in fresh produce and the benefits of eating seasonally.

• Changing bus routes so that housing estate residents could catch the bus to the shops.

• Promoting the establishment of supermarkets in newly developed areas. In some places the Council established an interim fruit and vegetable market.

• Working with local fruit and vegetable retailers to expand to other suburbs, and to establish fruit and vegetable home delivery.

Local supermarkets also agreed to subsidise delivery to disabled and housebound residents.

• Establishing a fruit and vegetable barrow at a local train station.

• Establishing a school garden, a breakfast program and a healthy canteen in a disadvantaged area.

• Providing facilities in local centres to make it easier for women to breastfeed.

• Improving the quality of food served to children in childcare services operated by Council.

• Working with local businesses to increase the number displaying a 'breastfeeding welcome here' sticker, and

• Ruling that all applications for public building development must now include parents' rooms to enable breastfeeding (this policy went on to be adopted as policy by the National Assembly of Local Governments).

Some of the changes may sound simple, but it often took a lot of effort to overcome multiple bureaucratic obstacles. 'It took one and a half years to get the train station barrow, and a couple of years to get the farm gate sales,' says Webb. 'Councils, like all government departments, are highly bureaucratic. You must learn how the bureaucracy works and how to work within it while not losing hope and oomph. One of the lessons is that collaboration takes sustained effort.'

Webb says research suggests that outside experts who try to implement changes in a community are more likely to be effective if the locals are genuinely involved in the process, even though this usually requires more time and effort. 'How you do things is important in terms of whether it is implemented or lasts,' she says. It seems that the Penrith Food Project had had a lasting impact. The Council and local health services continue to work on improving residents' opportunities to eat well, and similar projects have since sprung up

353

across Australia. All of which suggests that local councils can have a huge impact on their community's health, particularly if they're willing and able to team up with other groups.

Rewriting a familiar story

A familiar story is unfolding in the City of Casey, a growth corridor southeast of Melbourne. It is a story that is being played out on the rapidly developing fringes of cities around the country.

It involves housing developments eating up market gardens and other productive agricultural lands, and new communities being established without the infrastructure that is vital for their good health. It also involves young families growing up in large houses with small gardens and little room for play. They often find it easier and cheaper to buy takeaways than fresh produce. And, finally, it involves food grown locally being transported elsewhere for sale.

The City of Casey is trying to create a more positive ending for this common story. It is making nutrition one of its top public health priorities, through its Sprouting New Ideas project. Here is what the project is doing:

• A farmers' market has been set up.

• The Choosing Healthy Options in Casey Eateries (CHOICE) awards have been set up, to encourage local cafés and restaurants to improve the nutritional value of their fare. Outlets that go through a training and assessment process are then promoted as healthy places to eat.

• Casey and its neighbour, the Shire of Cardinia, have won funding for a joint project for improving their local food supply. It is likely to include a fruit and vegetable delivery service and having schoolchildren visit local farms. 'There's a lot of evidence that younger children don't know where food comes from,' says Kim

Carter, the Council's health promotion officer. 'They think it comes from supermarkets. They will incorporate what they learn at the farms into the school curriculum and setting up their own gardens.'

• Gardeners have been hired to work with children in family day care centres to establish their own gardens and grow their own vegetables.

• Existing community gardens are popular; most are full, and have waiting lists. Carter plans to lobby Council for new gardens and to ensure that new developments include space for community gardens.

• The Council has developed a nutrition and physical activity policy for preschools and other early childhood services.

Governments

Public health is the poor but powerful cousin of our health system. Historically it has been responsible for many of the major improvements to our health, such as those which have flowed from reducing smoking rates. But it receives a tiny fraction of the overall health budget—only 2.5 per cent of governments' health expenditure each year.[5] This wee drop in the bucket is stretched to cover everything from immunisation and breast and cervical cancer screening to drug abuse prevention and control of infectious diseases. Health promotion—which could play such an important role in helping families have healthier lifestyles and in preventing childhood obesity—accounts for less than a fifth of all public health spending. It's often said that an ounce of prevention is worth a pound of cure, but our health system is heavily weighted towards making sure that illness is treated rather than prevented. One public health academic has contrasted the $48 million spent on health promotion by the Federal

Government in 2004, with the more than $50 million spent by McDonald's in Australia that year on advertising.[6]

Boosting support for public health is, however, only one of the many ways in which federal, state and territory governments could do more for families and children's health. It could be argued that other portfolios—treasury, industrial relations, planning, transport or education—are at least as important in creating healthy environments. The statistics on childhood obesity, because they reflect the extent of the underlying problems of poor nutrition and inactivity, tell us that governments should be doing far more to promote healthy environments for families. Many strategies will be most effective if communities themselves develop and implement them. But governments need to take a lead, by providing funding and support and, where necessary, legislative change. As some researchers have put it, so powerfully: 'Confronting the powerful vested interests that shape our lives cannot be left to individuals.'[7] It is true that many of the projects mentioned in this book have been funded by governments at some level. But too often the funding is short term, leaving successful projects in the lurch or trapped in an unproductive cycle of chasing short-term grants.

Australia has been a leader in developing policies for tackling childhood obesity. But it has been far less effective at translating these policies into action. And given that there are so many uncertainties about which approaches will be most effective for which communities, it is also important that governments support careful evaluation of obesity control strategies. We need to know much more about what works and what does not. However, governments often seem to have put more energy into talking about the problems of childhood obesity than into doing anything about it. Experts say that researchers have been calling for action to tackle obesity since the 1970s, and recall the suggestion that the 1997 National Health and Medical Research Council document called 'Acting on Australia's Weight' would be more appropriately titled 'Waiting on Australia's Act'.[8] The Australasian Society for the Study of Obesity, and other experts, have criticised the Australian Government for failing to implement the recommendations of the National Obesity Task Force. Many believe the powerful food industry exerts an unhealthy influence on government policies and decision-making.

The Australian Government's top priority, according to many experts, should be a ban on junk food advertising to children. Nutritionist Dr Rosemary Stanton says that Australia is ideally placed to test the impact of such a ban because of our geographic location. Countries which have introduced such a ban, including Sweden, Norway and Quebec, are unable to stop ads being beamed in from neighbouring countries, she points out.[9] Some experts have called for a ban on all junk foods and soft drinks in publicly funded premises such as hospitals, as well as for fiscal policies making vegetables and fruit cheaper, relative to fatty or sweet foods.[10] Another suggestion is for all food and drink—including takeaways and restaurant meals—to carry a label indicating how much exercise would be required to burn it up. Dr Michael Booth, National Health and Medical Research Council Senior Research Fellow at the NSW Centre for Overweight and Obesity, believes this would help consumers understand the energy density of their food and drink. For example, the label may say 'Walk 30'—30 minutes of walking would be typically required to use up the energy from one serve of the food or drink. Foods and drinks targeted at children or adolescents could carry information related to their sorts of activities, such as 'Football 40' or 'Play 30'. Another hint for what governments might do comes from Britain, where all children in state schools between the ages of 4 and 6 are entitled to a free piece of fruit or vegetable each school day. This initiative, introduced in 2000, is a major undertaking, involving the distribution of millions of pieces of fruit to children in about 18,000 schools.[11]

Individual politicians too can have a major impact. In the United States, Arkansas has led the way in introducing initiatives to tackle childhood obesity which appear to be making a real difference. It is widely perceived that the personal experiences of two of the state's prominent politicians—the Democratic speaker of the house, Herschel Cleveland, suffered a heart attack, and the Republican governor, Mike Huckabee, was diagnosed with type 2 diabetes—contributed to public and bipartisan political support for changes. After his diagnosis, Governor Huckabee lost more than 45 kgs and became a champion for both healthy environments and healthy lifestyles.[12] It is unfortunate, to put it politely, that Australia's governments and politicians have been unable to develop a more constructive, bipartisan approach; too often, obesity has been used as a political football.[13]

The Finnish example

Fifty years ago, children growing up in the North Karelia region of eastern Finland often did not get a chance to know their grandparents. This was because so many people died so young—often in their fifties—from heart disease.

The area, famous for its rich dairy produce and its consumption of butter, cream and cheese, was notorious for having one of the world's highest rates of premature death from heart disease.

In the early 1970s, they decided to do something. The result was a pioneering project, which extended across the country after being piloted in North Karelia. It involved many sections of society and government—the Finns knew they had a health problem, but they also realised that the solutions would not come only from the health sector. Farmers and other food producers, health professionals, employers, schools and the media were enlisted. Here are some of the initiatives:

- Farmers made changes in their practices, including changing the fertilisers used, to boost the population's intake of selenium, a trace mineral important for health. A domestic vegetable oil industry was developed, and low-fat and skimmed milk were introduced.

- Taxation laws were changed so that low-fat spreads could compete with butter. Previously margarine had been taxed to keep its price equivalent to butter, to protect the local dairy industry.

- Health professionals, teachers, social workers and counsellors were trained to give advice on quitting smoking and healthy lifestyles. People were also encouraged to have their blood pressure and cholesterol monitored.

- Healthy lifestyle programs were introduced to workplaces. They included increasing the availability and affordability of fruit and vegetables in staff canteens.

- Television shows promoted healthy lifestyles.

- Cholesterol-lowering competitions were organised between villages in North Karelia.

- A peer education program was set up in which active community members were engaged in spreading the word about healthy lifestyles and lobbying local grocery stores to improve the variety of fruits and vegetables on sale.

- Tough antismoking legislation was introduced.
- Food manufacturers and retailers were encouraged to develop and promote low-fat dairy and meat products and to reduce salt content in foods.
- People were encouraged to grow berries, which thrive in the Finnish climate, and are a rich source of nutrients.

The impact was impressive. People changed their way of living significantly: they ate less saturated fats and more fruit and vegetables and stopped smoking. Their blood pressure, cholesterol and other risk factors improved, and death rates from coronary heart disease plummeted. Lung cancer deaths also fell. Many thousands of premature deaths were prevented. The project faced its share of difficulties, though. The national dairy industry, for example, went to great lengths to protect its market and resisted efforts to reduce butter consumption.[14]

The project, which ran for more than 20 years, is often cited as an example of how governments, working with all sectors of society, can help create healthier communities. It is also cited as an example of the need for sustained and comprehensive intervention. Long-term gain requires long-term effort and commitment.

Liveable Neighbourhoods

In Western Australia, the state government is actively supporting the development of neighbourhoods that make it easier for people to be active.

Liveable Neighbourhoods, a development control policy of the WA Planning Commission, stresses that streets and suburbs should be designed so that they promote walking and cycling, for both recreation and transport.

It recommends integrating residential and mixed business development, so that most residents live within walking distance of their daily needs: groceries, health care, train or bus connections, or recreation. Several other measures are recommended:

• Interconnected networks of streets mean safe, efficient and pleasant walking. Most people will consider walking up to 400 metres (about 5 minutes) to daily activities, or 800 metres (10 minutes) to a train station or town centre. A well-connected street network is defined as one where at least 60 per cent of the area is within a 400 metre radius of a destination, such as the shops or train station, (that is, it can be reached by a 400 metre walk).

• Where cul de sacs are created, they should be connected by a minor street or laneway that is clearly visible to local residents, and that gives safe pedestrian and bicycle access.

• Buildings should front onto streets. This boosts safety, especially for walkers, because it improves residents' surveillance of their local area.

• On major roads, traffic lights should be used instead of roundabouts, to improve pedestrians' opportunity to cross the road.

• Narrow pedestrian underpasses with poor visibility should be avoided, because they can be a security hazard.

• Safe routes to schools, bus stops, train stations and other services should be clearly marked.

Employers

Employers have a vested interest in the community's health, if for no other reason than their bottom line. Healthy employees are more likely to be productive and less likely to require time off work. There is some evidence that people who are obese are more likely to be absent and for longer periods.[15] With skill shortages affecting many sectors of the workforce, employers also have an interest in maintaining a supply of healthy, older workers.

Bicycle Victoria says cycle-friendly workplaces generally have greater morale, lower absenteeism and higher productivity as a result of improved fitness and mental health. It notes that building a new inner-city car parking space costs, on average, about $30,000, and that the same space will fit 12 bikes, at a cost of about $80 per bike. When DuPont Corporation (US) introduced a fitness program, there was a 14 per cent decline in the number of days off, which translated to 11,000 saved work days per year. Swedish researchers found that fit and healthy workers committed fewer errors than non-fit workers, and a Canadian study found that staff participating in an employee fitness program were more productive, felt more alert, had better rapport with co-workers and generally enjoyed their work more than those who did not.[16]

Bicycle Victoria has produced an excellent brochure detailing the steps employers can take to encourage people to cycle to work (available at http://www.bv.com.au). Apart from the obvious measures—such as providing secure storage, change and shower facilities, and a supportive culture—it cites the example of an English company that gives employees who ride to work extra holiday leave. Another option is to provide staff with interest-free loans to buy bicycles. It notes that several councils in Melbourne provide a bike pool or fleet for employees to use for short local trips.

Here are some other ways employers can help support the community's health:
• Provide safe, health-promoting working conditions.
• Offer family-friendly, flexible working arrangements.

- Support employees who want to breastfeed.
- Offer health promotion in the workplace; for example, provide programs to help employees quit smoking or to be active in their lunch breaks.
- Provide facilities to encourage activity; for example, showers and change rooms.
- Provide incentives for people to travel by public transport. These could be financial or take the form of extra leave or more flexible working arrangements.
- Through workplace design; for example, the Centers for Disease Control and Prevention in the United States increased its employees' use of the stairs by installing new carpet on the stairs, adding artwork to the stairwell walls, hanging motivational signs and playing music in the stairwell.[17]
- Make gym membership part of employee packages. Police officers in one area of the United States receive financial incentives for improving their physical fitness, and one company's employees accrue extra holidays by working out at the company's onsite fitness centre.[18]

Business

Any entrepreneur worth their salt knows that adversity often yields new opportunities. Already some businesses have found new markets as a result of the world's weight problem; meeting the demand, for example, for larger seats on toilets, airlines and buses. There are also new business opportunities in preventing obesity and promoting healthier environments for children. One company reportedly saw an opening in the move to healthier fundraising in schools, providing boxes of its toothpaste and toothbrushes to schools for fundraisers.[19] The Apple Slinky Machine is just one example of health-promoting profits. The food industry appears to be responding to concerns about its role in promoting globesity; healthy food and drinks for children and young people are projected to be among its most active and profitable new product categories in the next few years. One industry analysis found that 18 of the 24 fastest growing food categories internationally are perceived to be healthier.[20] However, there is still a glaring need for a more healthy balance in our food supply. Desperately needed is far more high-profile, clever marketing of vegetables and fruit, to make them at least as cool, funky and fun as anything the fast food outlets can offer.

After years of working in senior marketing and management positions at major corporations, Dr Ken Hudson struck out on his own, setting up an innovation consultancy business called The Idea Centre. One of his reasons for doing this was his belief that businesses should be looking to creativity and imagination to improve their bottom line, rather than to cost cutting. Another reason was that he wanted to spend more time with his young children. His interest in their health and wellbeing started him thinking about how business could get involved in tackling the childhood obesity problem. He had noticed in discussions with leaders of major food companies that many were defensive about the issue, rather than seeing it as a potential opportunity. 'I was struck by a sense that they were resisting it rather than trying to do anything meaningful about it', he says. 'They saw it as a threat to profits and marketing. I wanted to try to get people to try to change their mindset.'

Dr Hudson got a group of creative thinkers together to develop ideas for how business might get involved in improving children's health. Here are some of their suggestions:[21]

- Record companies or radio stations could sponsor dance competitions in school lunch breaks, for students, teachers and parents.
- A footwear manufacturer could sponsor Friday as 'walk to school day'. Children who participate build up points that lead to a special deal on new running shoes.
- Apple Computers could provide apples to schoolchildren.
- PlayStation could develop a game that requires kids to use large muscle groups to drive it.
- A health pay television station could be set up, dedicated to all aspects of kids' health—from exercise and cooking to dancing.
- Cereal manufacturers could begin incrementally reducing sugar content.

Health services

Health professionals and health services are often so flat out treating sick people that they have little time, energy or resources left for thinking about the bigger picture. However, their professional clout means they are ideally placed to take a leadership role in working with other sectors and the community on measures to improve children's health. Here are some examples of how this can be achieved.

Outside the square

When patients with diabetes or heart disease are referred to Beth O'Shannessy for counselling about their diet and lifestyle, they don't go to the local hospital or doctor's surgery. Instead, they head to their fitness centre. That's where they find Beth, a nurse who works as

Health Promotion and Community Development Co-ordinator for the Upper Murray Health and Community Services at Corryong, a picturesque town in the mountains of northwestern Victoria.

And it truly is *their* fitness centre. The health service bought the Community Health and Fitness Centre after extensive investigation of how locals wanted their health dollars spent. Several hundred people voted for the money to be spent on a fitness centre rather than on more traditional types of health services. The centre reflects the health service's commitment to improving the population's health—as well as to providing care for sick people, of course—and to having a democratic approach to decisions about local health priorities and services.

The facility opens seven days a week to all locals, who are simply asked to make a gold coin donation for entry. Doctors refer patients there for rehabilitation after heart surgery, for diabetes care, physiotherapy, activity programs and lifestyle counselling. Regular seminars on different health topics are also run. The centre makes a special effort to engage children and young people, and runs programs aimed at improving their physical skills, self-esteem and confidence. 'The kids are flocking in,' says Beth. 'What gets them in is that it's fun. It's the place to go.'

Which just goes to show that it's not only traditional health services that can provide a health service.

Doing a tonne

It began, as so many clever ideas do, over a cup of tea. A community nurse, a dietitian and a cardiac rehabilitation co-ordinator were chatting over a cuppa about their patients and their problems. And then it hit them: so many of their patients had one thing in problem—they needed to lose weight.

The picture gets bigger

One thing led to another, including some funding from the Australian Government, and the people of Wellington in central western New South Wales found themselves embarking on an ambitious project. The goal of the WellingTONNE Challenge was for the local community to collectively lose 1000 kilograms—1 tonne—in 12 weeks. It began with more than 450 overweight people registering at the official weigh-in. Many other locals participated without officially registering. Of the town's 9200 residents, around 2400 were considered overweight.

The challenge, which involved just about every section of the community, and had lots of components:

- Sports and recreation clubs offered special deals to encourage people to take part in physical activities, whether those activities were going to the gym, playing golf or line dancing.
- A regular exercise program was held in a public park. Family activities were also organised, including a family sports day. September was renamed 'Steptember', and pedometers were distributed.
- Food businesses offered healthy options at special prices. Hotel counter meals offered grills with salad instead of schnitzel and chips; fast food outlets offered a discount on healthy meals; and butchers had daily specials on low-fat cuts of meat.
- Enthusiastic coverage by the local media helped generate awareness, enthusiasm and support for the challenge.
- Supermarket tours showed people how to make healthy choices. Free public talks were also given by a nutritionist, a dietitian, a fitness instructor, a doctor, a physiotherapist and a psychologist.
- Cooking demonstrations were held with a particular focus on encouraging healthy school lunchboxes.

A set of scales was prominently displayed, showing the community's accumulated weight loss after regular weigh-ins. After 12 weeks, the goal had not quite been reached—only 772kg had been lost—so the challenge continued for an extra three months, until the town had done a tonne.

By then, the organisers, who had run the challenge on a shoestring budget of $27,000, on top of doing their usual jobs, were utterly exhausted. But all the effort was worth it in the end, says Debbie Bennett, a community nurse at the Wellington Community Health Centre, who was one of the tea-drinkers behind the challenge. And not just because people lost weight and the community generally became more aware of the importance of healthy eating, being physically active, behavioural change and the benefits of avoiding fad diets. She says:

> The community spirit was one of the big highlights of the challenge which we weren't expecting. It was a wonderful program to work on because of all the enthusiasm. It was really a very social and vibrant time. People were happy, and would be asking each other how much they'd lost. We were in the midst of a horrific drought and there was quite a bit of depression. Farmers and small businesses were doing it fairly tough. People saw the challenge as something they could achieve and have some control over, whereas they couldn't have any control over the drought.

In response to widespread interest from other communities, the WellingTONNE Challenge organisers prepared a step-by-step guide to planning and running the challenge. Thousands of the kits have been distributed. A free copy is available by writing to: National Mail and Marketing, PO Box 7077, Canberra BC ACT 2610. Quote the title: The WellingTONNE Challenge.

Advocacy

Many people make their living as professional advocates for the community's health; they might be employed as public health experts, anti-tobacco campaigners or academics. But parents and other concerned community members can also be influential advocates. The relatively simple act of writing a letter to a politician or newspaper, or meeting with a school principal or childcare centre manager, or organising a neighbourhood petition to your local council, can have a powerful impact. Cycling advocates, for example, have had significant results from their lobbying for cycling lanes and facilities in Melbourne's CBD—more people are now cycling.[22]

Health organisations are increasingly recognising the power of community advocacy (such as Parents Jury, a parent organisation pushing for tighter regulation of advertising to children—see Chapter 6). The Heart Foundation also plans to encourage people to get active—and not just in the physical sense. The foundation is developing an audit tool to help people rate their community's support of walking. According to the foundation's physical activity manager, Trevor Shilton, the audit will let residents and parents assess their neighbourhood, looking at things like access to parks and cycle ways, and whether or not local infrastructure is conducive to walking—for example, are the pavements cracked and are walking paths well lit at night? Shilton hopes the audit will encourage people to become active advocates for healthy communities.

Individuals and families can also take a stand through the decisions they make in their daily lives—for example, by supporting businesses that are trying to provide a healthy alternative. Spend up at the greengrocer. Support the café that

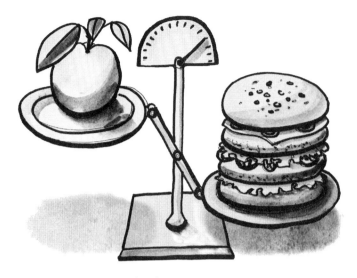

Tipping point

sells fresh healthy food. Buy toys that encourage active play. Nothing influences businesses more than the bottom line.

It's just a handful of decades ago that societies around the world began reaching a 'tipping point', where the big fat conspiracies of modern life combined to push their scales upwards. When enough individuals, communities, organisations, businesses and governments combine forces to tackle the big fat conspiracy head-on, we may reach another tipping point. Hopefully the reward will be better environments for children and their families—and healthier children.

Making a stand

Corinne Paterson was surprised when her 4-year-old son Damien recognised a box of Fruit Loops at the supermarket. She never bought them for her family because of their high sugar content and low nutritional value. The penny dropped when she realised that the children at the childcare centre Damien attended were being given Fruit Loops and Coco Pops for morning tea.

Corinne, from Lake Macquarie in New South Wales, decided to take a stand. She wrote a letter asking the centre and its parents' committee to consider supplying other cereals. She included an article from *CHOICE* magazine on breakfast cereals, and arranged for samples of one of the products the article rated highly to be sent to the centre. She also provided a list of other healthy options for morning tea.

The feedback was not immediately positive. Corinne felt she was being thought of as a troublemaker, someone who was making a mountain out of a molehill. A survey of other parents found few shared her concerns. 'That really shocked me,' says Corinne. 'At the time there was so much press about childhood obesity.' However, the centre was prompted to review its food policies. It now does not offer the high sugar cereals so often, and it no longer uses them in games—no more Fruit Loops on a string.

It isn't quite the victory Corinne would have liked. But it's a small win which she hopes might lead to bigger changes. Taking a stand was not easy, but she feels it was worthwhile. Corinne is now a member of Parents Jury. This gives her plenty of opportunity to interact with other parents who are also prepared to make a stand.

Are you one of them?

Appendices

Useful resources

There is a huge range of resources available to help parents, families, communities and other interested groups. This section is broken into the following broad categories to try to make your search easier:

Breastfeeding

The Australian Baby Friendly Hospital Initiative (information about hospitals and breastfeeding):
> http://www.bfhi.org.au

Australian Breastfeeding Association:
> http://www.breastfeeding.asn.au.

Community gardens

Cultivating Community, an organisation which promotes community gardens: http://www.cultivatingcommunity.org.au.

Community initiatives and issues (including town planning)

Active Living By Design (a US program to encourage physical activity through community design): http://www.activelivingbydesign.org.

The Victorian Health Promotion Foundation (VicHealth) has a wealth of resources to help communities improve health:
> http://www.vichealth.vic.gov.au.

'Challenging your community to better health: A healthy lifestyle
resource based on experiences from The Wellingtonne Challenge
[Funded by the Australian Government Department of Health and
Ageing. Macquarie Area Health Service, 2004]' (a guide to help
communities develop health promotion campaigns, based on the
experiences of the WellingTONNE Challenge). Free copies of the
toolkit are available (quote WellingTONNE Challenge) from
National Mail and Marketing, PO Box 7077, Canberra BC ACT
2610.

Eating well

Parental Guidance Recommended (PGR) manual (for conducting
community education on childhood nutrition, from the WA Cancer
Council):
   http://www.cancerwa.asn.au/resources/publications/index.shtml.
A manual providing practical advice on nutrition, health and physical
activity for services providing out of school hours care: Van
Herwerden, E. and Cooper, C., 2004, 'Eat Smart Play Smart: A
manual for out of school hours care', Heart Foundation, Victoria
(http://www.heartfoundation.com.au/eatsmartplaysmart).
A colourful, fun website for engaging children (and their parents) in
fresh fruit and veg, from Sydney and Brisbane Markets, with
games and quizzes as well as nutritional advice:
http://www.freshforkids.com.
A wealth of resources for families, schools and communities, from the
Centre for Health Promotion at the Women's and Children's
Hospital in Adelaide:
http://www.chdf.org.au.
The Centre for Community Child Health at the Royal Children's
Hospital in Melbourne:
http://www.rch.org.au/ccch/index.cfm?doc_id=427.
Community Foodies, a peer education program in South Australia: Liz
Sanders, Southern Adelaide Health Service, Noarlunga Health
Village, on (08) 8384 9266.
Dietitians Association of Australia:
http://www.daa.asn.au.

Rick Kausman's resources are at:

http://www.ifnotdieting.com.au/cpa/htm/htm_home.asp.

Eat Well Australia (Australia's national public health nutrition strategy):

http://www.health.gov.au/pubhealth/strateg/food/nphp.htm.

Family Feud Food (video produced by the Tasmanian Branch of Dietitians Association of Australia and the Community Nutrition Unit of the Department of Health and Human Services, Tasmania in 1999).

Food Standards Australia (for information about food labels): search http://www.foodstandards.gov.au.

The Community Guide (a US group which reviews the evidence on health interventions, including nutrition): http://www.thecommunityguide.org/.

The Toronto Food Policy Council (for information about Toronto's pioneering approach to food security issues): http://www.city.toronto.on.ca/health/tfpc_index.htm.

Fun not fuss with food (a Queensland Government resource for help with problem eating behaviours), available from Brisbane Southside Public Health Unit, on (07) 3000 9148, or search: http://www.health.qld.gov.au/.

General nutrition information from Nutrition Australia: http://wwwnutritionaustralia.org.

The Mai Wiru Stores Policy (how some Aboriginal communities are improving their food supply):

http://www.nganampahealth.com.au (look under programs).

The Food Alliance for Remote Australia (issues for rural and remote communities):

http://www.fara.bite.to.

Parenting SA (for practical information to help parents feed toddlers, children and teenagers):

http://www.parenting.sa.gov.au.

Queensland Government link page for resources on food and nutrition: http://www.health.qld.gov.au/health_professionals/ food_nutrition.asp#1.

What better food? (a Queensland Government publication stacked with practical food tips for parents and early childhood services): http://www.health.qld.gov.au/phs/Documents/shpu/6656.pdf.

Useless

Psychologist and educator Denise Greenaway takes a holistic approach
to encouraging healthy enjoyment of food:
http://www.rainbowfood.com.au.

The UK Health Education Authority and the National Food Alliance
Food Poverty Database (details of community food projects):
http://www.sustainweb.org/povdb_index.asp

Savenake, Jennifer, 2004, *Improving food security: Healthy eating for
people on low incomes* (training package for dietitians and
nutritionists), SA Government (Department of Human Services and
Womens and Children's Hospital), Adelaide.

Tooty Fruity Vegie project (how to increase primary school children's
fruit and vegetable consumption):
http://www.ncahs.nsw.gov.au/tooty-fruity.

General health information

An Australian Government initiative with information for schools,
families and communities:
http://www.healthyactive.gov.au.

A UK site for use by children, teachers and families:
http://www.welltown.gov.uk/teachers/pupilintro.html.

A WA Government website with a wide range of health information:
http://www.yourzone.com.au/index.htm.

Irwig, J. et al, 1999, *Smart Health Choices*, Allen & Unwin, Sydney.
This book gives readers the tools to critically assess health
information and advice. A revised and updated version will be
published in 2007 by Hammersmith (UK).

Credible information about how to improve the population's health,
from the US Centers for Disease Control and Prevention:
http://www.thecommunityguide.org.

Growth charts

In April 2006, the World Health Organization launched new charts
describing growth of children from birth to 5 years. Importantly,
these are based on the growth patterns associated with breastfeeding:
http://www.who.int/childgrowth.

Growth charts for calculating children's BMI from the US Centers for
Disease Control and Prevention:
http://www.cdc.gov/growthcharts.

Organisations

Cancer Council Australia:
http://www.cancer.org./
Diabetes Australia (freecall 1300 136 588):
http://www.diabetesaustralia.com.au.
National Heart Foundation (Heartline 1300 36 2787):
http://www.heartfoundation.com.au.
Strategic Inter-Government Forum on Physical Activity and Health
(SIGPAH):
http://www.nphp.gov.au/sigpah.
Strategic Inter-Governmental Nutritional Alliance (SIGNAL):
http://www.nphp.gov.au/signal/index.htm.

Overweight and obesity

General information from a NSW summit on obesity:
http://www.health.nsw.gov.au.
General information from Australian Sports Commission:
http://www.ausport.gov.au/aasc/about_aasc/facts.asp.
Guidelines for managing obesity in children, adolescents and adults
from the National Health and Medical Research Council:
http://www.obesityguidelines.gov.au.
US Surgeon General's healthy weight advice:
http://www.surgeongeneral.gov/topics/obesity.
The Big Girls' Group (a weight loss and lifestyle program from the
Royal Women's Hospital Melbourne): ph. (03) 9344 2372.
US Surgeon General's call to action to prevent and decrease overweight
and obesity:
http://www.surgeongeneral.gov/library.
US Centers for Disease Control and Prevention:
http://www.cdc.gov/nccdphp/dnpa/obesity.
Weight-control Information Network - An information service of the
National Institute of Diabetes and Digestive and Kidney Diseases:
http://win.niddk.nih.gov/

Parenting

Australian Childhood Foundation:
http://www.childhood.org.au/website/default.asp.

Early Childhood Australia: http://www.earlychildhoodaustralia.org.au.

Kids Help Line (a free, confidential, anonymous phone and online counselling service for children aged 5 to 18), on 1800 55 1800: http://www.kidshelp.com.au.

Tips from the Triple P positive parenting program: http://www1.triplep.net.

Physical activity

Australian Physical Activity Network has updates on latest research and developments:
http://auspanet.heartfoundation.com.au.

Australia's physical activity recommendations for children and young people: http://www.health.gov.au/internet/wcms/publishing.nsf/Content/health-pubhlth-strateg-active-recommend.htm.

Bicycle Victoria (including The Cycle Friendly Workplace):
http://www.bv.com.au.

Bluearth Institute, promoting active lives:
http://www.bluearth.org/home.cfm?id=1.

Canada's physical activity guidelines for children:
http://www.phac-aspc.gc.ca/pau-uap/paguide/child_youth/children/index.html.

Challenge your thinking about cars (more about the Brisbane inventor David Engwicht):
http://www.creative-communities.com; http://www.lesstraffic.com; http://www.mentalspeedbumps.com; http://www.traffictamers.com.

Sport and Recreation Queensland has a number of resources, including:
- *Move Baby Move* (activities for babies as they develop);
- *Active Alphabet* (a booklet for parents and toddlers);
- *Let's Get Moving* (a booklet for parents of preschoolers to encourage participation in regular movement activities);
- *Active Choices* (an online checklist for parents to select suitable sport and recreation clubs and groups for their children); and

379

•*Moving with Young Children* (workshops for early childhood
professionals to develop skills and knowledge on good quality
physical activity).
All at: http://www.sportrec.qld.gov.au.
Case studies from the WHO Regional Office for Europe (tips for making
physical activity part of your daily life):
http://www.who.dk/transport.
The Community Guide (a US group which reviews the evidence on
health interventions, including physical activity)
http://www.thecommunityguide.org/
US physical activity guidelines for infants and toddlers:
http://www.aahperd.org/naspe/template.cfm?template=
toddlers.htm.
Various websites with practical tips for making activity a
daily routine:
•http://www.10000steps.org.au
•http://www.find30.com.au
•http://www.travelsmart.gov.au
•http://www.human-race.org/community_new
•http://www.whi.org.uk
•http://www.goforyourlife.vic.gov.au
•http://www.cyh.com/HealthTopics/HealthTopicDetails.aspx?p=11
4&np=301&id=1977
•http://www.healthyactive.gov.au/initiative/tips.pdf
•http://www.health.qld.gov.au/phs/Documents/shpu/24719.pdf
•http://www.cdc.gov/youthcampaign
•http://www.verbnow.com
•http://www.womensport.com.au
•http://www.activeaustralia.org
•http://www.irisheart.ie/slinaslainte/default.htm
•http://www.fitness.gov
•http://www.cdc.gov/nccdphp/dnpa/index.htm
•http://www.pecentral.org
•http://www.humankinetics.com
•http://www.americaonthemove.org
•http://www.sportengland.org
•http://www.activeontario.org

Useful resources

- •http://www.healthycommunities.org
- •http://www.goforgreen.ca
- •http://www.opc.on.ca/sites.html
- •http://www.ncppa.org
- •http://www.dsr.nsw.gov.au
- •http://www.hillarsport.org.nz
- •http://www.beactive.com.au
- •http://www.smartplay.net.

VicFit Physical activity infoline: 1300 885 602

Schools

Active-Ate is a school program that aims to promote healthy eating and increased daily physical activity in primary schools: http://www.health.qld.gov.au/Active-Ate.

Advice about how to set up and promote walking school buses—contained in a guide produced by the Australian Greenhouse Office. Available at: www.greenhouse.gov.au.

Queensland Association of School Tuckshops (for healthy fundraising ideas and other resources): http://www.qast.org.au.

NSW's Canteen Menu Planning Guide: http://www.health.nsw.gov.au/obesity/adult/canteens.html, or order from http://www.det.nsw.edu.au/detsales.

Queensland Canteen Strategy: Smart Choices—the Healthy Food and Drink Supply Strategy for Queensland Schools: http://education.qld.gov.au/schools/healthy/food-drink-strategy.html.

SA Health Promoting Schools Network: http://www.sahps.net.

SA schools and preschool guidelines: http://www.decs.sa.gov.au/speced/pages/default/eatwellsa.

School gardens information: http://www.edibleschoolyard.org/homepage.html or http://www.stephaniealexander.com.au or http://www.collingwood.vic.edu.au.

Tasmanian School Canteen Association: http://www.tased.edu.au/tasonline/tsca.

The Crunch 'n Sip program in Western Australia:
    http://www.crunchandsip.com.au.
The International Walk to School website:
    http://www.iwalktoschool.org.
Travel Smart in Victoria has school travel planning reosurces:
    http://www.vichealth.vic.gov.au/walkingschoolbus.
WA school canteen information:
    http://www.waschoolcanteens.org.au.

Television and screen-related issues

A community education kit about food advertising and children:
    http://www.chdf.org.au/foodadstokids.
Child-friendly search engines:
    •http://www.askjeevesforkids.com
    •http://www.yahooligans.com.
    Young Media Australia (1800 700 357):
    http://www.youngmedia.org.au
    Other relevant websites:
    •http://www.mediadietforkids.com
    •http://www.getnetwise.org
    •http://www.kidsmart.org.uk
    •http://www.chatdanger.com
    •http://www.parentscentre.gov.uk
    •http://www.iwf.org.uk
    •http://www.fkbko.co.uk
    •http://www.bbc.co.uk (offers a webwise online course)
    •http://www.thinkuknow.co.uk
    •http://www.nch.org.uk
    •http://www.pin.org.uk
    •http://www.brainworks.co.uk
    •http://www.parentscentre.gov.uk
    •http://www.mediasmart.org.uk.

The slow movement

    •http://www.slowfood.com
    •http://www.farmersmarkets.net

•http://www.matogmer.no/slow_cities_citta_slow.html/
(slow cities Italy)
•http://www.homezones.org (UK)
•http://www.newurbanism.org
•http://www.swt.org (shorter work time group, US)
•http://www.worktolive.info
•http://www.employersforwork-lifebalance.org.uk
•http://www.worklessparty.ca
•http://www.timeday.org.

Treatment services

Australian Health Map (guide to health services throughout Australia):
http://www.abc.net.au/health/healthmap/default.htmASSO.
Australian General Practice Network:
http://www.adgp.com.au.
Australian Psychological Society:
http://www.psychology.org.au.
Community health centres in Victoria:
http://www.health.vic.gov.au/communityhealth/ch_centres.htm.
Dietitians Association of Australia:
http://www.daa.asn.au.

Bibliography

Introduction, Chapters 1, 2 and 3

Books

Dixon, J., and Broom, D.H. (eds) 2007. *The seven deadly sins of obesity: How the modern world is making us fat*. (manuscript). University of NSW Press. Sydney

Egger, G. and Swinburn, B. 1996, *The fat loss handbook. A guide for professionals*, Allen & Unwin, Sydney.

Egger, G. and Binns, A. 2001, *The experts' weight loss guide. For doctors, health professionals…and all those serious about their health*, Allen & Unwin, Sydney.

Gard, M. and Wright, J. 2005, *The obesity epidemic. Science, morality and ideology*, Routledge, London.

Hamilton, C. and Denniss, R. 2005, *Affluenza. When too much is never enough*, Allen & Unwin, Sydney.

Hamilton, C. 2003, *Growth Fetish*, Allen & Unwin, Sydney.

Honoré, C. 2004, *In praise of slow. How a worldwide movement is challenging the cult of speed*, Orion Books, London.

Johnson, C. 2004, *Healthy environments. 11 essays*, Government Architect's Publications, Sydney.

Kopelman, P.G., Caterson, I.D. and Dietz, W.H. 2005, *Clinical obesity in adults and children*, 2nd edn, Blackwell Publishing, Massachusetts.

Nestle, M. 2002, *Food politics. How the food industry influences nutrition and health*, University of California Press, California.

Nestle, M. and Dixon, B.L. 2004, *Taking sides. Clashing views on controversial issues in food and nutrition*, McGraw Hill/Dushkin, Connecticut.

O'Dea, J. 2005, *Positive food for kids. Healthy food, healthy children, healthy life*, Doubleday, Sydney.

Schlosser, E. 2002, *Fast Food Nation. What the all-American meal is doing to the world*, Penguin Books, London.

Shell, E.R. 2003, *Fat Wars. The inside story of the obesity industry*, Atlantic Books, London.

Stanton, R. and Hills, A. 2004, *A matter of fat. Understanding and overcoming obesity in kids*, University of New South Wales (UNSW) Press, Sydney.

Wahlqvist, M.L. 1997, *Australasia, Asia and the Pacific. Food and nutrition*, Allen & Unwin, Sydney.

Journal articles and reports

Astrup, A. et al. 2004, 'The cause of obesity: Are we barking up the wrong tree?' (editorial), *Obesity Reviews*, vol. 5, pp. 125–27.

Australian Institute of Criminology 2006, 'Crime facts info. Perception of crime trends', Australian Government, Canberra.

Australian Institute of Family Studies 2004, 'Growing up in Australia: The longitudinal study of Australian children—an Australian Government initiative. 2004 annual report', Australian Institute of Family Studies, Melbourne.

Australian Institute of Heath and Welfare (AIHW) 2005, 'A picture of Australia's children', cat. no. PHD 58, AIHW, Canberra.

Banwell, C. et al. 2005, 'Reflections on expert consensus: a case study of the social trends contributing to obesity', *The European Journal of Public Health*, vol. 15, no. 6, pp. 564–68.

Banwell, C. et al. 2006, 'Fast and slow food in the fast lane: automobility and the Australian diet', in Wilk, R. (ed.), *Fast food/slow food. The economic anthropology of the global food system*, Society of Economic Anthropology Monograph Series, vol. 24, AltaMira Press MD.

Bell, C. et al. 2002, 'The road to obesity or the path to prevention: Motorized transportation and obesity in China', *Obesity Research*, vol. 10, no. 4, pp. 277–83.

Booth, M.L. et al. 2003, 'Change in the prevalence of overweight and obesity among young Australians 1969–1997', *American Journal of Clinical Nutrition*, vol. 77, no. 1, pp. 29–36.

Booth, M. et al. 2006, *NSW Schools Physical Activity and Nutrition Survey (SPANS) 2004*, NSW Health, Sydney.

Brown, R. et al. 1999, '100 Minutes Project: Researching PE and sport in DETE schools', Flinders University, Adelaide.

Campbell, K. et al. 2006, 'Family food environment and dietary behaviours likely to promote fatness in 5–6-year-old children'. *International Journal of Obesity, vol.* 30, pp. 1272–280.

Choi, B.C.K., Hunter, D.J., Tsou, W. and Sainsbury, P. 2005. Diseases of comfort: primary cause of death in the 22nd century. *J Epidemiol Community Health*, vol. 59, pp.1030–34

Commission for Architecture and the Built Environment (CABE) 2005, 'What are we scared of? The value of risk in designing public space', CABE Space, London.

Dixon, J. et al. 2004, 'Exploring the intersectoral partnerships guiding Australia's dietary advice', *Health Promotion International*, vol. 19, no. 1, pp. 5–13.

Dollman, J. et al. 2005, 'Evidence for secular trends in children's physical activity behaviour', *British Journal of Sports Medicine*, vol. 39, pp. 892–97.

Dollman J. et al. 2006, 'The relationship between curriculum time for physical education and literacy and numeracy standards in South Australian primary schools', *European Physical Education Review*, (in press).

Drewnowski, A. and Specter, S.E. 2004, 'Poverty and obesity: The role of energy density and energy costs', *Am J Clin Nutr*, vol. 79, no. 1. pp6–16.

Eckersley, R. 2001, 'Losing the battle of the bulge: Causes and consequences of increasing obesity', *The Medical Journal of Australia (MJA)*, vol. 174, pp. 590–92.

Egger, G. 2001, 'Estimating historical changes in physical activity levels', *MJA*, vol. 175, pp. 635–36.

Giles-Corti, B. 2005, 'Increasing walking: How important is distance to, attractiveness and size of public open space?', *American Journal of Preventive Medicine*, vol. 28, pp. 169–76.

Bibliography

Gill, T. et al. 2004, 'Detailed review of intervention studies: How do we best address the issues of overweight, obesity and cardiovascular disease?', NSW Centre for Public Health Nutrition (on behalf of the National Heart Foundation), National Heart Foundation of Australia.

Gleeson, B. 2004, 'The future of Australia's cities: Making space for hope', professorial lecture, Griffith University, Brisbane, 19 February.

Harrison, M.S. 2007. The increasing cost of the basic foods required to promote health in Queensland. *MJA*, vol. 186. no.1 pp. 9–14.

Hill, J. et al. 2003, 'Viewpoint. Obesity and the environment: where do we go from here?', *Science*, vol. 299, issue 5608, pp. 853–55.

Institute of Medicine of the National Academies 2006. *Progress in Preventing Childhood Obesity. How Do We Measure Up?* The National Academies Press. Washington, DC. Available at: www.iom.edu/obesity

Kant, A.K. 2000, 'Consumption of energy-dense, nutrient poor foods by adult Americans: Nutritional and health implications. The Third National Health and Nutrition Examination Survey, 1988–1999', *Am J Clin Nutr*, vol. 72, no. 4, pp. 929–36.

Kunkel, D. et al. 2004, 'Report of the American Psychological Association Task Force on Advertising and Children. Section: Psychological issues in the increasing commercialisation of childhood', American Psychological Association, 20 February.

League, C.A. and Dearry, A. 2004, 'Obesity and the built enviornment: Improving pubic health through community design', National Institute of Environmental Health Sciences/National Institute of Heath, Division of Research Coordination, Planning and Translation, Research Triangle Park NC.

Lee, A.J. et al.1994, 'Apparent dietary intake in remote Aboriginal communities', *Australian Journal of Public Health*, vol. 18, no. 2, pp. 190–97.

Lee, A.J. et al. 1994, 'Survival tucker: Improved diet and health indicators in an Aboriginal community', *AJPH*, vol. 18, no. 3, pp. 277–85.

Lewis, N.R. and Dollman, J. (2007), 'Trends in physical activity behaviours and attitudes among young South Australian youth between 1985–2004', (draft).

Muñoz, K.A. et al. 1997, 'Food intakes of US children and adolescents compared with recommendations', *Pediatrics*, vol. 100, no. 3, pp. 323–29.

Naughton, J. et al. 1986, 'Animal foods in traditional Australian Aboriginal diets: polyunsaturated and low in fat', *Lipids*, vol. 21, no. 11, pp. 684–90.

National Heart Foundation of Australia (Victorian Division) 2003, 'Healthy eating and physical activity in early childhood services: Enhancing policy and practice in Victorian family day care and long day care', report to the *Eat Well Victoria Partnership*, Melbourne, July.

Nielsen, S.J. et al. 2002, 'Trends in energy intake in US between 1997 and 1996: Similar shifts seen across age groups', *Obesity Research*, vol. 10, pp. 370–78.

NSW Centre for Public Health Nutrition 2005, 'Best options for promoting healthy weight and preventing weight gain in NSW', NSW Centre for Public Health Nutrition, March.

NSW Department of Infrastructure, Planning and Natural Resources, Transport and Population Data Centre 2004, '2002 Household Travel Survey Summary report', NSW Government, Sydney.

NSW Childhood Obesity Summit Secretariat 2002, 'Childhood Obesity NSW Summit Background Paper', NSW Government, Sydney 28 August.

NSW Health 2005, 'Key findings from qualitative research into childhood overweight/obesity, health eating and physical activity', (working document), NSW Government, Sydney.

O'Brien P. 1995, 'Dietary shifts and implications for US agriculture', *Am J Clin Nutr*, vol. 61 (suppl.), pp. I390S–96S.

O'Dea, J.A. 2004, 'Prevention of child obesity: "First, do no harm"', *Health Education Research* (advance access).

O'Dea, K. et al. 1980, 'The effect of transition from traditional to urban lifestyle on the insulin secretory response in Australian Aborigines', *Diabetes Care*, vol. 3, no. 1, pp. 31–37.

O'Dea, K. 1984, 'Marked improvement in carbohydrate and lipid metabolism in diabetic Australian Aborigines after temporary reversion to traditional lifestyle', *Diabetes*, vol. 33, pp. 596–603.

Bibliography

O'Dea, K. et al. 1988, 'An investigation of nutrition-related risk factors in an isolated Aboriginal community in Northern Australia: Advantages of a traditionally orientated lifestyle', *MJA*, vol. 148, pp. 177–80.

O'Dea, K. 1991, 'Traditional diet and food preferences of Australian Aboriginal hunter-gatherers', *Philosophical Transactions of the Royal Society of London B (Phil. Trans. R. Soc. Lond. B)*, vol. 334, pp. 233–41.

—— 1992, 'Obesity and diabetes in "the land of milk and honey"', *Diabetes/Metabolism Reviews*, vol. 8, no. 4, pp. 373–88.

—— 1992, 'Review article. Diabetes in Australian Aborigines: Impact of the western diet and lifestyle', *Journal of Internal Medicine*, vol. 232, pp. 103–17.

—— 2003, 'Diet, nutrition and lifestyles in health promotion', in Elmadfa I. et al. (eds), 'Modern aspects of nutrition. Present knowledge and future perspectives', *Forum Nutr. Basel*, Karger, vol. 56, pp. 100–3.

Olds, T. and Harten, N. 2001, 'One hundred years of growth: The evolution of height, mass, and body composition in Australian children, 1899–1999', *Human Biology*, vol. 73, no. 5, pp. 727–38.

Oxford Vision 2020 Tobacco Working Group 2004, 'Learning from tobacco to address diet and nutrition more effectively', September (draft report).

Patton, G. et al. 2005, 'A picture of Australia's children', *MJA*, vol. 182, no. 8, pp. 437–38.

Queensland Government 2001, *The 2001 Healthy Food Access Basket (HFAB) Survey*, Queensland Government, Brisbane.

—— 2004, *The 2004 Healthy Food Access Basket (HFAB) Survey*, Queensland Government, Brisbane.

—— 2005, *Eat well, be active—healthy kids for life. The Queensland Government's first action plan 2005–2008*, Queensland Government, Brisbane.

Reynolds, J. 2005, 'Nutrition education in schools—the good, the bad and the ugly', *Food Chain*, Strategic Intergovernmental Nutrition Alliance, no. ??, February.

Salmon, J. et al. 2005, 'Trends in children's physical activity and weight status in high and low socio-economic status areas of Melbourne, Victoria, 1985–2001', *Australian and New Zealand Journal of Public Health*, vol. 29, pp. 337–42.

Sanigorski, A. et al. 2005, 'High childhood obesity in an Australian population', poster presentation at Australasian Society for the Study of Obesity 14th annual scientific meeting, Glenelg, SA 28–30 October.

Schwartz, M.B. 2003, 'Weight bias among health professionals specializing in obesity', *Obesity Research*, vol. 11, pp. 1033–39.

Silburn, S. 2003, 'Guest editorial: Improving the developmental health of Australian children', *Australian e-Journal for the Advancement of Mental Health*, vol. 2, no. 1, accessed at: 2http://auseinet.flinders.edu.au/journal/vol2iss1/Silburn.pdf.

Stanley, F. 2003, 'Kenneth Myer Lecture 2003. Before the bough breaks: Children in contemporary Australia', accessed at: http://www.nla.gov.au/events/seminars/kmyer03.html.

Stanton, R. 2006, 'Clinical update: Nutrition problems in an obesogenic environment', *MJA*, vol. 184, no. 2, pp. 76–79.

—— 2003, 'Ensuring a safe and healthy food supply', *Food Chain*, Strategic Intergovernmental Nutrition Alliance, no. 13, December.

Stettler, N. 2004, 'Comment: The global epidemic of childhood obesity: Is there a role for the paediatrician?', *Obesity Reviews*, vol. 5, suppl. 1, pp. 1–3.

Story, M. and French, S. 2004, 'Food advertising and marketing directed at children and adolescents', *The International Journal of Behavioral Nutrition and Physical Activity*, accessed at: http://www.ijbnpa.org/content/1/1/3.

Stubbs, Christina and Lee, Amanda 2004, 'The obesity epidemic: Both energy intake and physical activity contribute', *MJA*, vol. 181, no. 9, pp. 489–91.

Tomkinson, G.R et al. 2003, 'Review article. Secular trends in the performance of children and adolescents (1980–2000)', *Sports Medicine*, vol. 33, no. 4, pp. 285–300.

Tranter, P. and Doyle, J. 1996, 'Reclaiming the residential street as play space', *International Play Journal*, vol. 4, pp. 81–97.

Bibliography

Tranter, P.J. 1996, 'Children's independent mobility and urban form in Australasian, English and German cities', in Hensher, D. King, J. and Oum, T. (eds), *World Transport Research: Proceedings of the Seventh World Conference on Transport Research*, Volume 3: Transport Policy, pp. 31–44.

Tranter, P. and Pawson, E. 2001, 'Children's access to local environments: A case study of Christchurch, New Zealand', *Local Environment*, vol. 6, no.1, pp. 27–48.

Tranter, P. and Malone, K. 2003, 'Out of bounds: Insights from children to support a cultural shift towards sustainable and child-friendly cities', presentation to State of Australian Cities national conference, Parramatta (NSW), 3–5 December.

—— 2004, 'Geographies of environmental learning: An exploration of children's use of school grounds', *Children's Geographies*, vol. 2, no. 1, pp. 131–56.

Vaska V.L. and Volkmer, R. 2004, 'Increasing prevalence of obesity in South Australian 4-year-olds: 1995–2002', *Journal of Paediatric Child Health*, vol. 40, pp. 353–55.

Victorian Health Promotion Foundation 2005, *VicHealth Letter*, issue 24, Summer, Victorian Health Promotion Foundation, Melbourne.

—— 2003, *Food for all? Food insecurity community demonstration projects; Maribyrnong City Council and North Yarra Community Health. Case studies*, Victorian Health Promotion Foundation, accessed at: http://www.vichealth.vic.gov.au.

Volker, D. 2004, 'How much is on your plate?', *Nutrition Research Foundation Annual Report 2003–2004*, University of Sydney.

Young, C.E. and Kantor, L.S. 1999, 'Moving toward the food guide pyramid: Implications for US agriculture', US Department of Agriculture (USDA), Washington DC.

Young, L. and Nestle, M. 2002, 'The contribution of expanding portion sizes to the US obesity epidemic', *American Journal of Public Health*, vol. 92, no. 2, pp. 246–49.

WA Government 2003, *Results of Western Australian Child and Adolescent Physical Activity and Nutrition Survey 2003 (CAPANS)*, WA Government, Perth.

Western Australian Physical Activity Taskforce Research and
Evaluation Working Party 2001, 'Background and summary of
research', WA Government, Perth.

Media articles

Anon. 2004, 'Be a sport, pass me another Maccas', *Australian Medicine*,
15 March, p. 10.

Australian Food and Grocery Council 2002, 'Obesity media briefing',
4 September.

AIHW 2006, 'Half of all Australians not eating their fruit and veg',
press release, 22 February.

Australasian Society for the Study of Obesity 2001, 'The proportion of
young Australians who are overweight is not just increasing; it's
accelerating', media release, 8 September.

Coultan, M. 2005, 'Digestible democracy: Extra calories and fat all part
of having it your way', *The Sydney Morning Herald* (*SMH*), 23 July,
p. ??.

Dwyer, J. 2005, 'Beware the child glued to his handheld', *SMH*,
5 August, p. 13.

—— 2004, 'Sports sponsors are turning our kids into junk food
freaks', *SMH*, 12 May, p. 15.

Gooch, L. 2005, 'Children's freedoms reduced out of fear', *SMH*, 15
November, p. 3.

Horin, A. 2005, 'Like America, we're destined for big things', *SMH*,
8–9 October, p. 37.

—— 2005, 'Nursery crimes', *SMH*, 27–28 August, p. 33.

—— 2006, 'Tighten the belt on children's advertising', *SMH*, 14–16
April, p. 23.

—— 2006, 'A ritual worth bringing to the table', *SMH*, 22–23 April,
p. 31.

Kron, J. 2004, 'Weighing in on obesity', *Australian Doctor*, 9 July,
pp. 47–49.

Huxley, J. 2005, 'Sport dreams coddled in cotton wool', *SMH*, 27–28
August, p. 13.

Jacobson, G. 2005, 'What kids really need—and want', *SMH*,
2 February, p. 14.

Lemonick, M. D. 2004, 'How we grew so big', *Time*, 28 June, pp. 49–53.

Mathews, C. 2004, 'We're all part of the problem', *Australian Medicine*, 3 May.

Norrie, J. and Maley, J. 2005, 'Parents get serious: Junk the junk', *SMH*, 29 July, pp. 1–2.

O'Dea, J. 2005, 'A fat lot of good in chiding chubby children', *SMH*, 20 May, p. 15.

Smith, A. 2005, 'Students driven to school rain or shine', *SMH*, 2 May, p. 3.

Tabakoff, J. 2004, 'Heckler', *SMH*, 21 June, p. 18.

Chapter 4

Journal articles and reports

AIHW 2001, 'National Diabetes Register. Statistical profile, December 2001', cat. no. CVD 24 (Diabetes Series no. 4), AIHW, Canberra.

——Australian Institute of Health and Welfare 2002. Diabetes: Australian facts 2002. AIHW Cat. No. CVD 20 (Diabetes Series. No. 3) Canberra: AIHW

—— 2003, 'Indicators of health risk factors', cat. no. PHE 47, AIHW, Canberra.

Ball, K. et al. 2004, 'Longitudinal relationships among overweight, life satisfaction, and aspirations in young women', *Obesity Research*, vol. 12, no. 6, pp. 1019–30.

Batch, J.A. and Baur, L.A. 2005, 'Management and prevention of obesity and its complications in children and adolescents', *MJA*, vol. 182, no. 3, pp. 130–35.

Baur, L. and Denney-Wilson, E. 2006, 'Obesity in children and adolescents', draft.

Davison, K.K. et al. 2003, 'Percent body fat at age five predicts earlier pubertal development among girls at age nine', *Pediatrics*, vol. 111, no. 4, pp. 815–21.

Davison, K.K. and Birch, L.L. 2004, 'Predictors of fat stereotypes among 9 year old girls and their parents', *Obesity Research*, vol. 12, pp. 86–94.

Diabetes Australia 2004, 'What is diabetes?', Diabetes Australia.

Dietz, W.H. 1998, 'Health consequences of obesity in youth: Childhood predictors of adult disease', *Pediatrics*, vol. 101, no. 3, Suppl., pp. 518–25.

—— 1998, 'Childhood weight affects adult morbidity and mortality', *J Nutr*, vol. 128, no. 2, pp. 411S–14S.

—— 2001, 'The obesity epidemic in young children', *British Medical Journal*, vol. 322, pp. 313–14.

Dietz, W.H. et al. 2003, 'The relation of menarcheal age to obesity in childhood and adulthood: The Bogalusa heart study', *BMC Pediatrics*, vol. 3, p. 3.

Dixon, H. et al. 2005, *Body weight, nutrition, alcohol and physical activity: Key messages for the Cancer Council Australia*, Cancer Council Australia, February.

NSW Department of Health 2004, *Eat Well NSW: Strategic directions for public health nutrition 2003–2007*, NSW Department of Health, Sydney.

Field, A.E. et al. 2001, 'Impact of overweight on the risk of developing common chronic diseases during a 10-year period', *Archives of Internal Medicine*, vol. 161, pp. 1581–86.

Flegal, K.M. et al. 2005, 'Excess deaths associated with underweight, overweight, and obesity', *Journal of the American Medical Association*, vol. 293, pp. 1861–67.

Freedman, D.S. et al. 1999, 'The relation of overweight to cardiovascular risk factors among children and adolescents: The Bogalusa Heart Study', *Pediatrics*, vol. 103, no. 6, pp. 1175–82.

Freedman, D.S. et al. 2001, 'Relationship of childhood obesity to coronary heart disease risk factors in adulthood: The Bogalusa Heart Study', *Pediatrics*, vol. 108, pp. 712–18.

Freedman, D.S. et al. 2005, 'The relation of childhood BMI to adult adiposity: The Bogalusa Heart Study', *Pediatrics*, vol. 115, pp. 22–27.

Friedlander, S.L. et al. 2003, 'Decreased quality of life associated with obesity in school-aged children', *Archives of Pediatric and Adolescent Medicine*, vol. 157, no. 12, pp. 1206–11.

Galloway, A.T. et al. 2003, 'Predictors and consequences of food neophobic and pickiness in young girls', *Journal of the Anerican Dietetic Association*, vol. 103, no. 6, pp. 692–98.

Bibliography

Gortmaker, S.L. et al. 1992, 'Social and economic consequences of overweight in adolesence and young adulthood', *New England Journal of Medicine*, vol. 329, no. 14, pp. 1008–12.

Hawley, J. 2004, 'Exercise as a therapeutic intervention for the prevention and treatment of insulin resistance', *Diabetes/Metabolism Research and Reviews*, vol. 20, pp. 383–93.

Hayman, L.L. et al. 2004, 'American Heart Association Scientific Statement. Cardiovascular Health Promotion in the Schools. A statement for health and education professionals and child health advocates from the Committee on Atherosclerosis, Hypertension, and Obesity in Youth (AHOY) of the Council on Cardiovascular disease in the Young, American Heart Association', *Circulation*, vol. 110, pp. 2266–75.

Hesketh, K. et al. 2004, 'Body mass index and parent-reported self-esteem in elementary school children: Evidence for a causal relationship', *International Journal of Obesity*, vol. 28, pp. 1233–37.

Hesketh, K. et al. 2005, 'Stability of body mass index in Australian children: A prospective cohort study across the middle childhood years', *Public Health Nutrition*, vol. 7, no. 2, pp. 303–09.

Institute of Medicine of the National Academies 2006. Progress in Preventing Childhood Obesity. How Do We Measure Up? The National Academies Press. Washington, DC. Available at: www.iom.edu/obesity

Janssen I. et al. 2005, 'Utility of childhood BMI in the prediction of adult disease: Comparison of national and international references', *Obesity Research*, vol.13, pp. 1106–15.

Lobstein T. et al. 2004, 'Obesity in children and young people: A crisis in public health', *Obesity Reviews*, vol. 5, suppl. 1, pp. 4–85.

Ludwig, D.S. and Ebbeling, C.B. 2001, 'Type 2 diabetes mellitus in children: Primary care and public health considerations', *JAMA*, vol. 286, pp. 1427–30.

McMahon, S. et al. 2004, 'Increase in type 2 diabetes in children and adolescents in WA', *MJA*, vol. 180, no. 9, pp. 459–61.

Must, A. et al. 1992, 'Long-term morbidity and mortality of overweight adolescents: A follow-up of the Harvard Growth Study of 1922 to 1935', *NEJM*, vol. 327, no. 19, pp. 1350–55.

Nankervis, A.J. 2006, 'Obesity and reproductive health', *MJA*, vol. 184, no. 2, p. 51.

Redline, S. et al. 1999, 'Risk factors for sleep-disordered breathing in children: Associations with obesity, race and respiratory problems', *American Journal of Respiratory Critical Care Medicine*, vol. 159, no. 5, pp. 1527–32.

Strauss, R.S. 2000, 'Childhood obesity and self-esteem', *Pediatrics*, vol. 105, no. 1, p. 15.

Taplin C.E. et al. 2005, 'The rising incidenc of childhood type 1 diabetes in New South Wales, 1990–2002', *MJA*, vol. 183, no. 5, pp. 243–46.

US Surgeon General 1996, 'Physical activity and health. A report of the surgeon general', US Department of Health and Human Services. Available at: http://www.cdc.gov/nccdphp/sgr/summary.htm.

Wang, G. and Dietz, W.H. 2002, 'Economic burden of obesity in youths aged 6 to 17 years: 1979–1999', *Pediatrics*, vol. 109, no. 5, p. 81.

Waters, E.B. and Baur, L.A. 2003, 'Childhood obesity: modernity's scourge', *MJA*, vol. 178, no. 9, pp. 422–23.

Whitaker, R.C. et al. 1997, 'Predicting obesity in young adulthood from childhood and parental obesity', *NEJM*, vol. 337, no. 13, pp. 869–73.

Whitlock, E.P. 2005, 'Screening and interventions for childhood overweight: A summary of evidence for the US Preventive Services Task Force', *Pediatrics*, vol. 116, pp. 125–44.

Media articles

Chapman, M. 2004, 'Iron link to child obesity', *Australian Doctor*, 23 July, p. 5.

Hickman, B. 2004, '"Diabesity" the new epidemic', *The Australian*, 26–27 June , p. 7.

Kerin, J. 2005, 'Youths too stoned, too fat to join forces', *The Australian*, 12 December, pp. 1–4.

Chapter 5

Journal articles and reports

Baker, D. and Eyeson-Annan, M. 2003 year, 'Monitoring health behaviours and health status in NSW: Release of the adult health survey 2003. *NSW Public Health Bulletin*, vol. 16, nos 1–2, pp. 13–17.

Bibliography

Birch, L.L. and Fisher, J.O. 2000, 'Mothers' child-feeding practices influence daughters' eating and weight', *Am J Clin Nutr*, vol. 71, no. 5, pp. 1054–61.

Campbell, K.J. et al. (draft), 'Associations between the home food environment and obesity-promoting eating behaviours in adolescence'.

Fisher, J.O. 2001, 'Maternal milk consumption predicts the tradeoff between milk and soft drinks in young girls' diets', *J Nutr*, vol. 131, pp. 246–50.

Dal Grande, E. 2005, 'Obesity in South Australian adults—prevalence, projections and generational assessment over 13 years', *Aust NZ J Public Health*, vol. 29, pp. 343–48.

Davison K.K. et al. 2001, 'Weight status, parent reaction, and self-concept in five-year-old girls', *Pediatrics*, vol. 107, no. 1, pp. 46–53.

Davison K.K. et al. 2003, 'Parents' activity-related parenting practices predict girls' physical activity', *Med Sci Sports Exerc*, vol. 35, no. 9, pp. 1589–95.

Davison, K.K. and Birch L.L. 2004, 'Lean and weight stable: Behavioral predictors and psychological correlates', *Obesity Research*, vol. 12, pp. 1085–93.

Davison K.K., Campbell K.J. (in press), 'Opportunities to prevent obesity in children within families: An ecological approach', in Crawford, D. and Jeffery, R., *Obesity Prevention in the 21st Century: Public Health Approaches to Tackle the Obesity Pandemic*, Oxford University Press.

Greenberg, B.S., Eastin, M., Hofschire, L., Lachlan, K. and Brownell, K.D. 2003.

'Portrayals of overweight and obese individuals on commercial television'. *American Journal of Public Health,* vol. 93, no. 8, pp. 1342–1348

Jain, Anjali et al. 2001, 'Why don't low-income mothers worry about their preschoolers being overweight?', *Pediatrics*, vol. 107, pp. 1138–46.

Juel, A. 2001, 'Does size really matter? Weight and values in public health', *Perspectives in Biology and Medicine*, vol. 44, no. 2.

397

Sanders, M.R. et al. 2003, 'Theoretical, scientific and clinical foundations of the triple P Positive Parenting Program: A population approach to the promotion of parenting competence', *Parenting Research and Practice Monograph*, no. 1, The Parenting and Family Support Centre, University of Queensland, Brisbane.

Sanders, M. (undated), 'Top 10 tips for parents: Triple P Positive Parenting Program fact sheet', University of Queensland, Brisbane.

Shunk J.A. and Birch L.L. 2004, 'Girls at risk for overweight at age 5 are at risk for dietary restraint, disinhibited overeating, weight concerns, and greater weight gain from 5 to 9 years', *J Am Diet Assoc*, vol. 104, no. 7, pp. 1120–26.

Tranter, P. 2004, 'Effective speeds: Car costs are slowing us down', for the Australian Greenhouse Office, Department of the Environment and Heritage. Available at: http://www.greenhouse.gov.au/publications/.

Media articles

Anon. 2004, 'Obesity apathy alarming: AMA', *Australian Medicine*, 15 November, p. 4.

Lee, J. 2005, 'Concerns food firms distorting diet policy', *SMH*, 4 July, p. 5.

Chapter 6

Books

Sigman, Aric 2005, *Remotely controlled. How television is damaging our lives—and what we can do about it*, Vermilion, London.

Greene, Jane and Grant, Anthony M. 2003, *Solution-focused coaching. Managing people in a complex world*, Pearson Education Ltd, Harlow (England).

Orange, Teresa and O'Flynn, Louise 2005, *The media diet for kids. A parent's survival gide to TV & computer games*, Hay House, London.

Journal articles and reports

Barkin, S. et a. 2006, 'Parental media mediation styles for children aged 2 to 11 years', *Arch Pediatr Adolesc Med*, vol. 160, pp. 395–401.

Bibliography

Campbell, K. et al. 2002, 'Family food environments of 5–6-year-old children: Does socioeconomic status make a difference?', *Asia Pacific Journal of Clinical Nutrition*, vol. 11, pp. S553–61.

Christakis, D.A. and Zimmerman, F.J. 2006. Media as a Public Health Issue *Arch Pediatr Adolesc Med*, vol.160, pp. 445–446.

Royal Australasian College of Physicians (RACP) 1999, 'Getting in the picture. A parent's and carer's guide for the better use of television for children' (3rd edn), Division of Paediatrics, Health Policy Unit, RACP, Sydney.

Francis, L.A. et al. 2003, 'Parental weight status and girls' television viewing, snacking, and body mass indexes', *Obesity Research*, vol. 11, pp. 143–51.

Hardy, L.L. 2006. Descriptive epidemiology of small screen recreation among Australian adolescents. *Journal of Paediatrics and Child Health*, vol. 42, no.11. pp. 709–714.

Institute of Medicine of the National Academies 2006. Progress in Preventing Childhood Obesity. How Do We Measure Up? The National Academies Press. Washington, DC. Available at: www.iom.edu/obesity.

Lumeng, J.C. et al. 2006, 'Television exposure and overweight risk in preschoolers', *Arch Pediatr Adolesc Med*, vol. 160, pp. 417–22.

National Health and Medical Research Council 2003, *Clinical practice guidelines for the management of overweight and obesity in children and adolescents*, Australian Government, Canberra.

Salmon, J. et al. 2005, 'Reducing sedentary behaviour and increasing physical activity among 10-year-old children: Overview and process evaluation of the "Switch-Play" intervention', *Health Promotion International*, vol. 20, no. 1, pp. 7–17.

Salmon J. et al. 2006, 'Television viewing habits associated with obesity risk factors: A survey of Melbourne schoolchildren', *MJA*, vol. 184, no. 2, pp. 64–67.

Taylor J. et al. 2005, 'Determinants of healthy eating in children and youth', *Canadian Journal of Public Health*, vol. 96, S 3.

RACP 2004, 'Children and the media: Advocating for the future', Paediatrics and Child Health Division RACP, Sydney. Available at: http://www.racp.edu.au/hpu/paed/media/.

Young Media Australia fact sheet 2004, 'Mind over media: Developing healthy relationships'.

— 2004, 'Mind over media: Developing good social and emotional skills'.

Van Zutphen, Moniek et al. (draft), 'Screen time, television access and weight status in Australian children'.

Wake, M. et al. 2003, 'Television, computer use and body mass index in Australian primary school children', *J Paediatr Child Health*, vol. 39, no. 2, pp. 130–34.

Media articles

Anon. 1956, 'When Sydney began to glow in the dark', 22 September, reproduced in 2006, *Special Supplement: 175 years of the Sydney Morning Herald*, 18 April, p. 3.

Meade, Amanda and Sinclair, Lara 2005, 'Fat chance of taking food off kids' TV', *The Australian* (Media section), 29 September, p. 15.

Oberklaid, Frank and Efron, Daryl 2005, 'Mixed messages', *Australian Doctor*, Therapy Update, 3 June, pp. 35–36.

Rideout, Victoria J. (Vice President and Director, Program for the Study of Entertainment Media and Health, Henry J. Kaiser Family Foundation) 2004, 'The role of media in childhood obesity', statement before the Senate Committee on Commerce, Science and Transportation Subcommittee on Competition, Foreign Commerce and Infastructure, 2 March, Canberra. Available at http://www.kff.org/.

Chapters 7–9

Books

Kausman, R. 2004, *If not dieting, then what?*, Allen & Unwin, Sydney.

Satter, E. 1987, *How to get your kid to eat...but not too much. From birth to adolescence*, Bull Publishing Co., Colorado.

Satter, . 2000, *Child of mine. Feeding with love and good sense*, Bull Publishing Co., Colorado.

Journal articles and reports

Abramovitz, B.A. and Birch L.L. 2000, 'Five-year-old girls' ideas about dieting are predicted by their mothers' dieting', *J Am Diet Assoc*, vol. 100, no. 10, pp. 1157–63.

Baker, H. 2004, *Parental Guidance Recommended* (National Child Nutrition Program Project Final Report), Cancer Council WA, Perth.

Barkeling, B. et al. 1992, 'Eating behaviour in obese and normal weight 11-year-old children', *International Journal of Obesity*, vol. 16, pp. 355–60.

Birch, L.L.1998, 'Psychological influences on the childhood diet', *J Nutr*, vol. 128, no. 2, pp. 407S–10S.

Birch, L.L. and Fisher, J.O. 1998, 'Development of eating behaviours among children and adolescents', *Pediatrics*, vol. 101, no. 3, pp. S539–49.

Birch L.L. et al. 1990, 'Conditioned flavor preference in young children', *Physiology & Behavior*, vol. 47, no. 3, pp. 501–05.

Birch, L.L. et al. 1991, 'The variability of young children's energy intake', *NEJM*, vol. 324, no. 4, pp. 232–35.

Birch, L.L. et al. 1998, 'Infants' consumption of a new food enhances acceptance of similar foods', *Appetite*, vol. 30, no. 3, pp. 283–95.

Birch L.L. et al. 2003, 'Learning to overeat: Maternal use of restricting feeding practices promotes girls' eating in the absence of hunger', *Am J Clin Nutr*, vol. 78, no. 2, pp. 215–20.

Bjork, C.C. and Rossner, S. 1998, '"Extravagances" during weight reduction: An analysis of food preference and selection', *Appetite*, vol. 31, pp. 93–99.

Campbell, K. et al. (draft), 'Family food environment and dietary behaviours likely to promote fatness in 5–6-year-old children'.

Campbell, K. and Crawford, D. 2001, 'Family food environments as determinants of preschool-aged children's eating behaviours: Implications for obesity prevention policy. A review', *Aust J Nutr Diet*, vol. 58, no. 1, pp. 19–25.

Campbell, K.J. et al. 2005, 'The home environment and obesogenic eating in early adolescence', presentation to the International Society for Behavioral Nutrition and Physical Activity Annual Meeting, Amsterdam.

Campbell, K. et al. 2002, 'Family food environments of 5–6-year-old-children: Does socioeconomic status make a difference?', *Asia Pacific J Clin Nutr*, vol. 11, S553–61.

Carper J.L. et al. 2000, 'Young girls' emerging dietary restraint and disinhibition are related to parental control in child feeding', *Appetite*, vol. 35, no. 2, pp. 121–29.

American Academy of Pediatrics Committee on School Health Policy Statement 2004, 'Soft drinks in schools', *Pediatrics*, vol. 113, no. 1, pp. 152–54.

Cutting, T.M. et al. 1999, 'Like mother, like daughter: Familial patterns of overweight are mediated by mothers' dietary disinhibition', *Am J Clin Nutr*, vol. 69, no. 4, pp. 608–13.

Davison K.K. et al. 2003, 'A longitudinal examination of patterns in girls' weight concerns and body dissatifaction from ages 5 to 9 years', *International Journal of Eating Disorders*, vol. 33, no. 3, pp. 320–32.

Davison K.K. and Birch L.L. 2001, 'Child and parent characteristics as predictors of change in girls' body mass index', *International Journal of Obesity-related Metabolic Disorders*, vol. 25, no. 12, pp. 1834–42.

Drewnowski, A. and Darmon, N. 2005, 'The economics of obesity: Dietary energy density and energy cost', *Am J Clin Nutr*, vol. 82, pp. 265S–73S.

Drewnowski, A. and Gomez-Carneros, C. 2000, 'Bitter taste, phytonutrients, and the consumer: A review', *Am J Clin Nutr*, vol. 72, pp. 1424–35.

Drewnowski, A. and Levine, A.S. 2003, 'Sugar and fat—from genes to culture', presented as part of the symposium 'Sugar and fat—from genes to culture', given at the Experimental Biology Meeting in New Orleans, 23 April 2002, *J Nutr*, vol. 133, pp. 829S–30S.

Drewnowski, A. and Rolls, B. 2005, 'How to modify the food environment', *J Nutr*, vol. 135, pp. 898–99.

Fisher, J.O. 2003, 'Children's bite size and intake of an entrée are greater with large portions than with age-appropriate or self-selected portions', *Am J Clin Nutr*, vol. 77, no. 5, pp. 1164–70.

Fisher J.O. and Birch, L.L. 1999, 'Restricting access to palatable foods affects children's behavioral response, food selection, and intake', *Am J Clin Nutr*, vol. 69, pp. 1264–72.

Bibliography

Fisher, J.O. and Birch, L.L. 2000, 'Mothers' child-feeding practices influence daughters' eating and weight', *Am J Clin Nutr*, vol. 71, no. 5, pp. 1054–61.

Fisher, J.O. and Birch, L.L. 2000, 'Parents' restrictive feeding pratices are associated with young girls' negative self-evaluation of eating', *J Am Diet Assoc*, vol. 100, no. 11, pp. 1341–46.

Fisher, J.O. and Birch, L.L. 2002, 'Eating in the absence of hunger and overweight in girls from 5 to 7 years of age', *Am J Clin Nutr*, vol. 76, no 1, pp. 226–31.

Fisher J.O. et al. 2000, 'Breast-feeding through the first year predicts maternal control in feeding and subsequent toddler energy intakes', *J Am Diet Assoc*, vol. 100, no. 6, pp. 641–46.

Fisher, J.O. et al. 2002, 'Parental influences on young girls' fruit and vegetable, miconutrient and fat intakes', *J Am Diet Assoc*, vol. 102, no. 1, pp. 58–64.

Gabriel, R. et al. 2005, 'Infant and child nutrition in Queensland 2003', Queensland Health, Brisbane.

Gehling R.K. et al. 2005, 'Food-based recommendations to reduce fat intake: An evidence-based approach to the development of a family-focused child weight management programme', *Journal of Paediatric Child Health*, vol. 41, pp. 112–18.

Hesketh, K. et al. 2005, 'Healthy eating, activity and obesity prevention: A qualitative study of parent and child perceptions in Australia', *Health Promotion International*, vol. 20, no. 1, pp. 19–26.

Johnson, S.L. 2000, 'Improving preschoolers' self-regulation of energy intake', *Pediatrics*, vol. 106, no. 6, pp. 1429–35.

Magarey, A. et al. 2006, 'Evaluation of fruit and vegetable intakes of Australian adults: The National Nutrition Survey 1995', *Aust NZ J Public Health*, vol. 30, pp. 32–37.

Mannino, M.L. et al. 2004, 'The quality of girls' diets declines and tracks across middle childhood', *International Journal of Behavioral Nutrition and Physical Activity*, vol. 1, no. 5, 27 February.

NHMRC 2003, 'Dietary guidelines for children and adolescents in Australia incorporating the infant feeding guidelines for health workers (endorsed 10 April 2003)', NHMRC, Canberra.

NSW Centre for Public Health Nutrition (CPHN) 2003, 'Report on the consumption of vegetables and fruit in NSW', CPHN, Sydney. Available at: http://www.cphn.biochem.usyd.edu.au.
—— 2004, 'Overview of recent reviews of interventions to promote and support breastfeeding', CPHN, Sydney. Available at: http://www.cphn.biochem.usyd.edu.au.

Nutrition and Physical Activity Branch, WA Department of Health 2005, 'Crunch & Sip', WA Government, Perth.

O'Dea, J. 2003, 'Why do kids eat healthful foods? Perceived benefits of and barriers to healthful eating and physical activity among children and adolescents', *J Am Diet Assoc*, vol. 103, no. 4, pp. 497–500.

Picciano, M.F. et al. 2000, 'Nutritional guidance is needed during dietary transition in early childhood', *Pediatrics*, vol. 106, no.1 , pp. 109–14.

Polivy, J. and Herman, C.P. 2005, 'Mental health and eating behaviours: A bi-directional relation', *Canadian Journal of Public Health*, vol. 96, pp. S43–S46.

Rolls, B. et al. 2005, 'Changing the energy density of the diet as a strategy for weight management', *J Am Diet Assoc* (suppl.), vol. 105, no. 5, pp. S98–103.

Sanigorski, A.M. et al. 2005, 'Lunchbox contents of Australian school children: Room for improvement', *European Journal of Clinical Nutrition*, vol. 59, pp. 1310–16.

Savenake, J. 2004, 'Improving food security: Healthy eating for people on low incomes', training package for use by dietitians and nutritionists, SA Government, Department of Human Services, Womens and Children's Hospital, Adelaide.

Sherry, B. et al. 2004, 'Attitudes, practices and concerns about child feeding and child weight status among socioeconomically diverse white, Hispanic and African-American mothers', *J Am Diet Assoc*, vol. 104, no. 2, pp. 215–21.

Strategic Inter-Governmental Nutrition Alliance 2001, *Eat Well Australia. An agenda for action for public health nutrition 2000–2010*, National Public Health Partnership. Available at: http://www.health.vic.gov.au/nhpa/resources/nu_eatwell.htm.

—— 2003, 'Promoting healthy weight', *Food Chain*, no. 11.

—— 2004, 'Workforce development', *Food Chain*, no. 15.

Swinburn, B. and Egger, G. 2002, 'Preventive strategies against weight gain and obesity', *Obesity Reviews*, vol. 3, pp. 289–301.

Rosenbaum, M. and Leibel, R.L. 1998, 'The physiology of body weight regulation: relevance to the etiology of obesity in children', *Pediatrics*, vol. 101, no. 3, pp. S525–39.

Taveras, E.M. et al. 2004, 'Association of breastfeeding with maternal control of infant feeding at age 1 year', *Pediatrics*, vol. 114, no. 5, pp. 577–83.

Webb, K. et al. 2005, 'Guest editorial: Breast feeding and the public's health', *NSW Public Health Bulletin*, vol. 16, nos 3–4, pp. 37–41.

WA Country Health Service 2005, 'Improving parents and carers awareness of healthy food options for the lunch box', Nutrition articles for school newsletters, WA Health Department, Perth.

Williams, C.L. et al. 2002, '"Healthy-Start": Outcome of an intervention to promote a heart healthy diet in preschool children', *Journal of the American College of Nutrition*, vol. 21, no. 1, pp. 62–71.

Wood, K. et al. 2003, 'Hot topic: Breastfeeding and obesity', Lactation Resource Centre, Australian Breastfeeding Association. Available at: http://www.breastfeeding.asn.au/lrc/publications.html.

Zelman, K. and Kennedy, E. 2004, 'Naturally nutrient rich...putting more power on Americans' plates', *Nutrition Today*, vol. 40, no. 2, pp. 60–68.

Media articles

Alexander, Stephanie 2004, 'Fresh ideas the key to fighting obesity', *SMH*, 14 July, p. 11.

Gressor, Megan 2005, 'The alarming history of diets', *SMH* (Health and Science section), 12 May, pp. 4–5.

James, Tony 2003, 'Soft drink hard on health', *Australian Doctor*, 22 August, p. 12.

Stanton, Rosemary 2004, 'When children don't eat', *Australian Doctor*, 30 April, pp. 45–46.

Chapter 10

Books

Engwicht, David 2005, *Mental Speed Bumps: The smarter way to tame traffic*, Envirobook, Sydney.

Journal articles and reports

Ball, K. et al. 2000, 'Too fat to exercise? Obesity as a barrier to physical activity', *Aust NZ J Public Health*, vol. 24, no. 3, pp. 331–33.

Bauman. A.E. et al. 2001, 'The epidemiology of dog walking: An unmet need for human and canine health', *MJA*, vol. 175, pp. 632–34.

Beck, A.M. and Meyers, N.M. 1996, 'Health enhancement and companion animal ownership', *Annual Review of Public Health*, vol. 17, pp. 247–57.

Booth, M.L. et al. 2002, 'Epidemiology of physical activity participation among New South Wales school students', *Aust NZ J Public Health*, vol. 26, no. 4, pp. 371–74.

Booth, M.L. et al. 2004, 'Patterns of activity energy expenditure among Australian adolescents', *Journal of Physical Activity and Health*, vol. 1, pp. 246–58.

Brown, W. et al. 2006, '10,000 Steps Rockhampton: Evaluation of a whole community approach to improving population levels of physical activity', *Journal of Physical Activity and Health*, vol. 3, no. 1, pp. 1–14.

Brown, W. et al. 2003, '10,000 Steps Rockhampton: Establishing a multi-strategy physical activity promotion project in a community', *Health Promotion Journal of Australia*, vol. 14, no. 2, pp. 96–101.

Brownson, R.C. et al. 2001. Environmental and Policy Determinants of Physical Activity in the United States. Am J Pub Health, vol. 91, no. 1995–2003.

Bull, F.C. et al. 2003, 'Review of best practice and recommendations for interventions on physical activity', report for the Premier's physical activity taskforce on behalf of the Evaluation and Monitoring Group, WA Government, Perth.

Bibliography

Campbell, K. et al. 2001, 'Interventions for preventing obesity in childhood. A systematic review', *Obesity Reviews*, vol. 2, pp. 149–57.

Centers for Disease Control and Prevention (undated), 'Tips for parents: 60 play every day, any way', Youth Media Campaign. Available at: http://www.cdc.gov/youthcampaign/materials/adults/tips.htm.

Collins, D.C. and Kearns, R.A. 2005, 'Geographies of inequality: Child pedestrian injury and walking school buses in Auckland, New Zealand', *Social Science & Medicine*, vol. 60, no. 1, pp. 61–69.

Commonwealth Department of Health and Ageing 2004, 'Active kids are healthy kids. Australia's physical recommendations for 5–12-year-olds', Australian Government, Canberra.

——— 2004, 'Get out and get active. Australia's physical activity recommendations for 12–18-year-olds', Australian Government, Canberra.

Davison, K.K. et al. 2002, 'Participation in aesthetic sports and girls' weight concerns at ages 5 and 7 years', *Int J Eat Disord*, vol. 31, no. 3, pp. 312–17.

Dollman, J. et al. 2002, 'Anthropometry, fitness and physical activity of urban and rural South Australian children', *Pediatric Exercise Science*, vol. 14, no. 3, pp. 297–312.

Dwyer, T. et al. 1983, 'An investigation of the effects of daily physical activity on the health of primary school students in South Australia', *Int J Epidemiol*, vol. 12, no. 3, pp. 308–13.

Hume, C. et al. 2005, 'Children's perceptions of their home and neighborhood environments, and their association with objectively measured physical activity: A qualitative and quantitative study', *Health Education Research*, vol. 20, no. 1, pp. 1–13.

Institute of Medicine of the National Academies 2006. Progress in Preventing Childhood Obesity. How Do We Measure Up? The National Academies Press. Washington, DC. Available at: www.iom.edu/obesity.

McNicholas, J. and Collis, G.M. 2001, 'Children's representations of pets in their social networks', *Child: Care, Health and Development*, vol. 27, no. 3, pp. 279–94.

Morris, L. et al. 2003, 'Sport, physical activity and antisocial behaviour in youth', Australian Institute of Criminology Research and Public Policy Series, no. 49, Australian Government, Canberra.

Morrow, V. 1998, 'My animals and other family: Children's perspectives on their relationships with companion animals', *Anthrozoos*, vol. 11, no. 4, pp. 218–26.

Naughton, G. 2005, 'Children's activity and weight management', presentation, Graduate Certificate in Paediatric Nutrition Unit 1: Nutrition and Child Health, Australian Catholic University, Sydney.

Naughton, Geraldine 2005, 'Critical windows—industry partner report 2005', presentation to NSW Health, August, Sydney.

O'Brien, C. 2003, 'Transportation…that's actually good for the soul', National Center for Bicycling and Walking Forum, National Center for Bicycling and Walking (http://www.bikewalk.org).

Okley, A.D. and Booth, M.L. 2004, 'Mastery of fundamental movement skills among children in New South Wales: Prevalence and sociodemographic distribution', *Journal of Science and Medicine in Sports*, vol. 7, no.3, pp. 358–72.

Okley, A.D. et al. 2001, 'Relationship of cardiorespiratory endurance to fundamental movement skill proficiency among adolescents', *Pediatric Exercise Science*, vol. 13, pp. 380–91.

Okley, A.D. et al. 2001, 'Relationship of physical activity to fundamental movement skills among adolescents', *Medicine & Science in Sports & Exercise*, vol. 33, no. 11, pp. 1899–1904.

Okley, A.D. et al. 2004, 'Relationships between body composition and fundamental movement skills among children and adolescents', *Research Quarterly for Exercise and Sport*, vol. 75, no. 3, pp. 238–47.

Salmon J. 2003, 'Home and neighbourhood: The influence of the environment on children's physical activity', presentation to Royal Australasian College of Physicians 2003 Annual Scientific Meeting, 26–28 May, Hobart.

Salmon, J. et al. 2004, 'The Children's Leisure Activities Study. Summary Report', Centre for Physical Activity & Nutrition Research, Deakin University, Melbourne, July. Available at: http://www.deakin.edu.au/hbs/cpan/be.php.

Serpell, J. 1991, 'Beneficial effects of pet ownership on some aspects of human health and behaviour', *Journal of the Royal Society of Medicine*, vol. 84, pp. 717–20.

Bibliography

Site specific approaches to prevention or management of pediatric obesity conference 2004, 'Summary report', 14–15 July, Bethesda MD. Available at: http://www.niddk.nih.gov/fund/other/conferences-arch.htm

Southall, J.E. et al. 2004, 'Actual and perceived physical competence in overweight and non overweight children', *Pediatric Exercise Science*, vol. 16, pp. 15–24.

Spinks, A. 2006. Determinants of sufficient daily activity in Australian primary school children. *Journal of Paediatrics and Child Health*. vol. 42, no. 11, pp. 674–679.

Telford, A. et al. 2005, 'Quantifying and characterising physical activity among children in Australia: The Children's Leisure Activities Study (CLASS)', *Pediatric Exercise Science*, vol. 17, pp. 266–80.

Tranter, P.J. 2004, 'Effective speeds: Car costs are slowing us down', report for the Australian Greenhouse Office, Commonwealth Department of the Environment and Heritage. Available at: http://www.greenhouse.gov.au/tdm/publications/pubs/effectivespeeds.pdf.

—— 2006, 'Overcoming social traps: A key to creating child-friendly cities?', in Gleeson, B.J. and Sipe, N. (eds), *Creating Child-Friendly Cities*, Routledge, London (in press).

Tranter, P.J. and Malone, K. 2003, 'Out of bounds: Insights from children to support a cultural shift towards sustainable and child-friendly cities', State of Australian Cities National Conference, 3–5 December, University of Western Sydney, Urban Frontiers Program, Parramatta.

Tranter, P. and May, M. 2005, 'Questioning the need for speed: Can effective speed guide change in travel behaviour and transport policy?', *Proceedings of the 28th Australasian Transport Research Forum*, 28–30 September, Sydney.

TravelSmart Australia 2005, 'Walking School Bus. A guide for parents and teachers', Australian Greenhouse Office in the Commonwealth Department of the Environment and Heritage. Available at: http://www.travelsmart.gov.au/schools/schools2.html#download.

Trost, S.G. 1996, 'Gender differences in physical activity and determinants of physical activity in rural fifth grade children', *Journal of School Health*, vol. 66, no. 4, pp. 145–49.

—— 2001, 'Physical activity and determinants of physical activity in obese and non-obese children', *International Journal of Obesity*, vol. 25, pp. 822–29.

—— 2005, 'Discussion paper for the development of recommendations for children's and youths' participation in health promoting physical activity', Australian Government Department of Health and Ageing, Canberra.

Trost, S.G. et al. 1997, 'A prospective study of the determinants of physical activity in rural fifth grade children', *Preventive Medicine*, vol. 26, pp. 257–63.

Trost, S.G. et al. 1999, 'Correlates of objectively measured physical activity in preadolescent youth', *Am J Prev Med*, vol. 17, no. 2, pp. 120–26.

Trost S.G. et al. 2002, 'Evaluation of a pedometer-based, moderate-intensity physical activity program in obese children and adolescents', paper presented at the 11th Annual Scientific Meeting of the Australasian Society of the Study of Obesity, Melbourne.

Trost S.G. et al. 2003, 'Evaluating a model of parental influence on youth behavior', *Am J Prev Med*, vol. 25, pp. 277–82.

Veitch, J. et al. (in press), 'Where do children usually play? A qualitative study of parents' perceptions of influences on children's active free-play', *Health & Place*.

WA Premier's Physical Activity Taskforce (undated), A series of fact sheets and information bulletins about physical activity, WA Government, Perth. Available at: http://www.patf.dpc.wa.gov.au.

—— 2001, *Getting Western Australians More Active. A strategic direction report from the Premier's Physical Activity Taskforce*, WA Government, Perth.

Wood, L. et al. 2005, 'The pet connection: Pets as a conduit for social capital?', *Soc Sci Med*, vol. 61, pp. 1159–73.

Media articles

Magnay, Jacqueline 2005, 'Sporty girls can't get by without their mum', *SMH*, 17 Nov, 2003 p. 3.

Nixon, Sherrill 2006, 'Nature lessons make children smarter, fitter', *SMH*, 13 February, p. 2.

Tobler, Helen 2003, 'Your neighbourhood could be making you fat',
      The Weekend Australian, 6–7 September, p. 3.

Williams, L. 2006, 'Every move they make, mum's watching', *SMH*,
      11–12 February, pp.1–2.

Chapter 11

Journal articles and reports

Dietz, W.H. 1997, 'Periods of risk in childhood for the development of
      adult obesity—what do we need to learn?', presented as part of a
      symposium, 'Obesity: Common symptom of diverse gene-based
      metabolic dysregulations', American Society for Nutritional
      Sciences, Little Rock AR, 4 March, pp. 1884S–86S.

McCallum, Z. et al. 2005, 'Can Australian general practitioners tackle
      childhood overweight/obesity? Methods and processes from the
      LEAP (Live, Eat and Play) randomized controlled trial', *Journal of
      Paediatric Child Health*, vol. 41, pp. 488–94.

National Health and Medical Research Council (NHMRC) 2003, *Clinical
      practice guidelines for the management of overweight and obesity in
      children and adolescents*, Australian Government, Canberra.

—— 2003, *Overweight and obesity in children and adolescents: A guide
      for general practitioners*, Australian Government, Canberra.

O'Brien,P. et al. 2004, 'Obesity is a surgical disease: Overview of
      obesity and bariatric surgery', *Australian and New Zealand Journal
      of Surgery*, vol. 74, pp. 200–04.

O'Dea, J. 2002, 'Can body image education programs be harmful to
      adolescent females?', *Eating Disorders*, vol. 10, pp. 1–13.

—— 1999, 'Cross-cultural, body weight and gender differences in the
      body size, perceptions and body ideals of university students',
      Aust J Nutr Diet, vol. 56, no. 3, pp. 144–50.

Wake, M. and McCallum, Z. 2004, 'Secondary prevention of
      overweight in primary school children: What place for general
      practice?', *MJA*, vol. 181, no. 2, pp. 82–83.

Wake, M. et al. 2002, 'Parent-reported health status of overweight and
      obese Australian primary school children: A cross-sectional
      population survey', *International Journal of Obesity*, vol. 26,
      pp. 717–24.

Media articles

Harris, Francis 2005, 'Doctor censured for telling patient she is dangerously fat', *SMH*, 27–28 August, p. 19.

Chapters 12 and 13

Journal articles and reports

AIHW 2006, 'National public health expenditure report 2001–02 to 2003–04', Health and Welfare Expenditure Series No. 26, cat. no. HWE 33, AIHW, Canberra.

—— 2005, 'Obesity and workplace absenteeism among older Australians', Bulletin No. 31, cat. no. AUS 67, Canberra.

Ball, K. and Crawford, D. 2004, 'Healthy weight 2008: Still waiting on Australia to act?', *Nutrition & Dietetics*, vol. 61, no. 1, pp. 5–7.

Bell, C. and Swinburn, B. 2005, 'School canteens: Using ripples to create a wave of healthy eating', *MJA*, vol. 183, no. 1, pp. 5–6.

Bicycle Victoria 2003, 'The cycle-friendly workplace'. Available at http://www.bv.com.au.

Booth, M. (in press), 'Behavioural food labelling', *Int J Obesity*.

Macquarie Area Health Service 2004, 'Challenging your community to better health. A healthy lifestyle resource based on experiences from The Wellingtonne Challenge', Macquarie Area Health Service, Dubbo .

Brierley, A. et al. , 'Executive summary. Feasibility summary for a multistrategy nutrition project in Penrith LGA', Penrith City Council, Penrith.

Cheong, M.T. et al. 2002, 'School based intervention has reduced obesity in Singapore', *BMJ*, vol. 324, p. 427.

Colagiuri, R., Colagiuri, S. Yach, D. and Pramming, S. 2006. The Answer to Diabetes Prevention: Science, Surgery, Service Delivery or Social Policy? *Am J Pub Health*. Vol. 96, no. 9, pp. 1562–1569.

Daube, M. 2006. Public health needs a strong, well-planned advocacy program. *Aust NZ J Public Health,* vol. 30, no.5 pp. 405–406.

Garrard, J. et al. 2004, 'Planning for healthy communities: Reducing the risk of cardiovascular disease and type 2 diabetes through healthier environments and lifestyles', Victorian Government, Department of Human Services, Melbourne.

Bibliography

Hudson, K. 2006, 'A creative consumer panel report on kids' obesity'. Available at: http://www.ideacentre.com.au.

Institute of Medicine of the National Academies 2006. Progress in Preventing Childhood Obesity. How Do We Measure Up? The National Academies Press. Washington, DC. Available at: www.iom.edu/obesity

Miller, M. and Stafford, H. 2002, 'Selecting interventions to promote vegetables and fruit: Summary of current resources', NSW Centre for Public Health Nutrition, Sydney.

National Obesity Taskforce 2005, 'Overview'. Available at: http://www.healthyactive.gov.au/publications.htm.

Payet, J. et al. 2005, 'Gascoyne Growers Market: A sustainable health promotion activity developed in partnership with the community', *Australian Journal of Rural Health*, vol. 13, no. 5, pp. 309–14.

Premier's Physical Activity Taskforce 2006. How to: Promote Walking. A Guide for Local Government. WA Government, Perth.

Pietinen, P. 1996, 'Changes in diet in Finland from 1972 to 1992: Impact on coronary heart disease risk', *Prev Med*, vol. 25, no. 3, pp. 243–50.

—— 2001, 'Nutrition and cardiovascular disease in Finland since the early 1970s: A success story', *Journal of Nutrition, Health and Aging*, vol. 5, no. 3, pp. 150–54.

Puska, P. 2002, 'Successful prevention of non-communicable diseases: 25 year experiences with North Karelia Project', *Public Health Medicine*, vol. 4, no. 1, pp. 5–7.

Puska, P. et al. 1989, 'The North Karelia project: 15 years of community-based prevention of coronary heart disease', *Annals of Medicine*, vol. 21, no. 3, pp. 169–73.

Reay, L. and Webb, K. 1997, 'Penrith food project. Triennial report 1994–1997', Penrith City Council.

Ryan, K.W. Arkansas Fights Fat: Translating Research Into Policy To Combat Childhood And Adolescent Obesity. *Health Affairs*, vol. 25, no. 4, pp. 992–1004

Sach & Associates 2000, 'Multi-purpose services program evaluation (Victoria), November 2000', prepared for Commonwealth Department of Health and Aged Care and (Victorian) Department of Human Services.

Seppanen, S. (undated), 'Finland—a case study in healthy eating'.
Available at: http://www.irishhealth.com/clin/ffl/finland.html.

Shilton, S. and Naughton, G. 2001, 'Physical activity and children', for
the National Heart Foundation's National Physical Activity
Program Committee, May.

Tranter, P. and Malone, K. 'Geographies of environmental learning: An
exploration of children's use of school grounds', *Children's
Geographies*, vol. 2, no. 1, pp. 131–56.

Trust for America's Health 2006. F as in Fat: How Obesity Policies are
Failing in America. Issue Report. Available at:
www.healthyamericans.org.

Vartiainen, E. et al. 2000, 'Cardiovascular risk factor changes in Finland
1972–1997', *International Journal of Epidemiology*, vol. 29, pp.
49–56.

Washington State Department of Health 2005, 'Nutrition and physical
activity: A policy resource guide', Office of Community Wellness
and Prevention, Washington State. Available at:
http://www.doh.wa.gov/cfh/steps/default.

Webb, K. et al. 2001, 'Collaborative intersectoral approaches to
nutrition in a community on the urban fringe', *Health Education &
Behavior*, vol. 28, no. 3, pp. 306–19.

Zaccari, V. and Dirkis, H. 2003, 'Walking to school in inner Sydney',
Health Promotion Journal of Australia, vol. 14, no. 2, pp. 137–40.

Zimmet, P.Z., and James, W.P.T. 2006. The unstoppable Australian
obesity and diabetes juggernaut. What should politicians do? *MJA*,
Vol. 185, no. 4. pp. 187–188.

Media articles

Canning, Simon 2005, 'Chocolate fundraisers given the brush', *The
Australian* (Media section), 4 August, 2005. p. 18.

Franklin, Matthew 2006, 'States the 'villains' in battle of bulge', *The
Australian*, 24 October, p.5

Sinclair, Lara 2004, 'Healthier food hits school canteens', *The
Australian*, 22 July, p.19.

Stanton, R. 2006. 'Just say no', *Australian Doctor*. 22 Sept., pp. 33–34

Endnotes

Introduction

1 Rosenbaum, M. and Leibel, R.L. 1998, 'The physiology of body weight regulation: Relevance to the etiology of obesity in children', *Pediatrics*, vol. 101, no. 3, pp. S525–39.

2 Hesketh, K. et al. 2005, 'Healthy eating, activity and obesity prevention: A qualitative study of parent and child perceptions in Australia', *Health Promotion International*, vol. 20, no. 1, Advance access publication.

3 Hamilton, C. and Denniss, R. 2005, *Affluenza: When too much is never enough*, Allen & Unwin, Sydney.

Chapter 1

1 Egger, G. and Swinburn, B. 1996, *The fat loss handbook: A guide for professionals*, Allen & Unwin, Sydney.

2 WA Government 2003, *Results of Western Australian Child and Adolescent Physical Activity and Nutrition Survey 2003 (CAPANS)*, WA Government.

3 Shell, E.R. 2003, *Fat Wars: The inside story of the obesity industry*, Atlantic Books, London.

4 Kopelman, P.G., Caterson, I.D. and Dietz, W.H. 2005, *Clinical obesity in adults and children* (2nd edn), Blackwell Publishing, Massachusetts; Egger, G. and Binns, A. 2001, *The experts' weight loss guide. For doctors, health professionals…and all those serious about their health*, Allen & Unwin, Sydney.

5 Institute of Medicine of the National Academies 2006. Progress in Preventing Childhood Obesity. How Do We Measure Up? The National Academies Press. Washington, DC. Available at: www.iom.edu/obesity; Trust for America's Health 2006; Lobstein T. et al. 2004, 'Obesity in children and young people: a crisis in public health', *Obesity Reviews*, vol. 5, suppl. 1, pp. 4–85; Stettler, N. 2004, 'Comment: The global epidemic of childhood obesity: Is there a role for the paediatrician?', *Obesity Reviews*, vol. 5, suppl. 1, pp. 1–3.

6 Bell, C. et al. 2002, 'The road to obesity or the path to prevention: Motorized transportation and obesity in China', *Obesity Research*, vol. 10, no. 4, pp. 277–83.

7 Lobstein T. et al. 2004, 'Obesity in children and young people: A crisis in public health', *Obesity Reviews*, vol. 5, suppl. 1, pp. 4–85.

8 Egger, G. and Swinburn, B. 1996, *The fat loss handbook. A guide for professionals*, Allen & Unwin, Sydney.

9 O'Dea, K. 1991, 'Traditional diet and food preferences of Australian Aboriginal hunter-gatherers', *Philosophical Transactions of the Royal Society: Biological Sciences*, vol. 334, pp. 233–41.

10 Naughton, J. et al. 1986, 'Animal foods in traditional Australian Aboriginal diets: Polyunsaturated and low in fat', *Lipids*, vol. 21, no. 11, pp. 684–90.

11 O'Dea, K. et al. 1988, 'An investigation of nutrition-related risk factors in an isolated Aboriginal community in Northern Australia: Advantages of a traditionally orientated life-style', *The Medical Journal of Australia*, vol. 148, pp. 177–80.

12 National Health and Medical Research Council (NHMRC) 2003, 'Dietary Guidelines for Children and Adolescents in Australia, incorporating the Infant Feeding Guidelines for Health Workers, Endorsed 10 April 2003', NHMRC, Canberra.

13 Egger, G. 2001, 'Estimating historical changes in physical activity levels', *MJA*, vol. 175, pp. 635–36.

14 Kopelman, P.G., Caterson, I.D. and Dietz, W.H. 2005, *Clinical obesity in adults and children* (2nd edn), Blackwell Publishing, Massachusetts.

15 Dollman J. et al. 2006, 'The relationship between curriculum time for physical education and literacy and numeracy standards in

Endnotes

South Australian primary schools', *European Physical Education Review* (in press).

16 Tranter, P.J. 2006, 'Overcoming social traps: A key to creating child-friendly cities?', in Gleeson, B.J. and Sipe, N. (eds), *Creating child-friendly cities*, Routledge, London (in press).

17 Australian Institute of Family Studies 2004, *Growing up in Australia: The longitudinal study of Australian children—an Australian Government initiative. 2004 Annual Report*, Australian Institute of Family Studies, Melbourne.

18 Honoré, C. 2004, *In praise of slow: How a worldwide movement is challenging the cult of speed*, Orion Books, London.

19 Cited in Stanton, R. and Hills, A. 2004, *A matter of fat: Understanding and overcoming obesity in kids*, University of New South Wales (UNSW) Press, Sydney.

20 Shell, E.R. 2003, *Fat wars: The inside story of the obesity industry*, Atlantic Books, London.

21 Naughton, Geraldine 2005, 'Critical windows—Industry partner report 2005', presentation to NSW Health, August.

22 National Heart Foundation of Australia (Victorian Division) 2003, *Healthy eating and physical activity in early childhood services: Enhancing policy and practice in Victorian family day care and long day care*, report to the Eat Well Victoria Partnership, Melbourne, July.

23 Australian Institute of Criminology 2006, *Crime facts info: Perception of crime trends*, Australian Government, Canberra.

24 Commission for Architecture and the Built Environment (CABE) 2005, 'What are we scared of? The value of risk in designing public space', CABE Space, London.

25 Veitch, J. et al. (in press), 'Where do children usually play? A qualitative study of parents' perceptions of influences on children's active free play', *Health & Place*.

26 National Heart Foundation of Australia (Victorian Division) 2003, *Healthy eating and physical activity in early childhood services: Enhancing policy and practice in Victorian family day care and long day care*, report to the Eat Well Victoria Partnership, Melbourne, July.

27 Tranter, P.J. 2006, 'Overcoming social traps: A key to creating child-friendly cities?', in Gleeson, B.J. and Sipe, N. (eds), *Creating child-friendly cities*, Routledge, London (in press).

417

28 Patton, G. et al. 2005, 'A picture of Australia's children', *MJA*, vol. 182, no. 8, pp. 437–38.

29 Choi, B.C.K., Hunter, D.J., Tsou, W. and Sainsbury, P. 2005. Diseases of comfort: primary cause of death in the 22nd century. *J Epidemiol Community Health*, vol. 59, pp. 1030–34.

30 NSW Department of Infrastructure, Planning and Natural Resources, Transport and Population Data Centre 2004, *2002 Household Travel Survey Summary Report*, NSW Government.

31 Tranter, P.J. (1996) 'Children's independent mobility and urban form in Australasian, English and German cities', in Hensher, D., King, J. and Oum, T. (eds) *World Transport Research: Proceedings of the Seventh World Conference on Transport Research*, Volume 3: Transport Policy, pp. 31–44; Tranter, P. and Pawson, E. 2001, 'Children's access to local environments: A case study of Christchurch, New Zealand', *Local Environment*, vol. 6, no. 1, pp. 27–48.

32 Banwell, C. et al. 2005, 'Reflections on expert consensus: A case study of the social trends contributing to obesity', *The European Journal of Public Health*, vol. 15, no. 6, pp. 564–68.

Chapter 2

1 Kunkel, D. et al. 2004, 'Report of the American Psychological Association Task Force on Advertising and Children. Section: Psychological issues in the increasing commercialisation of childhood', American Psychological Association, 20 February.

2 Shell, E.R. 2003, *Fat wars: The inside story of the obesity industry*, Atlantic Books, London.

3 Hamilton, C. and Denniss, R. 2005, *Affluenza: When too much is never enough*, Allen & Unwin, Sydney.

4 Schlosser, E. 2002, *Fast food nation: What the all-American meal is doing to the world*, Penguin Books, London.

5 Shell, E.R. 2003, *Fat wars: The inside story of the obesity industry*, Atlantic Books, London.

6 Kunkel, D. et al. 2004, 'Report of the American Psychological Association Task Force on Advertising and Children. Section: Psychological issues in the increasing commercialisation of childhood', American Psychological Association, 20 February.

7   Story, M. and French, S. 2004, 'Food advertising and marketing directed at children and adolescents', *The International Journal of Behavioral Nutrition and Physical Activity*. Available at: http://www.ijbnpa.org/content/1/1/3.

8   Victoria J. Rideout (Vice-President and Director, Program for the Study of Entertainment Media and Health, Henry J. Kaiser Family Foundation) 2004, 'The role of media in childhood obesity', statement made before the Senate Committee on Commerce, Science and Transportation Subcommittee on Competition, Foreign Commerce and Infastructure, 2 March.

9   Cited in NSW Department of Health 2004, *Eat Well NSW: Strategic directions for public health nutrition 2003–2007*, NSW Department of Health, Sydney.

10 Story, M. and French, S. 2004, 'Food advertising and marketing directed at children and adolescents', *The International Journal of Behavioral Nutrition and Physical Activity*. Available at: http://www.ijbnpa.org/content/1/1/3.

11 Campbell, K. et al. 2006, 'Family food environment and dietary behaviours likely to promote fatness in 5–6-year-old children'. *International Journal of Obesity*, vol. 30, pp. 1272–80.

12 Victoria J. Rideout (Vice-President and Director, Program for the Study of Entertainment Media and Health, Henry J. Kaiser Family Foundation) 2004, 'The role of media in childhood obesity', statement made before the Senate Committee on Commerce, Science and Transportation Subcommittee on Competition, Foreign Commerce and Infastructure, 2 March.

13 Story, M. and French, S. 2004, 'Food advertising and marketing directed at children and adolescents', *The International Journal of Behavioral Nutrition and Physical Activity*. Available at: http://www.ijbnpa.org/content/1/1/3.

14 Story, M. and French, S. 2004, 'Food advertising and marketing directed at children and adolescents', *The International Journal of Behavioral Nutrition and Physical Activity*. Available at: http://www.ijbnpa.org/content/1/1/3.

15 Reynolds, Janet 2005, 'Nutrition education in schools—the good, the bad and the ugly', *Food Chain*, Strategic Inter-Governmental Nutrition Alliance, February.

16 Norrie, Justin and Maley, Jacqueline 2005, 'Parents get serious: Junk the junk', *The Sydney Morning Herald (SMH)*, 29 July, pp. 1–2.

17 Bell, C. and Swinburn, B. 2005, 'School canteens: Using ripples to create a wave of healthy eating', *MJA*, vol. 183, no. 1, pp. 5–6.

18 Author un-named 2005, 'Nutrition in schools', *Food Chain*, Strategic Inter-Governmental Nutrition Alliance, February.

19 Hesketh, K. et al. 2005, 'Healthy eating, activity and obesity prevention: A qualitative study of parent and child perceptions in Australia', *Health Promotion International*, vol. 20, no. 1, pp. 19–26.

20 Anon. 2004, 'Be a sport, pass me another Maccas', *Australian Medicine*, 15 March, p. 10.

21 Wahlqvist, M.L. 1997, *Australasia, Asia and the Pacific: Food and nutrition*, Allen & Unwin, Sydney.

22 Stanton, R. and Hills, A. 2004, *A matter of fat: Understanding and overcoming obesity in kids*, UNSW Press, Sydney.

23 Kopelman, P.G., Caterson, I.D. and Dietz, W.H. 2005, *Clinical obesity in adults and children* (2nd edn), Blackwell Publishing, Massachusetts.

24 Nestle, M. 2002, *Food politics: How the food industry influences nutrition and health*, University of California Press, California.

25 Kant, A.K. 2000, 'Consumption of energy-dense, nutrient-poor foods by adult Americans: Nutritional and health implications. The Third National Health and Nutrition Examination Survey, 1988–1999', *American Journal of Clinical Nutrition*, vol. 72, no. 4, pp. 929–36.

26 Dixon, J. et al. 2004, 'Exploring the intersectoral partnerships guiding Australia's dietary advice', *Health Promotion International*, vol. 19, no. 1, pp. 5–13.

27 Nestle, M. 2002, *Food politics: How the food industry influences nutrition and health*, University of California Press, California.

28 O'Brien P. 1995, 'Dietary shifts and implications for US agriculture', *Am J Clin Nutr*, vol. 61 (suppl.), pp. I390S–96S; Young. C.E. and Kantor, L.S. 1999, 'Moving toward the food guide pyramid: Implications for US Agriculture', US Department of Agriculture (USDA), Washington, DC.

29 NSW Centre for Public Health Nutrition 2005, 'Best options for promoting healthy weight and preventing weight gain in NSW', NSW Centre for Public Health Nutrition, March.

30 Young, L. and Nestle, M. 2002, 'The contribution of expanding portion sizes to the US obesity epidemic', *American Journal of Public Health*, vol. 92, no. 2, pp. 246–49.

31 Volker, D. 2004, 'How much is on your plate?', Nutrition Research Foundation Annual Report 2003–2004, University of Sydney.

32 NSW Centre for Public Health Nutrition 2005, 'Best options for promoting healthy weight and preventing weight gain in NSW', NSW Centre for Public Health Nutrition, March.

33 Tabakoff, Jenny 2004, 'Heckler', *SMH*, 21 June, p. 18.

34 Cited in Fisher, J.O. 2003, 'Children's bite size and intake of an entrée are greater with large portions than with age-appropriate or self-selected portions', *Am J Clin Nutr*, vol. 77, no. 5, pp. 1164–70.

35 Hamilton, C. and Denniss, R. 2005, *Affluenza: When too much is never enough*, Allen & Unwin, Sydney.

36 Gleeson, Brendan 2004, The future of Australia's cities: Making space for hope. Professorial Lecture, Griffith University, 19 February.

37 Stanton, R. 2003, 'Ensuring a safe and healthy food supply', *Food Chain*, Strategic Intergovernmental Nutrition Alliance, no. 13, December.

38 Drewnowski, A. and Rolls, B. 2005, 'How to modify the food environment', *J Nutr*, vol. 135, pp. 898–99; Drewnowski, A. and Darmon, N. 2005, 'The economics of obesity: Dietary energy density and energy cost', *Am J Clin Nutr*, vol. 82, pp. 265S–73S.

39 Australian Institute of Family Studies 2004, *Growing up in Australia: The longitudinal study of Australian children—an Australian Government initiative. 2004 Annual Report*, Australian Institute of Family Studies, Melbourne.

40 Victorian Health Promotion Foundation 2003, 'Food for all? Food insecurity community demonstration projects: Maribyrnong City Council and North Yarra Community Health. Case studies', Victorian Health Promotion Foundation. Available at: http://www.vichealth.vic.gov.au.

421

41 Harrison, M.S. et al. 2007. The increasing cost of the basic foods required to promote health in Queensland. *MJA*. Vol. 186. no. 1 pp. 9–14.

42 Drewnowski, A. and Darmon, N. 2005, 'The economics of obesity: Dietary energy density and energy cost', *Am J Clin Nutr*, vol. 82, pp. 265S–73S.

Chapter 3

1   Cited in Dixon, H. et al. 2005, 'Body weight, nutrition, alcohol and physical activity: Key messages for the Cancer Council Australia', Cancer Council Australia, February.

2   Cited in Denney-Wilson, E. 2005. Metabolic risk factors in overweight adolescents. PhD thesis. University of Sydney.

3. Cited in Stubbs, C. and Lee, A. 2004, 'The obesity epidemic: Both energy intake and physical activity contribute', *MJA*, vol. 181, no. 9, pp. 489–91.

4   Cited in Stubbs, C. and Lee, A. 2004, 'The obesity epidemic: Both energy intake and physical activity contribute', *MJA*, vol. 181, no. 9, pp. 489–91.

5   Cited in Dixon, H. et al. 2005, 'Body weight, nutrition, alcohol and physical activity: Key messages for the Cancer Council Australia', Cancer Council Australia, February; Stubbs, C. and Lee, A. 2004, 'The obesity epidemic: Both energy intake and physical activity contribute', *MJA*, vol. 181, no. 9, pp. 489–91.

6   NSW Department of Health 2004, *Eat Well NSW: Strategic directions for public health nutrition 2003–2007*, NSW Department of Health, Sydney.

7   WA Government 2003, *Results of Western Australian Child and Adolescent Physical Activity and Nutrition Survey 2003 (CAPANS)*, WA Government, Perth.

8   Naughton, Geraldine 2005, 'Critical windows—Industry partner report 2005', presentation to NSW Health, August.

9   Booth, M. et al. 2006, *NSW Schools Physical Activity and Nutrition Survey (SPANS) 2004*, NSW Health, Sydney.

10 WA Government 2003, *Results of Western Australian Child and Adolescent Physical Activity and Nutrition Survey 2003 (CAPANS)*, WA Government, Perth.

Endnotes

11 Australian Institute of Family Studies 2004, *Growing up in Australia: The longitudinal study of Australian children—an Australian Government initiative. 2004 Annual Report*, Australian Institute of Family Studies, Melbourne.

12 NSW Department of Health 2004, *Eat Well NSW: Strategic directions for public health nutrition 2003–2007*, NSW Department of Health, Sydney.

13 O'Dea, J. 2005, *Positive food for kids: Healthy food, healthy children, healthy life*, Doubleday, Sydney.

14 WA Government 2003, *Results of Western Australian Child and Adolescent Physical Activity and Nutrition Survey 2003 (CAPANS)*, WA Government, Perth.

15 Cited in Denney-Wilson, E. 2005. Metabolic risk factors in overweight adolescents. PhD thesis. University of Sydney.

16 NSW Department of Health 2004, *Eat Well NSW: Strategic directions for public health nutrition 2003–2007*, NSW Department of Health, Sydney.

17 NSW Department of Health 2004, *Eat Well NSW: Strategic directions for public health nutrition 2003–2007*, NSW Department of Health, Sydney.

18 Muñoz, K.A. et al. 1997, 'Food intakes of US children and adolescents compared with recommendations', *Pediatrics*, vol. 100, no. 3, pp. 323–29.

19 Booth, M. et al. 2006, *NSW Schools Physical Activity and Nutrition Survey (SPANS) 2004*, NSW Health, Sydney.

20 Queensland Government 2005, *Eat well, be active—healthy kids for life. The Queensland Government's first action plan, 2005–2008*, Queensland Government, Brisbane.

21 Australian Institute of Family Studies 2004, *Growing up in Australia: The longitudinal study of Australian children—an Australian Government initiative. 2004 Annual Report*, Australian Institute of Family Studies, Melbourne.

22 NSW Department of Health 2004, *Eat Well NSW: Strategic directions for public health nutrition 2003–2007*, NSW Department of Health, Sydney.

23 WA Physical Activity Taskforce Research and Evaluation Working Party 2001, 'Background and Summary of Research', WA Government.

24 Tranter, P.J. and Malone, K. 2003, 'Out of bounds: Insights from children to support a cultural shift towards sustainable and child-friendly cities', State of Australian Cities National Conference, 3–5 December, University of Western Sydney, Urban Frontiers Program, Parramatta.

25 Lewis, N.R. and Dollman, J. (in press), 'Trends in physical activity behaviours and attitudes among young South Australian youth 1985–2004'.

26 Booth, M. et al. 2006, *NSW Schools Physical Activity and Nutrition Survey (SPANS) 2004*, NSW Health, Sydney.

27 Salmon, J. et al. 2005, 'Trends in children's physical activity and weight status in high and low socio-economic status areas of Melbourne, Victoria, 1985–2001', *Australian and New Zealand Journal of Public Health*, vol. 29, pp. 337–42.

28 WA Physical Activity Taskforce Research and Evaluation Working Party 2001, 'Background and Summary of Research', WA Government.

29 Tomkinson, G.R. et al. 2003, 'Secular trends in the performance of children and adolescents (1980–2000). Review Article', *Sports Medicine*, vol. 33, no. 4, pp. 285–300.

30 Booth, M. et al. 2006, *NSW Schools Physical Activity and Nutrition Survey (SPANS) 2004*, NSW Health, Sydney.

31 Australasian Society for the Study of Obesity 2001, 'Media release. The proportion of young Australians who are overweight is not just increasing: It's accelerating', 8 September.

32 WA Government 2003, *Results of Western Australian Child and Adolescent Physical Activity and Nutrition Survey 2003 (CAPANS)*, WA Government.

33 Olds, T. and Harten, N. 2001, 'One hundred years of growth: The evolution of height, mass, and body composition in Australian children, 1899–1999', *Human Biology*, vol. 73, no. 5, pp. 727–38.

34 Vaska V.L. and Volkmer, R. 2004, 'Increasing prevalence of obesity in South Australian 4-year-olds: 1995–2002', *Journal of Paediatric Child Health*, vol. 40, pp. 353–55.

35 Sanigorski, A. et al. 2005, 'High childhood obesity in an Australian population', poster presentation at Australasian Society for the Study of Obesity 14th Annual Scientific Meeting, Glenelg, SA, 28–30 October; Booth, M. 2000, speech at the 9th Scientific Meeting of the Australasian Society for the Study of Obesity; Booth, M.L. et al. 2003, 'Change in the prevalence of overweight and obesity among young Australians, 1969–1997', *Am J Clin Nutr*, vol. 77, no. 1, pp. 29–36.

36 Booth, M. et al. 2006, *NSW Schools Physical Activity and Nutrition Survey (SPANS) 2004*, NSW Health, Sydney.

37 Australasian Society for the Study of Obesity 2001, 'Media release. The proportion of young Australians who are overweight is not just increasing: It's accelerating', 8 September; Booth, M.L. et al. 2003, 'Change in the prevalence of overweight and obesity among young Australians, 1969–1997', *Am J Clin Nutr*, vol. 77, no. 1, pp. 29–36.

Chapter 4

1 Wang, G. and Dietz, W.H. 2002, 'Economic burden of obesity in youths aged 6 to 17 years: 1979–1999', *Pediatrics*, vol. 109, no. 5, p. 81.

2 Kerin, John 2005, 'Youths too stoned, too fat to join forces', *The Australian*, 12 December, pp. 1–4.

3 Australian Institute of Health and Welfare 2005, 'Obesity and workplace absenteeism among older Australians', Bulletin No. 31, AIHW Cat. No. AUS 67, Canberra.

4 Hesketh, K. et al. 2005, 'Stability of body mass index in Australian children: A prospective cohort study across the middle childhood years', *Public Health Nutrition*, vol. 7, no. 2, pp. 303–09.

5 Freedman, D.S. et al. 2001, 'Relationship of childhood obesity to coronary heart disease risk factors in adulthood: The Bogalusa Heart Study', *Pediatrics*, vol. 108, pp. 712–18. Freedman, D.S. et al. 2005, 'The relation of childhood BMI to adult adiposity: The Bogalusa Heart Study', *Pediatrics*, vol. 115, pp. 22–27.

6 Whitaker, R.C. et al. 1997, 'Predicting obesity in young adulthood from childhood and parental obesity', *New England Journal of Medicine*, vol. 337, no. 13, pp. 869–73.

7   Redline, S. et al. 1999, 'Risk factors for sleep-disordered breathing in children. Associations with obesity, race and respiratory problems', *American Journal of Respiratory Critical Care Medicine*, vol. 159, no. 5, pp. 1527–32.

8   Baur, L. and Denney-Wilson, E. 'Obesity in children and adolescents', draft.

9   Freedman, D.S. et al.1999, 'The relation of overweight to cardiovascular risk factors among children and adolescents: The Bogalusa Heart Study', *Pediatrics*, vol. 103, no. 6, pp. 1175–82.

10 Australian Institute of Health and Welfare 2002. Diabetes: Australian facts 2002. AIHW Cat. No. CVD 20 (Diabetes Series. No. 3) Canberra: AIHW.

11 Cited in Kopelman, P.G., Caterson, I.D. and Dietz, W.H. 2005, *Clinical obesity in adults and children* (2nd edn), Blackwell Publishing, Massachusetts.

12 Institute of Medicine of the National Academies 2006. Progress in Preventing Childhood Obesity. How Do We Measure Up? The National Academies Press. Washington, DC. Available at: www.iom.edu/obesity.

13 Lobstein, T. et al. 2004, 'Obesity in children and young people: A crisis in public health', *Obesity Reviews*, vol. 5, suppl. 1, pp. 4–85.

14 Lobstein, T. et al. 2004, 'Obesity in children and young people: A crisis in public health', *Obesity Reviews*, vol. 5, suppl. 1, pp. 4–85.

15 McMahon, S. et al. 2004, 'Increase in type 2 diabetes in children and adolescents in WA', *MJA*, vol. 180, no. 9, pp. 459–61.

16 Hickman, Belinda 2004, '"Diabesity" the new epidemic', *The Australian*, 26–27 June , p. 7.

17 Booth, M. et al. 2006, *NSW Schools Physical Activity and Nutrition Survey (SPANS) 2004*, NSW Health, Sydney.

18 Lobstein T. et al. 2004, 'Obesity in children and young people: a crisis in public health', *Obesity Reviews*, vol. 5, suppl. 1, pp. 4–85.

19 Ludwig, D.S. and Ebbeling, C.B. 2001, 'Type 2 diabetes mellitus in children: Primary care and public health considerations', *Journal of the American Medical Association*, vol. 286, pp. 1427–30.

20 Taplin, C.E. et al. 2005, 'The rising incidence of childhood type 1 diabetes in New South Wales, 1990–2002', *MJA*, vol. 183, no. 5, pp. 243–46.

Endnotes

21 Lobstein, T. et al. 2004, 'Obesity in children and young people: A crisis in public health', *Obesity Reviews*, vol. 5, suppl. 1, pp. 4–85.

22 Davison, K.K. et al. 2003, 'Percent body fat at age five predicts earlier pubertal development among girls at age nine', *Pediatrics*, vol. 111, no. 4, pp. 815–21.

23 Davison, K.K. et al. 2003, 'Percent body fat at age five predicts earlier pubertal development among girls at age nine', *Pediatrics*, vol. 111, no. 4, pp. 815–21.

24 Cited in Davison, K.K. and Birch, L.L. 2004, 'Predictors of fat stereotypes among 9 year old girls and their parents', *Obesity Research*, vol. 12, pp. 86–94.

25 Lobstein, T. et al. 2004, 'Obesity in children and young people: A crisis in public health', *Obesity Reviews*, vol. 5, suppl. 1, pp. 4–85.

26 Davison, K.K. et al. 2003, 'Percent body fat at age five predicts earlier pubertal development among girls at age nine', *Pediatrics*, vol.111, no. 4, pp. 815–21.

27 Dietz, W.H. 1998, 'Health consequences of obesity in youth: Childhood predictors of adult disease', *Pediatrics*, vol. 101, no. 3, Suppl., pp. 518–25.

28 Dietz, W.H. 1998, 'Health consequences of obesity in youth: Childhood predictors of adult disease', *Pediatrics*, vol. 101, no. 3, Suppl., pp. 518–25.

29 Hesketh, K. et al. 2004, 'Body mass index and parent-reported self-esteem in elementary school children: Evidence for a causal relationship', *International Journal of Obesity*, vol. 28, pp. 1233–37.

30 Gortmaker, S.L. et al. 1992, 'Social and economic consequences of overweight in adolesence and young adulthood', *NEJM*, vol. 329, no. 14, pp. 1008–12.

31 Cited in Kopelman, P.G., Caterson, I.D. and Dietz, W.H. 2005, *Clinical obesity in adults and children* (2nd edn), Blackwell Publishing, Massachusetts.

32 Cited in Davison, K.K. and Birch, L.L. 2004, 'Predictors of fat stereotypes among 9 year old girls and their parents', *Obesity Research*, vol. 12, pp. 86–94.

33 Ball, K. et al. 2004, 'Longitudinal relationships among overweight, life satisfaction, and aspirations in young women', *Obesity Research*, vol. 12, no. 6, pp. 1019–30.

34 Ball, K. et al. 2004, 'Longitudinal relationships among overweight, life satisfaction, and aspirations in young women', *Obesity Research*, vol. 12, no. 6, pp. 1019–30.

35 Lobstein T. et al. 2004, 'Obesity in children and young people: a crisis in public health', *Obesity Reviews*, vol. 5, suppl. 1, pp. 4–85.

36 NSW Department of Health 2004, *Eat Well NSW: Strategic Directions for Public Health Nutrition 2003–2007*, NSW Department of Health, Sydney.

37 Nankervis, A.J. 2006, 'Obesity and reproductive health', *MJA*, vol. 184, no. 2, p. 51.

38 NSW Department of Health 2004, *Eat Well NSW: Strategic Directions for Public Health Nutrition 2003–2007*, NSW Department of Health, Sydney.

39 Cited in Lobstein T. et al. 2004, 'Obesity in children and young people: A crisis in public health', *Obesity Reviews*, vol. 5, suppl. 1, pp. 4–85.

40 Dietz, W.H. 1998, 'Childhood weight affects adult morbidity and mortality', *J Nutr*, vol. 128, no. 2, pp. 411S–14S.

41 Must, A. et al. 1992, 'Long-term morbidity and mortality of overweight adolescents: A follow-up of the Harvard Growth Study of 1922 to 1935', *NEJM*, vol. 327, no. 19, pp. 1350–55.

42 Freedman, D.S. et al. 2001, 'Relationship of childhood obesity to coronary heart disease risk factors in adulthood: The Bogalusa Heart Study', *Pediatrics*, vol. 108, pp. 712–18.

43 Field, A.E. et al. 2001, 'Impact of overweight on the risk of developing common chronic diseases during a 10-year period', *Archives of Internal Medicine*, vol. 161, pp. 1581–86.

44 Flegal, K.M. et al. 2005, 'Excess deaths associated with underweight, overweight, and obesity', *JAMA*, vol. 293, pp. 1861–67.

45 Cited in Kron, John 2004, 'Weighing in on obesity', *Australian Doctor*, 9 July, pp. 47–49.

46 Denney-Wilson, E. 2005. Metabolic risk factors in overweight adolescents. PhD thesis. University of Sydney.

47 Hawley, J. 2004, 'Exercise as a therapeutic intervention for the prevention and treatment of insulin resistance', *Diabetes/Metabolism Research and Reviews*, vol. 20, pp. 383–93.

48 Dixon, H. et al. 2005, 'Body weight, nutrition, alcohol and physical activity: Key messages for the Cancer Council Australia', Cancer Council Australia.

49 WA Government 2003, *Results of Western Australian Child and Adolescent Physical Activity and Nutrition Survey 2003 (CAPANS)*, WA Government.

50 Baker, H. 2004, 'Parental guidance recommended', *National Child Nutrition Program Project Final Report*, Cancer Council WA.

51 US Surgeon General 1996, *Physical activity and health. A report of the surgeon general*, US Department of Health and Human Services. Available at: http://www.cdc.gov/nccdphp/sgr/summary.htm

52 Gleeson, Brendan 2004, 'The future of Australia's cities: making space for hope', Professorial Lecture, 19 February, Griffith University.

53 Queensland Government 2005, *Eat well, be active—healthy kids for life. The Queensland Government's first action plan 2005–2008*, Queensland Government.

Chapter 5

1   Jain, Anjali et al. 2001, 'Why don't low-income mothers worry about their preschoolers being overweight?', *Pediatrics*, vol. 107, pp. 1138–46; Anon. 2004, 'Obesity apathy alarming: AMA', *Australian Medicine*, 15 November, p. 4; Hesketh, K. et al. 2005, 'Healthy eating, activity and obesity prevention: A qualitative study of parent and child perceptions in Australia', *Health Promotion International*, vol. 20, no. 1, pp. 19–26.

2   Eckersley, R. 2001, 'Losing the battle of the bulge: Causes and consequences of increasing obesity', *MJA*, vol. 174, pp. 590–92.

3   Rosenbaum, M. and Leibel, R.L. 1998, 'The physiology of body weight regulation: Relevance to the etiology of obesity in children', *Pediatrics*, vol. 101, no. 3, pp. S525–39.

4   Egger, G. and Binns, A. 2001, *The experts' weight loss guide. For doctors, health professionals...and all those serious about their health*, Allen & Unwin, Sydney.

5   Campbell, K. et al. 2006, 'Family food environment and dietary behaviours likely to promote fatness in 5–6-year-old children'. *International Journal of Obesity*, vol. 30, pp. 1272–1280.

6   Campbell, K. et al. 2006, 'Family food environment and dietary behaviours likely to promote fatness in 5–6-year-old children'. *International Journal of Obesity,*.vol. 30, pp.1272–1280.

7   Baker, D. and Eyeson-Annan, M. 2003, 'Monitoring health behaviours and health status in NSW: Release of the adult health survey 2003', *NSW Public Health Bulletin*, vol. 16, nos 1–2, pp. 13–17.

8   Fisher, J.O. 2001, 'Maternal milk consumption predicts the tradeoff between milk and soft drinks in young girls' diets', *J Nutr*, vol. 131, pp. 246–50.

9   Campbell K. J. et al. (draft), 'Associations between the home food environment and obesity-promoting eating behaviours in adolescence'.

10 Baker, D. and Eyeson-Annan, M. 2003, 'Monitoring health behaviours and health status in NSW: release of the adult health survey 2003', *NSW Public Health Bulletin*, vol. 16, nos 1–2, pp. 13–17.

11 WA Physical Activity Taskforce Research and Evaluation Working Party 2001, 'Background and summary of research', WA Government, Perth.

12 Egger, G. and Binns, A. 2001, *The experts' weight loss guide. For doctors, health professionals...and all those serious about their health*, Allen & Unwin, Sydney.

13 Birch, L.L. and Fisher, J.O. 2000, 'Mothers' child-feeding practices influence daughters' eating and weight', *Am J Clin Nutr*, vol. 71, no. 5, pp. 1054–61.

14 Birch, L.L. and Fisher, J.O. 1998, 'Development of eating behaviours among children and adolescents', *Pediatrics*, vol. 101, no. 3, pp. S539–49.

15 Juel, A. 2001, 'Does size really matter? Weight and values in public health', *Perspectives in Biology and Medicine*, vol. 44, no. 2.

16 Strauss, R.S. 2000, 'Childhood obesity and self-esteem', *Pediatrics*, vol. 105, no. 1, p. 15.

17 Cited in Satter, E. 2000, *Child of mine. Feeding with love and good sense*, Bull Publishing Co., Colorado.

Endnotes

18 Davison K.K. and Birch L.L. 2001, 'Child and parent characteristics as predictors of change in girls' body mass index', *Int J Obes Related Metab Disord*, vol. 25, no. 12, pp. 1834–42.

19 Shunk J.A. and Birch L.L. 2004, 'Girls at risk for overweight at age 5 are at risk for dietary restraint, disinhibited overeating, weight concerns, and greater weight gain from 5 to 9 years', *J Am Diet Assoc*, vol. 104, no. 7, pp. 1120–26.

20 Davison K.K. et al. 2001, 'Weight status, parent reaction, and self-concept in five-year-old girls', *Pediatrics*, vol. 107, no. 1, pp. 46–53.

21 Abramovitz, B.A., Birch L.L. 2000, 'Five-year-old girls' ideas about dieting are predicted by their mothers' dieting', *J Am Diet Assoc*, vol. 100, no. 10, pp. 1157–63.

22 Cited in Dietz, W.H. 1998, 'Health consequences of obesity in youth: Childhood predictors of adult disease', *Pediatrics*, vol. 101, no. 3 (suppl.), pp. 518–25.

23 Davison, K.K. and Birch L.L. 2004, 'Lean and weight stable: Behavioral predictors and psychological correlates', *Obesity Research*, vol. 12, pp. 1085–93.

24 Fisher, J.O. and Birch, L.L. 2000, 'Mothers' child-feeding practices influence daughters'eating and weight', *Am J Clinical Nutrition*, vol. 71, no. 5, pp. 1054–61.

25 Satter, E. 1987, *How to get your kid to eat…but not too much. From birth to adolescence*, Bull Publishing Co., Colorado.

26 Satter, E. 2000, *Child of mine. Feeding with love and good sense*, Bull Publishing Co., Colorado.

27 Baker, H. 2004, 'Parental Guidance Recommended', *National Child Nutrition Program Project Final Report*, Cancer Council WA, Perth.

28 Kopelman, P.G., Caterson, I.D. and Dietz, W.H. 2005, *Clinical obesity in adults and children* (2nd edn), Blackwell Publishing, Massachusetts.

29 Hill, James et al. 2003, 'Viewpoint. Obesity and the environment: Where do we go from here?', *Science*, vol. 299, issue 5608, pp. 853–55.

30 Hesketh, K et al. 2004, 'Body mass index and parent-reported self-esteem in elementary school children: Evidence for a causal relationship', *Int J Obes*, vol. 28, pp. 1233–37.

31 Sanders, M. (undated), 'Top 10 Tips for Parents. Triple P Positive Parenting Program fact sheet', University of Queensland, Brisbane.

32 Australian Childhood Foundation website: http://www.childhood.org.au/website/default.asp.

Chapter 6

1 Sigman, Aric 2005, *Remotely Controlled. How television is damaging our lives—and what we can do about it*, Vermilion, London.

2 Royal Australasian College of Physicians (RACP), Division of Paediatrics, Health Policy Unit 1999, *Getting in the picture. A parent's and carer's guide for the better use of television for children* (3rd edn), RACP, Sydney.

3 Cited in NHMRC 2003, *Dietary Guidelines for Children and Adolescents in Australia incorporating the Infant Feeding Guidelines for Health Workers (endorsed 10 April 2003)*, NHMRC, Canberra.

4 Christakis, D.A. and Zimmerman, F.J. 2006. Media as a Public Health Issue *Arch Pediatr Adolesc Med*, vol.160, pp.445–446.

5 Campbell, K. et al. 2006, 'Family food environment and dietary behaviours likely to promote fatness in 5–6-year-old children'. *International Journal of Obesity,*.vol. 30, pp.1272–80.

6 Gill, Tim et al. 2004, 'Detailed review of intervention studies: How do we best address the issues of overweight, obesity and cardiovascular disease?', NSW Centre for Public Health Nutrition (on behalf of the National Heart Foundation), Sydney; Kopelman, P.G., Caterson, I.D. and Dietz, W.H. 2005, *Clinical obesity in adults and children* (2nd edn), Blackwell Publishing, Massachusetts. Egger, G. and Swinburn, B. 1996, *The fat loss handbook. A guide for professionals*, Allen & Unwin, Sydney.

7 Young Media Australia factsheets 2004, 'Mind over media: Developing healthy relationships', 'Mind over media: Developing good social and emotional skills'.

8 Young Media Australia factsheets 2004, 'Mind over media: Developing healthy relationships', 'Mind over media: Developing good social and emotional skills'.

Endnotes

9   Australian Institute of Family Studies 2004, 'Growing up in
     Australia: The longitudinal study of Australian children—an
     Australian Government initiative. 2004 annual report', Australian
     Institute of Family Studies, Melbourne.

10   Wake, M. et al. 2003, 'Television, computer use and body mass
     index in Australian primary school children', *J. Paediatr Child
     Health*, vol. 39, no. 2, pp. 130–34.

11   NSW Department of Health 2004, *Eat Well NSW: Strategic
     directions for public health nutrition 2003–2007*, NSW Department
     of Health, Sydney.

12   NSW Department of Health 2004, *Eat Well NSW: Strategic
     directions for public health nutrition 2003–2007*, NSW Department
     of Health, Sydney.

13   WA Government 2003, *Results of Western Australian Child and
     Adolescent Physical Activity and Nutrition Survey 2003 (CAPANS)*,
     WA Government, Perth.

14   Hardy, L.L. et al. 2006. Descriptive epidemiology of small screen
     recreation among Australian adolescents. *Journal of Paediatrics and
     Child Health*, vol. 42, no.11. pp. 709–14.

15   Victorian Health Promotion Foundation 2005, *VicHealth Letter*,
     issue 24, Summer.

16   RACP, Paediatrics & Child Health Division 2004, 'Children and the
     media: Advocating for the future', RACP, Sydney. Available at:
     http://www.racp.edu.au/hpu/paed/media.

17   Victorian Health Promotion Foundation 2005, *VicHealth Letter*,
     issue 24, Summer.

18   Victorian Health Promotion Foundation 2005, *VicHealth Letter*,
     issue 24, Summer.

19   Van Zutphen, Moniek et al. (draft), 'Screen time, television access
     and weight status in Australian children'.

20   Campbell, K. et al. 2002, 'Family food environments of 5–6-year-
     old-children: Does socioeconomic status make a difference?', *Asia
     Pacific J Clin Nutr*, vol. 11, pp. S553–61.

21   Denney-Wilson, E. 2005. Metabolic risk factors in overweight
     adolescents. PhD thesis. University of Sydney.

22 RACP, Division of Paediatrics, Health Policy Unit 1999, *Getting in the picture. A parent's and carer's guide for the better use of television for children* (3rd edn), RACP, Sydney.

23 RACP, Division of Paediatrics, Health Policy Unit 1999, *Getting in the picture. A parent's and carer's guide for the better use of television for children* (3rd edn), RACP, Sydney.

24 Institute of Medicine of the National Academies 2006. Progress in Preventing Childhood Obesity. How Do We Measure Up? The National Academies Press. Washington, DC. Available at: www.iom.edu/obesity.

25 Barkin, S. et al. 2006, 'Parental media mediation styles for children aged 2 to 11 years', *Arch Pediatr Adolesc Med*, vol. 160, pp. 395–401.

26 Lumeng, J.C. et al. 2006, 'Television exposure and overweight risk in preschoolers', *Arch Pediatr Adolesc Med*, vol. 160, pp. 417–22.

27 Salmon, J. et al. 2006, 'Television viewing habits associated with obesity risk factors: A survey of Melbourne schoolchildren', *MJA*, vol. 184, no. 2, pp. 64–67.

28 Rideout, Victoria J. (Vice-President and Director, Program for the Study of Entertainment Media and Health, Henry J. Kaiser Family Foundation) 2004, 'The role of media in childhood obesity', statement made before the Senate Committee on Commerce, Science and Transportation Subcommittee on Competition, Foreign Commerce and Infastructure, 2 March, Washington DC.

29 Van Zutphen, Moniek et al. (draft), 'Screen time, television access and weight status in Australian children'.

30 Egger, G. and Binns, A. 2001, *The experts' weight loss guide. For doctors, health professionals...and all those serious about their health*, Allen & Unwin, Sydney.

31 Cited in NHMRC 2003, *Dietary Guidelines for Children and Adolescents in Australia incorporating the Infant Feeding Guidelines for Health Workers (endorsed 10 April 2003)*, NHMRC, Canberra.

32 Sigman cites Reilly J. et al. 2004, 'Total energy expenditure and physical activity in young Scottish children: Mixed longitudinal study', *The Lancet*, vol. 363, pp. 211–12.

33 Rideout, Victoria J. (Vice-President and Director, Program for the Study of Entertainment Media and Health, Henry J. Kaiser Family

Endnotes

Foundation) 2004, 'The role of media in childhood obesity', statement made before the Senate Committee on Commerce, Science and Transportation Subcommittee on Competition, Foreign Commerce and Infastructure, 2 March, Washington DC.

34 Sigman cites Stroebele, N. and De Castro, J.I. 2004, 'Effect of ambience on food intake and food choice', *Nutrition*, vol. 20, no. 9, pp. 821–38.

35 Denney-Wilson, E. 2005. Metabolic risk factors in overweight adolescents. PhD thesis. University of Sydney.

36 RACP, Paediatrics & Child Health Division 2004, 'Children and the media: Advocating for the future', RACP, Sydney. Available at: http://www.racp.edu.au/hpu/paed/media.

37 Rideout, Victoria J. (Vice-President and Director, Program for the Study of Entertainment Media and Health, Henry J. Kaiser Family Foundation) 2004, 'The role of media in childhood obesity', statement made before the Senate Committee on Commerce, Science and Transportation Subcommittee on Competition, Foreign Commerce and Infastructure, 2 March, Washington DC.

38 Sigman cites Becker, A.E. et al. 2002, 'Eating behaviours and attitudes following prolonged exposure to television among ethnic Fijian adolescent girls', *British Journal of Psychiatry*, vol. 180, pp. 509–14.

39 RACP, Paediatrics & Child Health Division 2004, 'Children and the media: Advocating for the future', RACP, Sydney. Available at: http://www.racp.edu.au/hpu/paed/media.

40 Meade, Amanda and Sinclair, Lara 2005, 'Fat chance of taking food off kids' TV', *The Australian* (Media section), 29 September, p. 15.

41 Young Media Australia factsheets 2004, 'Mind over media: Developing healthy relationships', 'Mind over media: developing good social and emotional skills'.

42 RACP, Paediatrics & Child Health Division 2004, 'Children and the media: Advocating for the future', RACP, Sydney. Available at: http://www.racp.edu.au/hpu/paed/media.

43 Sigman cites Hancox, R.L. 2005, 'Association of television viewing during childhood with poor educational achievement', *Arch Pediatr Med*, vol. 159, pp. 614–18.

435

44 Anon. 1956, 'When Sydney began to glow in the dark', 22 September, reproduced in 2006, *175 years of the Sydney Morning Herald* (Special supplement), *SMH*, 18 April, p. 3.

45 RACP, Paediatrics & Child Health Division 2004, 'Children and the media: Advocating for the future', RACP, Sydney. Available at: http://www.racp.edu.au/hpu/paed/media.

46 RACP, Paediatrics & Child Health Division 2004, 'Children and the media: Advocating for the future', RACP, Sydney. Available at: http://www.racp.edu.au/hpu/paed/media.

47 American Academy of Pediatrics 2000. Joint Statement on the Impact of Entertainment Violence on Children Congressional Public Health Summit July 26, 2000. Available at: www.aap.org/advocacy/releases/jstmtevc.htm http://www.aap.org/advocacy/releases/jstmtevc.htm.

48 Orange, T. and O'Flynn, L. 2005, *The media diet for kids. A parent's survival gide to TV & computer games*, Hay House, London.

49 Sigman cites Centerwall, B.S. 1989, 'Exposure to television as a risk factor for violence', *Am J Epidemiol*, vol. 129, pp. 642–52, and Centerwall, B.S. 1992, 'Television and violence: The scale of the problem and where to go from here', *JAMA*, vol. 267, no. 22, pp. 3059–63.

50 RACP, Paediatrics & Child Health Division 2004, 'Children and the media: Advocating for the future', RACP, Sydney. Available at: http://www.racp.edu.au/hpu/paed/media.

51 RACP, Division of Paediatrics, Health Policy Unit 1999, *Getting in the picture. A parent's and carer's guide for the better use of television for children* (3rd edn), RACP, Sydney.

52 Satter, E. 2000, *Child of mine. Feeding with love and good sense*, Bull Publishing Co., Colorado.

53 Rideout, Victoria J. (Vice-President and Director, Program for the Study of Entertainment Media and Health, Henry J. Kaiser Family Foundation) 2004, 'The role of media in childhood obesity', statement made before the Senate Committee on Commerce, Science and Transportation Subcommittee on Competition, Foreign Commerce and Infastructure, 2 March, Washington DC.

54 Salmon, J. et al. 2005, 'Reducing sedentary behaviour and increasing physical activity among 10-year-old children: Overview and process evaluation of the 'Switch-Play' intervention', *Health Promotion International*, vol. 20, no. 1, pp. 7–17.

55 Satter, E. 2000, *Child of mine. Feeding with love and good sense*, Bull Publishing Co., Colorado.

56 RACP, Paediatrics & Child Health Division 2004, 'Children and the media: Advocating for the future', RACP, Sydney. Available at: http://www.racp.edu.au/hpu/paed/media.

57 Cited in NHMRC 2003, *Dietary Guidelines for Children and Adolescents in Australia incorporating the Infant Feeding Guidelines for Health Workers (endorsed 10 April 2003)*, NHMRC, Canberra.

Chapter 7

1 Taylor J. et al. 2005, 'Determinants of healthy eating in children and youth', *Canadian Journal of Public Health*, vol. 96, S 3.

2 Lobstein, T. et al. 2004, 'Obesity in children and young people: A crisis in public health', *Obesity Reviews*, vol. 5, suppl. 1, pp. 4–85.

3 Birch L.L. et al. 1990, 'Conditioned flavor preference in young children', *Physiol Behav*, vol. 47, no. 3, pp. 501–05.

4 Rosenbaum, M. and Leibel, R.L. 1998, 'The physiology of body weight regulation: Relevance to the etiology of obesity in children', *Pediatrics*, vol. 101, no. 3, pp. S525–39.

5 Kopelman, P.G., Caterson, I.D. and Dietz, W.H. 2005, *Clinical obesity in adults and children* (2nd edn), Blackwell Publishing, Massachusetts.

6 Birch, L.L. and Fisher, J.O. 1998, 'Development of eating behaviours among children and adolescents', *Pediatrics*, vol. 101, no. 3, pp. S539–49.

7 Fisher, J.O. and Birch, L.L. 2002, 'Eating in the absence of hunger and overweight in girls from 5 to 7 years of age', *Am J Clin Nutr*, vol. 76, no. 1, pp. 226–31.

8 Batch, J.A. and Baur, L.A. 2005, 'Management and prevention of obesity and its complications in children and adolescents', *MJA*, vol. 182, no. 3, pp. 130–35.

9 Birch, L.L. and Fisher, J.O. 1998, 'Development of eating behaviours among children and adolescents', *Pediatrics*, vol. 101, no. 3, pp. S539–49.

10 Birch, L.L. and Fisher, J.O. 2000, 'Mothers' child-feeding practices influence daughters' eating and weight', *Am J Clin Nutr*, vol. 71, no. 5, pp. 1054–61.

11 Carper J.L. et al. 2000, 'Young girls' emerging dietary restraint and disinhibition are related to parental control in child feeding', *Appetite*, vol. 35, no. 2, pp. 121–29.

12 Cited by Satter, *Child of Mine, 2000.*

13 Davison K.K. and Campbell K.J. (in press), 'Opportunities to prevent obesity in children within families: An ecological approach', in D. Crawford and R. Jeffery, *Obesity Prevention in the 21st Century: Public health approaches to tackle the obesity pandemic*, Oxford University Press, Oxford.

14 Fisher, J.O. and Birch, L.L. 2002, 'Eating in the absence of hunger and overweight in girls from 5 to 7 years of age', *Am J Clin Nutr*, vol. 76, no. 1, pp. 226–231.

15 Barkeling, B. et al. 1992, 'Eating behaviour in obese and normal weight 11-year-old children', *Int J Obes*, vol. 16, pp. 355–60.

16 Johnson, S.L. 2000, 'Improving preschoolers' self-regulation of energy intake', *Pediatrics*, vol. 106, no. 6, pp. 1429–35.

17 Sanigorski, A.M. et al. 2005, 'Lunchbox contents of Australian school children: Room for improvement', *EJCN*, vol. 59, pp. 1310–16.

18 Naughton, G. 2005, 'Critical windows—industry partner report 2005', presentation to NSW, August.

19 Birch, L.L. and Fisher, J.O. 1998, 'Development of eating behaviours among children and adolescents', *Pediatrics*, vol. 101, no. 3, pp. S539–49; Fisher J.O. and Birch, L.L. 1999, 'Restricting access to palatable foods affects children's behavioral response, food selection, and intake', *Am J Clin Nutr*, vol. 69, pp. 1264–72; cited in Fisher, J.O. and Birch, L.L. 2002, 'Eating in the absence of hunger and overweight in girls from 5 to 7 years of age', *Am J Clin Nutr*, vol. 76, no. 1, pp. 226–31; Fisher, J.O. and Birch, L.L. 2000, 'Parents' restrictive feeding practices are associated with young girls' negative self-evaluation of eating', *J Am Diet Assoc*, vol. 100, no. 11, pp. 1341–46.

20 Satter, E. 1987, *How to get your kid to eat...but not too much. From birth to adolescence*, Bull Publishing Co., Colorado.

Chapter 8

1   Nestle, M. 2002, *Food politics. How the food industry influences nutrition and health*, University of California Press, California.

2   James, Tony 2003, 'Soft drink hard on health', *Australian Doctor*, 22 August, p. 12.

3   NHMRC 2003, *Dietary Guidelines for Children and Adolescents in Australia incorporating the Infant Feeding Guidelines for Health Workers (endorsed 10 April 2003)*, NHMRC, Canberra.

4   Kopelman, P.G., Caterson, I.D. and Dietz, W.H. 2005, *Clinical obesity in adults and children* (2nd edn), Blackwell Publishing, Massachusetts.

5   WA Department of Health 2005, Nutrition and Physical Activity Branch, 'Crunch & Sip', WA Government, Perth.

6   Drewnowski, A. and Levine, A.S. 2003, 'Sugar and fat—from genes to culture', presented as part of the American Society for Nutritional Sciences symposium, 'Sugar and fat—from genes to culture', given at the Experimental Biology Meeting in New Orleans, 23 April 2002; *J Nutr*, vol. 133, pp. 829S–30S.

7   Drewnowski, Adam and Specter, SE. 2004, 'Poverty and obesity: The role of energy density and energy costs', *Am J Clin Nutr*, vol. 79, no. 1.

8   Rolls, B. et al. 2005, 'Changing the energy density of the diet as a strategy for weight management', *J Am Diet Assoc* (suppl.), vol. 105, no. 5, pp. S98–103.

9   Drewnowski, A. and Gomez-Carneros, C. 2000, 'Bitter taste, phytonutrients, and the consumer: A review', *Am J Clin Nutr*, vol. 72, pp. 1424–35.

10 Cited in Dixon, H. et al. 2005, 'Body weight, nutrition, alcohol and physical activity: Key messages for the Cancer Council Australia', Cancer Council Australia, Sydney.

11 Magarey, A. et al. 2006, 'Evaluation of fruit and vegetable intakes of Australian adults: The National Nutrition Survey 1995', *Aust NZ J Public Health*, vol. 30, pp. 32–37.

12 Lobstein, T. et al. 2004, 'Obesity in children and young people: A crisis in public health', *Obesity Reviews*, vol. 5, suppl. 1, pp. 4–85.

13 O'Dea, J. 2005, *Positive food for kids. Healthy food, healthy children, healthy life*, Doubleday, Sydney.

14 Campbell, K.J. et al. 2005, 'The home environment and obesogenic eating in early adolescence', presentation to the International Society for Behavioral Nutrition and Physical Activity Annual Meeting, Amsterdam.

15 Campbell, K.J. et al. 2005, 'The home environment and obesogenic eating in early adolescence', Presentation to the International Society for Behavioral Nutrition and Physical Activity Annual Meeting, Amsterdam.

16 NHMRC 2003, *Dietary Guidelines for Children and Adolescents in Australia incorporating the Infant Feeding Guidelines for Health Workers (endorsed 10 April 2003)*, NHMRC, Canberra.

17 Fisher, J.O, 2003, 'Children's bite size and intake of an entrée are greater with large portions than with age-appropriate or self-selected portions', *Am J Clin Nutr*, vol. 77, no. 5, pp. 1164–70.

Chapter 9

1   NHMRC 2003, *Dietary Guidelines for Children and Adolescents in Australia incorporating the Infant Feeding Guidelines for Health Workers (endorsed 10 April 2003)*, NHMRC, Canberra.

2   Wood, K. et al. 2003, 'Hot topic: Breastfeeding and obesity', Lactation Resource Centre, Australian Breastfeeding Association. Available at: http://www.breastfeeding.asn.au/lrc/publications.html; Strategic Inter-Governmental Nutrition Alliance 2003, 'Promoting healthy weight', *Food Chain*, no. 11.

3   Taveras, E.M. et al. 2004, 'Association of breastfeeding with maternal control of infant feeding at age 1 year', *Pediatrics*, vol. 114, no. 5, pp. 577–83; Dietz, W.H. 2001, 'The obesity epidemic in young children', *BMJ*, vol. 322, pp. 313–14.

4   Birch, L.L., Fisher, J.O. 1998, 'Development of eating behaviours among children and adolescents', *Pediatrics*, vol. 101, no. 3, pp. S539–49.

5   Wood, K. et al. 2003, 'Hot topic: Breastfeeding and obesity', Lactation Resource Centre, Australian Breastfeeding Association, available at: http://www.breastfeeding.asn.au/lrc/publications.html.

6   Wood, K. et al. 2003, 'Hot topic: Breastfeeding and obesity', Lactation Resource Centre, Australian Breastfeeding Association, available at: http://www.breastfeeding.asn.au/lrc/publications.html.

7   Dixon, J., and Broom, D.H. (eds) 2007. The seven deadly sins of
    obesity: How the modern world is making us fat. (manuscript).
    University of NSW Press. Sydney

8   Wahlqvist, M.L. 1997, *Australasia, Asia and the Pacific: Food and
    nutrition*, Allen & Unwin. Sydney; Wood, K. et al. 2003, 'Hot
    topic: Breastfeeding and obesity', Lactation Resource Centre,
    Australian Breastfeeding Association. Available at:
    http://www.breastfeeding.asn.au/lrc/publications.html.

9   Gabriel, R. et al. 2005, 'Infant and child nutrition in Queensland
    2003', Queensland Health, Brisbane.

10 Webb, K. et al. 2005, 'Guest editorial: Breastfeeding and the
    public's health', *NSW Public Health Bulletin*, vol. 16, nos 3–4, pp.
    37–41.

11 Australian Institute of Family Studies 2004, 'Growing up in
    Australia: The longitudinal study of Australian children—an
    Australian Government initiative. 2004 annual report', Australian
    Institute of Family Studies, Melbourne.

12 AIHW 2005. 'A picture of Australia's children', cat. no. PHD 58,
    AIHW, Canberra.

13 NHMRC 2003, *Dietary Guidelines for Children and Adolescents in
    Australia incorporating the Infant Feeding Guidelines for Health
    Workers (endorsed 10 April 2003)*, NHMRC, Canberra.

14 Kopelman, P.G., Caterson, I.D. and Dietz, W.H. 2005, *Clinical
    obesity in adults and children* (2nd edn), Blackwell Publishing,
    Massachusetts.

15 Lobstein, T. et al. 2004, 'Obesity in children and young people:
    A crisis in public health', *Obesity Reviews*, vol. 5, suppl. 1,
    pp. 4–85.

16 Mannino, M.L. et al. 2004, 'The quality of girls' diets declines and
    tracks across middle childhood', *Int J Behav Nutr Phys Act*, vol. 1,
    no. 5, 27 February.

17 Satter, E. 1987, *How to get your kid to eat…but not too much. From
    birth to adolescence*, Bull Publishing Co., Colorado.

18 Cited in Campbell, K. and Crawford, D. 2001, 'Family food
    environments as determinants of preschool-aged children's eating
    behaviours: Implications for obesity prevention policy. A review',
    Aust J Nutr Diet, vol. 58, no. 1, pp. 19–25.

19 Satter, E. 1987, *How to get your kid to eat...but not too much. From birth to adolescence*, Bull Publishing Co., Colorado.

20 Picciano, M.F. et al. 2000, 'Nutritional guidance is needed during dietary transition in early childhood', *Pediatrics*, vol. 106, no. 1, pp. 109–14; NHMRC 2003, *Dietary Guidelines for Children and Adolescents in Australia incorporating the Infant Feeding Guidelines for Health Workers (endorsed 10 April 2003)*, NHMRC, Canberra.

21 WA Country Health Service 2005, 'Improving parents' and carers' awareness of healthy food options for the lunch box', Nutrition articles for school newsletters, WA Health Department, Perth.

22 Wahlqvist, M.L. 1997, *Australasia, Asia and the Pacific. Food and nutrition*, Allen & Unwin. Sydney.

23 WA Government 2003, *Results of Western Australian Child and Adolescent Physical Activity and Nutrition Survey 2003 (CAPANS)*, WA Government, Perth.

24 Cited in Kopelman, P.G., Caterson, I.D. and Dietz, W.H. 2005, *Clinical obesity in adults and children* (2nd edn), Blackwell Publishing, Massachusetts.

25 Cited in Kopelman, P.G., Caterson, I.D. and Dietz, W.H. 2005, *Clinical obesity in adults and children* (2nd edn), Blackwell Publishing, Massachusetts.

26 Campbell, K.J. et al. 2005, 'The home environment and obesogenic eating in early adolescence', presentation to the International Society for Behavioral Nutrition and Physical Activity Annual Meeting, Amsterdam.

Chapter 10

1 NSW Health 2005, 'Key findings from qualitative research into childhood overweight/obesity, health eating and physical activity', working document NSW Health, Sydney.

2 Trost, S.G. 2005, 'Discussion paper for the development of recommendations for children's and youths' participation in health-promoting physical activity', Commonwealth Department of Health and Ageing, Canberra.

3 Shilton, S. and Naughton, G. 2001, 'Physical activity and children', for the National Heart Foundation's National Physical Activity Program Committee, May, Sydney; Trost, S.G. 2005, 'Discussion

paper for the development of recommendations for children's and youths' participation in health-promoting physical activity', Commonwealth Department of Health and Ageing, Canberra.

4   Morris, L. et al. 2003, 'Sport, physical activity and antisocial behaviour in youth', Australian Institute of Criminology Research and Public Policy Series, no. 49, Australian Government, Canberra.

5   Conference report 2004, 'Site specific approaches to prevention or management of pediatric obesity, 14–15 July, Hyatt Regency Bethesda MD. Available at: http://www.niddk.nih.gov/fund/other/conferences-arch.htm.; Trost, S.G. 2005, 'Discussion paper for the development of recommendations for children's and youths' participation in health promoting physical activity', Commonwealth Department of Health and Ageing, Canberra.

6   Dwyer, T. et al. 1983, 'An investigation of the effects of daily physical activity on the health of primary school students in South Australia', *Int J Epidemiol.*, vol. 12, no. 3, pp. 308–13.

7   Trost, S.G. 2005, 'Discussion paper for the development of recommendations for children's and youths' participation in health-promoting physical activity', Commonwealth Department of Health and Ageing, Canberra.

8   Trost, S.G. 2005, 'Discussion paper for the development of recommendations for children's and youths' participation in health-promoting physical activity', Commonwealth Department of Health and Ageing, Canberra.

9   Shilton, S. and Naughton, G. 2001, 'Physical activity and children', for the National Heart Foundation's National Physical Activity Program Committee, May, Sydney.

10 Morris, L. et al. 2003, 'Sport, physical activity and antisocial behaviour in youth', Australian Institute of Criminology Research and Public Policy Series, no. 49, Australian Government, Canberra.

11 Trost, S.G. 2005, 'Discussion paper for the development of recommendations for children's and youths' participation in health-promoting physical activity', Commonwealth Department of Health and Ageing, Canberra.

12 Davison, K.K. et al. 2002, 'Participation in aesthetic sports and girls' weight concerns at ages 5 and 7 years', *Int J Eat Disord*, vol.

31, no. 3, pp. 312–17; Trost, S.G. 2005, 'Discussion paper for the development of recommendations for children's and youths' participation in health-promoting physical activity', Commonwealth Department of Health and Ageing, Canberra.

13 Williams, L. 2006, 'Every move they make, Mum's watching', *SMH*, 11–12 February, pp. 1–2.

14 Trost, S.G. 2001, 'Physical activity and determinants of physical activity in obese and non-obese children', *Int J Obes*, vol. 25, pp. 822–29.

15 Shilton, S. and Naughton, G. 2001, 'Physical activity and children', for the National Heart Foundation's National Physical Activity Program Committee, May, Sydney.

16 Trost, S.G. 2005, 'Discussion paper for the development of recommendations for children's and youths' participation in health-promoting physical activity', Commonwealth Department of Health and Ageing, Canberra.

17 Davison K.K., and Campbell K.J. (in press), 'Opportunities to prevent obesity in children within families: An ecological approach', in D. Crawford and R. Jeffery, *Obesity Prevention in the 21st Century: Public health approaches to tackle the obesity pandemic*, Oxford University Press, Oxford.

18 O'Dea, J. 2003, 'Why do kids eat healthful foods? Perceived benefits of and barriers to healthful eating and physical activity among children and adolescents', *J Am Diet Assoc*, vol. 103, no. 4, pp. 497–500.

19 Trost, S.G. et al. 1999, 'Correlates of objectively measured physical activity in preadolescent youth', *Am J Prev Med*, vol. 17, no. 2, pp. 120–26.

20 Trost, S.G. 1996, 'Gender differences in physcial activity and determinants of physical activity in rural fifth grade children', *Journal of School Health*, vol. 66, no. 4, pp. 145–49.

21 Trost, S.G. 2001, 'Physical activity and determinants of physical activity in obese and non-obese children', *Int J Obes*, vol. 25, pp. 822–29.

22 Davison K.K. et al. 2003, 'Parents' activity-related parenting practices predict girls' physcial activity', *Med Sci Sports Exerc*, vol. 35, no. 9, pp. 1589–95.

23 Salmon J. 2003, 'Home and neighbourhood: the influence of the environment on children,s physical activity', presentation to RACP Annual Scientific Meeting, 26–28 May, Hobart.

24 Giles-Corti, B. 2005, 'Increasing walking. How important is distance to, attractiveness and size of public open space?' *Am J Prev Med*, vol. 28, pp. 169–76.

25 Swinburn, B. and Egger, G. 2002, 'Preventive strategies against weight gain and obesity', *Obesity Reviews*, vol. 3, pp. 289–301.

26 Tranter, P.J. 2004, 'Effective Speeds: Car costs are slowing us down', report for the Australian Greenhouse Office, Commonwealth Department of the Environment and Heritage. Available at: http://www.greenhouse.gov.au/tdm/publications/pubs/effectivespee ds.pdf.

27 Tranter, P. and May, M. 2005, 'Questioning the need for speed: Can 'effective speed' guide change in travel behaviour and transport policy?', proceedings of the 28th Australasian Transport Research Forum, 28–30 September, Sydney.

28 Tranter, P.J. and Malone, K. 2003, 'Out of bounds: Insights from children to support a cultural shift towards sustainable and child-friendly cities', State of Australian Cities National Conference, 3–5 December, University of Western Sydney, Urban Frontiers Program, Parramatta.

29 Tranter, P. and Doyle, J. 1996, 'Reclaiming the residential street as play space', *International Play Journal*, vol. 4, pp. 81–97.

30 Tranter, P.J. 2004, 'Effective Speeds: Car costs are slowing us down', report for the Australian Greenhouse Office, Commonwealth Department of the Environment and Heritage. Available at: http://www.greenhouse.gov.au/tdm/publications/pubs/effectivespee ds.pdf.

31 Cited in Veitch, J. et al. (in press), 'Where do children usually play? A qualitative study of parents' perceptions of influences on children's active free-play', *Health & Place*.

32 Naughton, G. 2005, 'Critical windows—industry partner report 2005', presentation to NSW Health, August.

33 Tranter, P. and Pawson, E. 2001, 'Children's access to local environments: A case study of Christchurch, New Zealand', *Local Environment*, vol. 6, no. 1, pp. 27–48.

34 NSW Centre for Public Health Nutrition 2005, 'Best options for promoting healthy weight and preventing weight gain in NSW', NSW Centre for Public Health Nutrition, Sydney.

35 Okley, A.D. and Booth, M.L. 2004, 'Mastery of fundamental movement skills among children in New South Wales: Prevalence and sociodemographic distribution', *J Sci Med Sport*, vol. 7, no. 3, pp. 358–72; Okley, A.D. et al. 2001, 'Relationship of cardiorespiratory endurance to fundamental movement skill proficiency among adolescents', *Pediatric Exercise Science*, vol. 13, pp. 380–91.

36 Okley, A.D et al. 2004, 'Relationships between body composition and fundamental movement skills among children and adolescents', *Research Quarterly for Exercise and Sport*, vol. 75, no. 3, pp. 238–47.

37 Okley, A.D. and Booth, M.L. 2004, 'Mastery of fundamental movement skills among children in New South Wales: Prevalence and sociodemographic distribution', *J Sci Med Sport*, vol. 7, no. 3, pp. 358–72.

38 Okley, A.D. et al. 2001, 'Relationship of cardiorespiratory endurance to fundamental movement skill proficiency among adolescents', *Pediatric Exercise Science*, vol. 13, pp. 380–91; Okley, A.D. et al. 2001, 'Relationship of physical activity to fundamental movement skills among adolescents', *Med Sci Sports Exerc*, vol. 33, no. 11, pp. 1899–1904.

39 Southall, J.E. et al. 2004, 'Actual and perceived physical competence in overweight and non overweight children', *Pediatric Exercise Science*, vol. 16, pp. 15–24.

40 Victorian Health Promotion Foundation 2005, *VicHealth Letter*, issue 24, Summer.

41 Victorian Health Promotion Foundation 2005, *VicHealth Letter*, issue 24, Summer.

42 Tranter, P.J. and Malone, K. 2003, 'Out of bounds: Insights from children to support a cultural shift towards sustainable and child-friendly cities', State of Australian Cities National Conference, 3–5 December, University of Western Sydney, Urban Frontiers Program, Parramatta.

Endnotes

43 Collins, D.C. and Kearns, R.A. 2005, 'Geographies of inequality: Child pedestrian injury and walking school buses in Auckland, New Zealand', *Soc Sci Med*, vol. 60, no. 1, pp. 61–69.

44 Telford, A. et al. 2005, 'Quantifying and characterising physical activity among children in Australia: The Children's Leisure Activities Study (CLASS)', *Pediatric Exercise Science*, vol. 17, pp. 266–80.

45 Cited in WA Government 2003, *Results of Western Australian Child and Adolescent Physical Activity and Nutrition Survey 2003 (CAPANS)*, WA Government, Perth.

46 O'Dea, J. 2003, 'Why do kids eat healthful foods? Perceived benefits of and barriers to healthful eating and physical activity among children and adolescents', *J Am Diet Assoc*, vol. 103, no. 4, pp. 497–500.

47 Magnay, J. 2005, 'Sporty girls can't get by without their mum', *SMH*, p. 3.

48 Booth, M.L. et al. 2002, 'Epidemiology of physical activity participation among New South Wales school students', *ANZ J Public Health*, vol. 26, no. 4, pp. 371–74.

49 Booth, M.L. et al. 2004, 'Patterns of activity energy expenditure among Australian adolescents', *Journal of Physical Activity and Health*, vol. 1, pp. 246–58.

50 Dollman, J. et al. 2002, 'Anthropometry, fitness and physical activity of urban and rural South Australian children', *Pediatric Exercise Science*, vol. 14, no. 3, pp. 297–312.

51 Institute of Medicine of the National Academies 2006. Progress in Preventing Childhood Obesity. How Do We Measure Up? The National Academies Press. Washington, DC. Available at: www.iom.edu/obesity

52 Naughton, G. 2005, 'Critical windows—industry partner report 2005', presentation to NSW Health, August.

53 Bauman. A.E. et al. 2001, 'The epidemiology of dog walking: An unmet need for human and canine health', *MJA*, vol. 175, pp. 632–34.

54 Salmon, J. et al. 2004, 'The Children's Leisure Activities Study: Summary report', Centre for Physical Activity & Nutrition Research, Deakin University, Melbourne, July. Available at: http://www.deakin.edu.au/hbs/cpan/be.php.

447

55 Wood, L. et al. 2005, 'The pet connection: Pets as a conduit for social capital?', *Soc Sci Med*, vol. 61, pp. 1159–73.

56 Beck, A.M. and Meyers, N.M. 1996, 'Health enhancement and companion animal ownership', *Annual Review of Public Health*, vol. 17, pp. 247–57; Morrow, V. 1998, 'My animals and other family: Children's perspectives on their relationships with companion animals', *Anthrozoos*, vol. 11, no. 4, pp. 218–26.

57 McNicholas, J. and Collis, G.M. 2001, 'Children's representations of pets in their social networks', *Child: Care, Health and Development*, vol. 27, no. 3, pp. 279–94.

58 Brown, W. et al. 2006, '10,000 Steps Rockhampton: Evaluation of a whole community approach to improving population levels of physical activity', *Journal of Physical Activity and Health*, vol. 3, no. 1, pp. 1–14.

Chapter 11

1 Australian Institute of Family Studies 2004, 'Growing up in Australia: The longitudinal study of Australian children—an Australian Government initiative. 2004 annual report', Australian Institute of Family Studies, Melbourne.

2 O'Dea, J. 1999, 'Cross-cultural, body weight and gender differences in the body size, perceptions and body ideals of university students', *Aust J Nutr Diet*, vol. 56, no. 3, pp. 144–50.

3 Lobstein, T. et al. 2004, 'Obesity in children and young people: A crisis in public health', *Obesity Reviews*, vol. 5, suppl. 1, pp. 4–85.

4 Kopelman, P.G., Caterson, I.D. and Dietz, W.H. 2005, *Clinical obesity in adults and children* (2nd edn), Blackwell Publishing, Massachusetts.

5 Dietz, W.H. 1997, 'Periods of risk in childhood for the development of adult obesity—what do we need to learn?', presented as part of an American Society for Nutritional Sciences symposium, 'Obesity: Common symptom of diverse gene-based metabolic dysregulations', Little Rock AR, 4 March, pp. 1884S–86S.

6 NHMRC 2003, *Dietary Guidelines for Children and Adolescents in Australia incorporating the Infant Feeding Guidelines for Health Workers (endorsed 10 April 2003)*, NHMRC, Canberra.

Endnotes

7   NHMRC 2003, *Dietary Guidelines for Children and Adolescents in Australia incorporating the Infant Feeding Guidelines for Health Workers (endorsed 10 April 2003)*, NHMRC, Canberra.

8   NHMRC 2003, *Dietary Guidelines for Children and Adolescents in Australia incorporating the Infant Feeding Guidelines for Health Workers (endorsed 10 April 2003)*, NHMRC, Canberra.

9   Dietz, W.H. 1997, 'Periods of risk in childhood for the development of adult obesity—what do we need to learn?', presented as part of an American Society for Nutritional Sciences symposium, 'Obesity: Common symptom of diverse gene-based metabolic dysregulations', Little Rock AR, 4 March, pp. 1884S–86S.

10 Lobstein, T. et al. 2004, 'Obesity in children and young people: a crisis in public health', *Obesity Reviews*, vol. 5, suppl. 1, pp. 4–85.

11 Dietz, W.H. 1997, 'Periods of risk in childhood for the development of adult obesity—what do we need to learn?', presented as part of an American Society for Nutritional Sciences symposium, 'Obesity: Common symptom of diverse gene-based metabolic dysregulations', Little Rock AR, 4 March, pp. 1884S–86S.

12 Lobstein T. et al. 2004, 'Obesity in children and young people: a crisis in public health', *Obesity Reviews*, vol. 5, suppl. 1, pp. 4–85.

13 NHMRC 2003, *Dietary Guidelines for Children and Adolescents in Australia incorporating the Infant Feeding Guidelines for Health Workers (endorsed 10 April 2003)*, NHMRC, Canberra.

14 Wake, M., McCallum, Z. 2004, 'Secondary prevention of overweight in primary school children: What place for general practice?', *MJA*, vol. 181, no. 2, pp. 82–83.

15 Lobstein, T. et al. 2004, 'Obesity in children and young people: a crisis in public health', *Obesity Reviews*, vol. 5, suppl. 1, pp. 4–85.

16 Wahlqvist, M.L. 1997, *Australasia, Asia and the Pacific. Food and nutrition*, Allen & Unwin. Sydney.

17 Dietz, W.H. 1998, 'Health consequences of obesity in youth: Childhood predictors of adult disease', *Pediatrics*, vol. 101, no. 3 (suppl.), pp. 518–25.

449

18 Dietz, W.H. 1997, 'Periods of risk in childhood for the development of adult obesity—what do we need to learn?', presented as part of an American Society for Nutritional Sciences symposium, 'Obesity: Common symptom of diverse gene-based metabolic dysregulations', Little Rock AR, 4 March, pp. 1884S–86S.

19 NHMRC 2003, *Dietary Guidelines for Children and Adolescents in Australia incorporating the Infant Feeding Guidelines for Health Workers (endorsed 10 April 2003)*, NHMRC, Canberra.

20 NHMRC 2003, *Dietary Guidelines for Children and Adolescents in Australia incorporating the Infant Feeding Guidelines for Health Workers (endorsed 10 April 2003)*, NHMRC, Canberra.

21 Kopelman, P.G., Caterson, I.D. and Dietz, W.H. 2005, *Clinical obesity in adults and children* (2nd edn), Blackwell Publishing, Massachusetts.

22 Batch, J.A. and Baur, L.A. 2005, 'Management and prevention of obesity and its complications in children and adolescents', *MJA*, vol. 182, no. 3, pp. 130–35.

23 Lobstein, T. et al. 2004, 'Obesity in children and young people: A crisis in public health', *Obesity Reviews*, vol. 5, suppl. 1, pp. 4–85.

24 Whitaker, R.C. et al. 1997, 'Predicting obesity in young adulthood from childhood and parental obesity', *NEJM*, vol. 337, no. 13, pp. 869–73.

25 Kopelman, P.G., Caterson, I.D., Dietz, W.H. 2005, *Clinical obesity in adults and children* (2nd edn), Blackwell Publishing, Massachusetts.

26 National Health and Medical Research Council 2003, *Dietary Guidelines for Children and Adolescents in Australia incorporating the Infant Feeding Guidelines for Health Workers, Endorsed 10 April 2003*, NHMRC, Canberra.

27 NHMRC 2003, *Dietary Guidelines for Children and Adolescents in Australia incorporating the Infant Feeding Guidelines for Health Workers (endorsed 10 April 2003)*, NHMRC, Canberra; Lobstein, T. et al. 2004, 'Obesity in children and young people: A crisis in public health', *Obesity Reviews*, vol. 5, suppl. 1, pp. 4–85.

28 Adapted from NHMRC 2003, *Dietary Guidelines for Children and Adolescents in Australia incorporating the Infant Feeding Guidelines for Health Workers (endorsed 10 April 2003)*, NHMRC, Canberra.

29 NSW Health 2004, *Eat Well NSW: Strategic directions for public health nutrition 2003–2007*, NSW Department of Health, Sydney.

30 Egger, G. and Binns, A. 2001, *The experts' weight loss guide. For
doctors, health professionals...and all those serious about their
health*, Allen & Unwin, Sydney.

31 Satter, E. 2000, *Child of mine. Feeding with love and good sense*, Bull
Publishing Co., Colorado.

32 Kopelman, P.G., Caterson, I.D. and Dietz, W.H. 2005, *Clinical
obesity in adults and children* (2nd edn), Blackwell Publishing,
Massachusetts.

33 Satter, E. 2000, *Child of mine. Feeding with love and good sense*, Bull
Publishing Co., Colorado.

Chapter 12

1 Booth, M. et al. 2006, *NSW Schools Physical Activity and Nutrition
Survey (SPANS) 2004*, NSW Health, Sydney.

2 Washington State Department of Health 2005, 'Nutrition and
physical activity: A policy resource guide', Office of Community
Wellness and Prevention, Washington State. Available at:
http://www.doh.wa.gov/cfh/steps/default.

3 Bell, C. and Swinburn, B. 2005, 'School canteens: Using ripples to
create a wave of healthy eating', *MJA*, vol. 183, no. 1, pp. 5–6.

4 Washington State Department of Health 2005, 'Nutrition and
physical activity: A policy resource guide', Office of Community
Wellness and Prevention, Washington State. Available at:
http://www.doh.wa.gov/cfh/steps/default.

5 Hamilton, C., and Denniss, R. 2005, *Affluenza. When too much is
never enough*, Allen & Unwin, Sydney.

6 Washington State Department of Health 2005, 'Nutrition and
physical activity: A policy resource guide', Office of Community
Wellness and Prevention, Washington State. Available at:
http://www.doh.wa.gov/cfh/steps/default.

7 Trust for America's Health 2006. F as in fat: How obesity policies
are failing in America. Issue Report. Available at:
www.healthyamericans.org.

8 Payet, J. et al. 2005, 'Gascoyne Growers Market: A sustainable
health promotion activity developed in partnership with the
community', *Australian Journal of Rural Health*, vol. 13, no. 5, pp.
309–14.

Chapter 13

1   Washington State Department of Health 2005, 'Nutrition and physical activity: A policy resource guide', Office of Community Wellness and Prevention, Washington State. Available at: http://www.doh.wa.gov/cfh/steps/default.

2. Premier's Physical Activity Taskforce 2006. How to: Promote Walking. A Guide for Local Government. WA Government, Perth.

3. Premier's Physical Activity Taskforce, factsheets and information bulletins about physical activity, WA Government, Perth. Available at: http://www.patf.dpc.wa.gov.au; Shilton, S. and Naughton, G. 2001, 'Physical activity and children', for the National Heart Foundation's National Physical Activity Program Committee, May, Sydney.

4   Brierley, A. et al., 'Executive summary. Feasibility summary for a multistrategy nutrition project in Penrith LGA', Penrith City Council, Penrith.

5   AIHW 2006, 'National public health expenditure report 2001–02 to 2003–04', Health and Welfare Expenditure Series No. 26, cat. no. HWE 33, AIHW, Canberra.

6   Daube, M. 2006. Public health needs a strong, well-planned advocacy program. *Aust NZ J Public Health,* vol. 30, no.5 pp. 405–406.

7   Choi, B.C.K., Hunter, D.J., Tsou, W. and Sainsbury, P. 2005. Diseases of comfort: primary cause of death in the 22nd century, *J Epidemiol Community Health*, vol. 59, pp. 1030–1034.

8   Ball, K. and Crawford, D. 2004, 'Healthy weight 2008: Still waiting on Australia to act?' *Nutrition & Dietetics*, vol. 61, no. 1, pp. 5–7.

9   Stanton, R. 2006. 'Just say no', *Australian Doctor*, 22 Sept. pp. 33–34

10 Zimmet, P.Z., and James, W.P.T. 2006. The unstoppable Australian obesity and diabetes juggernaut. What should politicians do? *MJA*, Vol. 185, no. 4. pp. 187–188.

11 Cited in NSW Centre for Public Health Nutrition 2005, 'Best options for promoting healthy weight and preventing weight gain in NSW', NSW Centre for Public Health Nutrition, March.

12 Ryan, K.W., Card-Higginson, P., McCarthy, S.G., Justus, M.B. and Thompson, J.W. 2006. Arkansas Fights Fat: Translating Research

Into Policy To Combat Childhood And Adolescent Obesity. *Health Affairs*, vol. 25, no. 4, pp. 992–1004.

13   Franklin, Matthew 2006, 'States the 'villains' in battle of bulge', *The Australian*, 24 October, p.5.

14   Puska, P. 2002, 'Successful prevention of non-communicable diseases: 25 year experiences with North Karelia Project', *Public Health Medicine*, vol. 4, no. 1, pp. 5–7; Vartiainen, E. et al. 2000, 'Cardiovascular risk factor changes in Finland 1972–1997', *Int J Epidemiol*, vol. 29, pp. 49–56; Pietinen, P. 1996, 'Changes in diet in Finland from 1972 to 1992: Impact on coronary heart disease risk', *Prev Med*, vol. 25, no. 3, pp. 243–50.

15   AIHW 2005, 'Obesity and workplace absenteeism among older Australians', Bulletin No. 31, cat. no. AUS 67, AIHW, Canberra.

16   Bicycle Victoria 2003, 'The Cycle-Friendly Workplace'. Available at: http://www.bv.com.au.

17   Washington State Department of Health 2005, 'Nutrition and physical activity: A policy resource guide', Office of Community Wellness and Prevention, Washington State. Available at: http://www.doh.wa.gov/cfh/steps/default.

18   Washington State Department of Health 2005, 'Nutrition and physical activity: A policy resource guide', Office of Community Wellness and Prevention, Washington State. Available at: http://www.doh.wa.gov/cfh/steps/default.

19   Canning, Simon 2005, 'Chocolate fundraisers given the brush', *The Australian* (Media section), August.

20   Institute of Medicine of the National Academies 2006. Progress in Preventing Childhood Obesity. How Do We Measure Up? The National Academies Press. Washington, DC. Available at: www.iom.edu/obesity

21   Hudson, K. 2006, 'A creative consumer panel report on kids' obesity'. Available at: http://www.ideacentre.com.au.

22   Garrard, J. et al. 2004, 'Planning for healthy communities: Reducing the risk of cardiovascular disease and type 2 diabetes through healthier environments and lifestyles', Victorian Government Department of Human Services, Melbourne.

Index

Index

Index

Index

Acknowledgements

I have researched and written this book from the perspective of a longstanding health writer and journalist. I am not a parent myself. But I am acutely aware of the pressures that parents face, and the last thing I want is for this book to add to them; parenting can be demanding enough as it is. I have tried to make the book as relevant as possible, and for helping me with this I thank the many parents who contributed, whether by giving time for interviews or by reading drafts and providing a 'reality check'.

I would also like to acknowledge my wonderful partner, Mitchell Ward, for both his personal support and his quirky illustrations. Thanks also to my agent, Deborah Callaghan, ABC Books, and the patience and care of TBFC's editor, Jody Lee. My appreciation also to Sarah Shrubb for her copyediting, and to the University of Sydney's library.

And a big fat thanks to those who provided feedback on drafts, including Louise Baur, Lorna Cameron, Sue Cameron, Jennifer Cooke, Linda Doherty, Miranda Harman, Bronwyn Marshall, Marge Overs, Matt Sweet, and Jacqui Tully

Many thanks also to those who gave so generously of their time and expertise with interviews: Jane Adams, Jenni Adams,

The big fat conspiracy

Tim Adams, Stephanie Alexander, Sarah Anderson, Helen Baker, Helen Barnard, Kylie Ball, Trent Ballard, Helen Barnard, Alan Barclay, Fran Baum, Adrian Bauman, Louise Baur, Debbie Bennett, Barbara Biggins, Colin Bell, Helen Berry, Catriona Bonfiglioli, Michael Booth, Leah Brennan, Graeme Brims, Karen Campbell, Michele Campbell, Kim Carter, Ian Caterson, John Catford, Kathy Chapman, Mark Coulton, Jane Cleary, Clare Collins, David Crawford, Elizabeth Denney-Wilson, Monique Desmarchalier, Elizabeth Develin, Jane Dixon, Jim Dollman, Josie Duncan, Terry Dwyer, Garry Egger, David Engwicht, Lyn Flegg, David Freeman, Janette Gale, Billie Giles-Corti, Tim Gill, John Given, Tony Grant, Suzy Green, Denise Greenaway, Beth Hands, Kate Hawkings, John Hawley, Kylie Hesketh, Justine Hodge, Peter Holt, Ken Hudson, Tamara Johnston, Virginia Jackson, Nicki Kajons, Annette Katelaris, Rick Kausman, Ian Kett, Alastair King, David Laing, Mark Lawrence, Sharon Laurence, Stephen Leeder, Dympna Leonard, Sandra Lilburn, Tim Lobstein, Zoe McCallum, Louise Mathews, Jess McEachen, Kaye Mehta, Liz Millen, Phil Morgan, Ben Neil, Geraldine Naughton, Kevin Norton, Sue Nunn, Paul O'Brien, Stan Oakley, Tony Okley, Jenny O'Dea, Kerin O'Dea, Chris Ogden, Tim Olds, Rhonda O'Sign, Marge Overs, Doug Paling, Nadine Paull, Jenny Payet, Joanne Paynter, Mary Pekin, Michelle Powers, Stephan Rainow, Helen Read, Janet Reynolds, Chris Rissel, Ann Roche, Lyn Roberts, Rose Romeo, Louise Roufeil, Jo Salmon, Liz Sanders, Matt Sanders, Liz Sanzaro, Jennifer Savenake, Lynne Saville, Trevor Shilton, Terry Slevin, Maxine Smith, Rosemary Stanton, Kate Steinbeck, Boyd Swinburn, Lyndal Taylor, Paul Tranter, Doug Tutt, Bob Volkmer, Melissa Wake, Scott Walker, Jeff Walkley, Janet Warren, Karen Webb, Felicity West, Julie Williams, Paul Zimmet.

Acknowledgements

And to class 6W at the Wilkins Public School in Sydney, the Parents, Jury members, Community Foodies and other parents, including: Lyn Abraham, John Allin, Tania Andrusiak, Glenn Austin, Liz Broad, Cathy Banwell, Sarah Breckenridge, Pip Budgen, Tanya Calderwood, Adele Chapman, David Frazer, Jackie De Koning, Liz Doherty, Alex Donaldson, Ralph Douglas, Karen Drayton, Sarah Grosvenor, Margaret Harrap, Gillian Hehir, Libby Hocking, Paul Jones, Julie Leask, Mary Mallett, Jane Martin, Lisa Newey, Corinne Paterson, Christine Robertson, Beth O'Shannessy, Michelle Prak, Rebecca Shaw, Karen Sims, Deborah Smith, Gail Smith, Jody Smith, Kerry Smith, Sarah Smith, Sharyn Spezzano, Gillian Street, Carol Roseberg, Ben Ross, Amanda Russell, Sandy Tindall, Jodie Weerasekera, Nancy Wyles.